1000 MCQs for **Davidson's**
Principles and Pr
Medicine

CW01020408

For Churchill Livingstone

Commissioning Editor Laurence Hunter
Project Development Manager Sarah Keer-Keer
Project Controller Frances Affleck
Designer Erik Bigland

1000 MCQs for Davidson's
Principles and Practice of
Medicine

M.J. Ford MD FRCPE
Consultant Physician, Western General Hospital, Edinburgh
Honorary Senior Lecturer, Edinburgh University, Edinburgh

A.T. Elder MB ChB FRCPE
Consultant Physician, Western General Hospital, Edinburgh
Honorary Senior Lecturer, Edinburgh University, Edinburgh

FOURTH EDITION

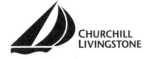
CHURCHILL
LIVINGSTONE

EDINBURGH LONDON NEW YORK PHILADELPHIA ST LOUIS SYDNEY TORONTO 1999

CHURCHILL LIVINGSTONE
An imprint of Harcourt Publishers Limited

First edition   1980
Second edition   1991
Third edition   1997
Fourth edition   1999

First edition by P. R. Fleming

Standard edition ISBN 0 443 06399 0

International Student Edition ISBN   0 443 06400 8

British Library Cataloguing in Publication Data
A catalogue record for this book is available from the British
Library

Library of Congress Cataloging in Publication Data
A catalog record for this book is available from the Library of
Congress

Note
Medical knowledge is constantly changing. As new
information becomes available, changes in treatment,
procedures, equipment and the use of drugs become
necessary. The authors and the publishers have, as far as it
is possible, taken care to ensure that the information given in
this text is accurate and up to date. However, readers are
strongly advised to confirm that the information, especially
with regard to drug usage, complies with the latest
legislation and standards of practice.

The
Publisher's
policy is to use
**paper manufactured
from sustainable forests**

Typeset by IMH (Catrif), Loanhead, Scotland
Printed by Bell & Bain Ltd., Glasgow

Contents

Introduction

Since the first edition of this book of multiple choice questions supplementing *Davidson's Principles and Practice of Medicine* by Dr P.R. Fleming was first published, medical knowledge has continued to grow at an exponential rate. MCQ companion books to medical textbooks remain both popular and useful methods of self-assessment for medical undergraduates and postgraduates. The aim of this book, like that of its predecessor, is to help students efficiently acquire the factual knowledge necessary for good medical practice. The questions have been arranged to correspond with the chapters of *Davidson's Principles and Practice of Medicine*, 18th edition, and, in addition, annotated answers have been compiled to enhance the educational value of the book.

The principles and technique

Multiple choice questions are widely used for examination purposes as a reliable and discriminatory test of factual knowledge. Lack of familiarity with the MCQ format may result in unexpected failure, although more usually failure is attributable to a lack of adequate reading and understanding of clinical medicine and the basic sciences. Familiarity with the technique of MCQ examinations is no substitute for the systematic study required to achieve a thorough understanding of medicine.

- Read each stem question and the five items carefully. The questions have been worded to avoid ambiguity and have not been designed to trick the unwary.
- Identify the items which you can answer with confidence and record the answer 'TRUE' or 'FALSE' as appropriate.
- Identify those items to which you do not know the answers. Do not guess the answer if you know nothing about the subject matter. Record the answer 'DO NOT KNOW' and move to the next item.
- There will be items the answers to which you may feel you know but lack confidence. After due consideration, record your answer, providing this is not a blind guess but informed and intuitive reasoning.
- Concentrate on each stem and item in turn rather than passing quickly from question to question. It is easier to concentrate on the problem in hand than to juggle with several unrelated questions simultaneously.

How to use this book

Students preparing themselves for examinations are recommended to read the appropriate chapters of the textbooks and then to assess themselves using the MCQ technique described.

Record your answers and your reasoning before checking the correct answer. Then return to the appropriate section of a medical textbook and read the relevant text for a more detailed explanation.

PART 1
QUESTIONS

1 THE MOLECULAR AND CELLULAR BASIS OF DISEASE

ANSWERS PAGE 154

1
In humans
Ⓐ somatic cell nuclei contain 22 pairs of homologous autosomes
Ⓑ gamete nuclei are haploid with a single X or Y chromosome
Ⓒ the haploid male cell (sperm) contains 22 autosomes and a Y chromosome
Ⓓ pairing of homologous chromosomes occurs during mitosis
Ⓔ both X chromosomes in females are genetically active

2
In the chromosomal disorders
Ⓐ aneuploidy is the addition or loss of a chromosome
Ⓑ deletions arise from the loss of a segment of a chromosome
Ⓒ the majority of affected conceptions result in miscarriage
Ⓓ identical deletions produce the same effects whether inherited from father or mother
Ⓔ translocation is the exchange of segments between chromosomes

3
In cellular protein synthesis
Ⓐ each tRNA molecule carries one anticodon
Ⓑ each tRNA molecule carries one amino acid
Ⓒ peptidyl transferase catalyses amino acid polymerisation
Ⓓ one of seven different stop codons is necessary to terminate amino acid polymerisation
Ⓔ recognition of the mRNA start codon occurs after binding to the small 40S ribosomal subunit

4
With regard to DNA
Ⓐ the mutation rate in genomic DNA is around 10^{-3} to 10^{-6}
Ⓑ single base coding errors are always replicated to daughter strand DNA
Ⓒ the most frequent single base mutation is a C to T substitution
Ⓓ deamination initiates mutation
Ⓔ ionising radiation induces breakage of double stranded DNA

5
In the human cell
Ⓐ the genome is separated from the cytoplasm by a nuclear membrane
Ⓑ the endoplasmic reticulum has a role in cellular calcium metabolism
Ⓒ the golgi apparatus facilitates aerobic metabolism
Ⓓ mitochondria have their own genome
Ⓔ mitochondrial disease states are associated with myopathy

6
In cellular protein metabolism
Ⓐ most protein synthesis occurs on the large ribosomal subunit
Ⓑ ubiquitin facilitates protein degradation in the cytoplasm
Ⓒ a protein's final conformation is determined by its peptide sequence (primary structure) alone
Ⓓ v-SNAREs participate in exchange of proteins between intracellular vesicles
Ⓔ integral cellular proteins are responsible for protein sorting and transport

7

In the cell cycle

Ⓐ DNA replication occurs during the G1 phase

Ⓑ chromatids are joined at the telomere

Ⓒ chromatid segregation occurs twice in meiosis

Ⓓ DNA recombination in meiosis occurs via chiasmata

Ⓔ telomere shortening is associated with cellular ageing

8

With regard to transport of molecules into cells

Ⓐ passive diffusion directly through the lipid bilayer cannot occur

Ⓑ movement of molecules can only occur down osmotic or concentration gradients

Ⓒ ion channels are always open for ion transport

Ⓓ endocytosis is responsible for internalising larger particles

Ⓔ acetylcholine binds to a cellular receptor which facilitates potassium influx

9

With regard to receptor-regulated cellular transport

Ⓐ each ligand–receptor interaction has a specific cellular response

Ⓑ receptors become 'resistant' to repeated ligand stimulation

Ⓒ ligand–receptor interactions control transcellular ionic movement

Ⓓ G-protein coupled receptors stimulate transmembrane adenyl cyclase

Ⓔ phosphorylation is a frequent component of signalling cascades

10

With regard to the cell cycle and cell death

Ⓐ cyclin-dependent kinases regulate the progression of the cell cycle

Ⓑ transient arrest of the cycle at the G1-S checkpoint is associated with an increased chance of malignant cellular transformation

Ⓒ the process of differentiation allows a cell to withdraw from the cell cycle

Ⓓ apoptosis (programmed cell death) usually occurs when cells are in G1-S phase

Ⓔ apoptotic cells discharge damaging enzymatic contents to the exterior

11

The following cancers are of infective origin

Ⓐ Burkitt's lymphoma

Ⓑ cervical carcinoma

Ⓒ thyroid carcinoma

Ⓓ Kaposi's sarcoma

Ⓔ ovarian carcinoma

12

Oncogenes

Ⓐ are genes which protect a cell from cancerous change

Ⓑ exert their effect by mimicking persistent growth factor stimulation

Ⓒ exert their effect by producing loss of a cellular protective mechanism

Ⓓ exert their effect by increasing cellular susceptibility to apoptosis

Ⓔ arise from single or multiple mutations

13

The following may be features of malignant cells

Ⓐ increased frequency of replication

Ⓑ loss of capacity to differentiate

Ⓒ failure of chromosomal separation pre-division

Ⓓ down-regulation of cell surface receptor molecules

Ⓔ synthesis of angiogenic factors

14

In the inflammatory response

Ⓐ neutrophils have a half-life of 24–48 hours

Ⓑ neutrophils arrive earliest at the site of inflammation

Ⓒ macrophages cannot synthesise cytokines

Ⓓ eosinophils have a specific role in defence against viruses

Ⓔ macrophages have a role in tissue repair

15

Excessive or inappropriate inflammation is a feature of

Ⓐ acute respiratory distress syndrome

Ⓑ Alzheimer's disease

Ⓒ bronchial asthma

Ⓓ multiple sclerosis

Ⓔ rheumatoid arthritis

16

In acute lobar streptococcal pneumonia

Ⓐ neutrophils appear in the spaces within 30 minutes

Ⓑ peak monocyte migration into alveoli occurs at 18–24 hours

Ⓒ there is local vasoconstriction to facilitate leucocyte adhesion to endothelial cells

Ⓓ integrin molecules facilitate leucocyte adhesion to endothelial cells

Ⓔ some bacterial products act directly as neutrophil chemotaxins

17

In the innate immune system

Ⓐ neutrophil leucocytes phagocytose particulate antigens

Ⓑ monocytes develop into tissue macrophages

Ⓒ natural killer cells produce interferons

Ⓓ acute phase proteins bind complement to enhance opsonisation

Ⓔ macrophage-derived interleukin-1 mediates the febrile response

18

In the adaptive immune system

Ⓐ small granular lymphocytes transform into killer cells

Ⓑ T lymphocytes produce helper, suppressor and cytotoxic cells

Ⓒ helper cells facilitate B cell-mediated killer cell activity

Ⓓ delayed hypersensitivity reactions are mediated by T cells

Ⓔ interleukin-2 is a lymphokine stimulating B cell proliferation

19

The following statements about immunoglobulins are true

Ⓐ they are secreted by transformed T lymphocytes

Ⓑ IgA is produced by B cells in the lamina propria of the gut

Ⓒ IgG is the only immunoglobulin to cross the placental barrier

Ⓓ IgA comprises 75% of the immunoglobulins in normal serum

Ⓔ IgD is mainly found on the surface of B lymphocytes

20

Pathophysiological functions of immunoglobulins shown below include

Ⓐ IgG—neutralisation of soluble toxins

Ⓑ IgA—agglutination of bacteria

Ⓒ IgM—complement activation to produce cell lysis

Ⓓ IgD—protection against viruses

Ⓔ IgE—major regulator of B cell functions

21

In immediate (anaphylactic) hypersensitivity reactions

Ⓐ eosinophils release histaminase to suppress inflammation

Ⓑ the severity depends on the antigen's portal of entry

Ⓒ most manifestations are due to mast cell degranulation

Ⓓ parenteral adrenaline therapy should be given for severe reactions

Ⓔ urticaria is always induced by foreign antigen

22
In delayed hypersensitivity reactions
Ⓐ T cells recruit macrophages in the development of the response
Ⓑ the provoking infectious agents are typically extracellular
Ⓒ antigen within the macrophage occasionally persists undestroyed
Ⓓ contact eczema is usually caused by haptens such as nickel
Ⓔ Langerhans cells in the dermis present the antigen in eczema

23
The deposition of immune complexes
Ⓐ produces a vasculitis within vessel walls
Ⓑ in tissues depends upon their size and local haemodynamics
Ⓒ produces an Arthus reaction in the skin 10 days after exposure
Ⓓ in serum sickness results in tissue damage within 12–24 hours
Ⓔ in extrinsic allergic alveolitis is caused by IgA antibodies

24
The following diseases are associated with the named immune response
Ⓐ allergic rhinitis—type I hypersensitivity
Ⓑ Graves' disease—type II hypersensitivity
Ⓒ systemic lupus erythematosus—type III hypersensitivity
Ⓓ rheumatoid arthritis—type III hypersensitivity
Ⓔ contact dermatitis—type IV hypersensitivity

25
Aetiological factors in the development of the spectrum of autoimmune disorders include
Ⓐ loss of suppressor T cell control of helper T cells
Ⓑ immunological exposure to sequestrated antigens
Ⓒ bacterial mimicry of tissue antigen producing a cross-reaction
Ⓓ drug-induced immune complexes activating complement
Ⓔ genetic variations in the major histocompatibility complex

26
In primary hypogammaglobulinaemia
Ⓐ cell mediated immunity is also abnormal
Ⓑ B lymphocytes are usually present
Ⓒ treatment with immunoglobulins each month is effective
Ⓓ isolated IgA deficiency is associated with gluten enteropathy
Ⓔ susceptibility to fungal infections is increased

27
In primary thymic hypoplasia (Di George's syndrome)
Ⓐ fungal and viral infections invariably occur
Ⓑ serum immunoglobulin concentrations are normal
Ⓒ there is severe lymphopenia
Ⓓ hypoparathyroidism may be associated
Ⓔ neonatal death is usual

28
In acquired immunodeficiency syndrome (AIDS)
Ⓐ the infectious agent is a retrovirus containing DNA
Ⓑ the virus infects helper T lymphoctes
Ⓒ B lymphocytes are activated to produce hypergammaglobulinaemia
Ⓓ monocytes with the T4 surface antigen are also infected
Ⓔ immune-mediated thrombocytopenia is common

29

The following statements about drug effects on the immune system are true

Ⓐ Chlorpheniramine blocks all histamine receptors

Ⓑ Sodium cromoglycate inhibits the degranulation of mast cells

Ⓒ Adrenaline blocks the T cell release of lymphokines

Ⓓ Corticosteroids inhibit neutrophil adherence to endothelium

Ⓔ Cyclosporin suppresses B cells and T helper cells

30

In immunisation

Ⓐ passive immunisation provides only temporary protection

Ⓑ tetanus protection is achieved using a live attenuated vaccine

Ⓒ diphtheria protection is achieved using an inactivated toxin

Ⓓ acute demyelinating encephalomyelitis is a complication of passive immunisation

Ⓔ BCG protects against tuberculosis in HIV positive individuals

31

In transplantation and graft rejection

Ⓐ humorally mediated immune responses are the principal cause of rejection

Ⓑ ABO antigen groups have a major role in rejection pathogenesis

Ⓒ antigen typing is best undertaken on donor blood lymphocytes

Ⓓ the chance of a close HLA match between unrelated people is about 1 in 100

Ⓔ transplanted bone marrow T lymphocytes react against the recipient

32

The following are autoimmune diseases

Ⓐ Goodpasture's syndrome

Ⓑ atrophic gastritis

Ⓒ myasthenia gravis

Ⓓ Graves' disease

Ⓔ primary biliary cirrhosis

33

A polymorphism is

Ⓐ the same as a mutation

Ⓑ a DNA sequence change resulting in disease

Ⓒ strictly defined on the basis of a 1% population prevalence

Ⓓ silent if located in non-coding DNA

Ⓔ likely to result in a functionally similar but novel amino acid

34

In autosomal dominant inheritance

Ⓐ affected individuals are usually heterozygotes

Ⓑ affected individuals rarely have an affected parent

Ⓒ male offspring are more likely to be affected than female

Ⓓ unaffected children of an affected parent have a 50% chance of transmitting the condition

Ⓔ clinical disease is always found in genetically affected individuals

35

Given the marriage of two heterozygotes carrying the same gene transmitting an autosomal recessive disorder

Ⓐ all of their healthy children will carry the gene

Ⓑ only male children will be affected

Ⓒ each of their children has a 1 in 4 chance of being affected

Ⓓ 75% of families with an only child will have a healthy child

Ⓔ 1 in 16 of their grandchildren will be affected

36
The genetic terms below are defined as follows

Ⓐ dominant: a trait expressed in a heterozygote

Ⓑ allele: alternative forms of a gene at a given locus

Ⓒ proband: the person who first attracted medical attention to the family

Ⓓ penetrance: frequency of expression of a gene

Ⓔ mosaic: cells of different genotype in a person

37
Given a husband with haemophilia and his unaffected wife

Ⓐ none of their sons will be affected

Ⓑ all of their daughters will carry the haemophilic gene

Ⓒ a daughter with Turner's syndrome may also have haemophilia

Ⓓ all of his sisters will be carriers

Ⓔ his maternal grandfather could have had haemophilia

38
The following disorders are transmitted in an autosomal dominant mode

Ⓐ phenylketonuria

Ⓑ polyposis coli

Ⓒ achondroplasia

Ⓓ cystic fibrosis

Ⓔ Marfan's syndrome

39
The following disorders are transmitted in an X-linked recessive mode

Ⓐ vitamin D resistant rickets

Ⓑ Christmas disease

Ⓒ nephrogenic diabetes insipidus

Ⓓ haemochromatosis

Ⓔ Duchenne muscular dystrophy

40
The following disorders are transmitted in an autosomal recessive mode

Ⓐ albinism

Ⓑ acute intermittent porphyria

Ⓒ Friedreich's ataxia

Ⓓ Wilson's disease

Ⓔ Gilbert's syndrome

41
The following disorders are caused by single gene disorders

Ⓐ cleft lip

Ⓑ sickle-cell anaemia

Ⓒ Alzheimer's disease

Ⓓ cystic fibrosis

Ⓔ familial hypercholesterolaemia

42
The human immunodeficiency virus (HIV)

Ⓐ has an RNA genome

Ⓑ displays marked genetic variability

Ⓒ recognises susceptible host cells via the CD4+ antigen

Ⓓ requires a co-receptor (e.g. CCR5) to permit viral to host membrane fusion

Ⓔ causes identical clinical effects in infected hosts

43
With regard to prion diseases

Ⓐ they have a characteristically short incubation period

Ⓑ they are caused by DNA containing virus like particles

Ⓒ prions occur due to mutations in the PrP gene

Ⓓ the infectious agent is predominantly protein

Ⓔ disease occurs when the PrP protein is rendered insoluble in tissue

44
The karyotype of a
Ⓐ human is usually identified using bone marrow cells
Ⓑ female with Down's syndrome is 46,XX,–21
Ⓒ male with Klinefelter's syndrome is 47,XXY
Ⓓ female with Turner's syndrome is 45,XO
Ⓔ male with Trisomy 18 (Edwards' syndrome) is 47,XX,+18

45
In the laboratory analysis of DNA
Ⓐ restriction endonucleases are used to join small segments of DNA
Ⓑ gene probes must be single stranded to be of use in hybridisation
Ⓒ the polymerase chain reaction is used to amplify small segments of genomic DNA
Ⓓ restriction fragment length polymorphisms are useful in gene tracking
Ⓔ a low recombination fraction suggests that a gene and its marker are closely linked

46
In Down's syndrome
Ⓐ non-disjunction of chromosome 21, producing trisomy 21, is the usual cause
Ⓑ translocation accounts for 25% of those affected
Ⓒ translocations often involve chromosomes 21 and 13, 14 or 15
Ⓓ the majority of siblings have chromosomal abnormalities
Ⓔ the commonest chromosomal abnormality is polyploidy

47
Characteristic features of Klinefelter's syndrome include
Ⓐ Fallot's tetralogy
Ⓑ mental retardation
Ⓒ short stature
Ⓓ normal gonadotrophin levels
Ⓔ gynaecomastia

48
The risk of a child developing congenital pyloric stenosis is greater if
Ⓐ the child is female rather than male
Ⓑ the mother rather than the father had the disorder
Ⓒ two siblings rather than one sibling had the disorder
Ⓓ the mother is aged 40 than if she is aged 20
Ⓔ a brother was severely affected rather than mildly affected

49
In screening for genetic disorders
Ⓐ congenital hypothyroidism is detected by measurement of neonatal thyroxine
Ⓑ asymptomatic carriers of cystic fibrosis can now be identified
Ⓒ the identification of homocystinuria is treated by dietary methionine restriction
Ⓓ haemoglobin electrophoresis is useful in the detection of haemophilia A
Ⓔ ophthalmoscopy is useful in screening the relatives of individuals with familial polyposis coli

50
The following conditions and genetic markers are associated
Ⓐ ankylosing spondylitis (AS) and HLA B27
Ⓑ peptic ulcer disease and blood group A
Ⓒ atherosclerosis and apolipoprotein A-1
Ⓓ insulin-dependent diabetes mellitus and HLA B8
Ⓔ Reiter's disease and HLA B27

DISEASES DUE TO INFECTION

ANSWERS PAGE 160

1

The infections listed below are transmitted in the following manner

Ⓐ meningococcal infection—faecal-oral spread

Ⓑ legionellosis—water aerosols

Ⓒ giardiasis—faecal-oral spread

Ⓓ listeriosis—ingestion of cheese

Ⓔ gonococcal infection—transplacental spread

2

The diagnostic techniques listed below are useful in the following infections

Ⓐ rectal scrape microscopy—*Entamoeba histolytica*

Ⓑ lung biopsy—*Pneumocystis carinii*

Ⓒ bone marrow culture—Pneumococcal infection

Ⓓ rising titre of IgM antibodies—*Mycobacterium tuberculosis*

Ⓔ delayed hypersensitivity skin testing—histoplasmosis

3

Diseases typically acquired from animals include

Ⓐ leptospirosis

Ⓑ *Myobacterium tuberculosis*

Ⓒ Q fever

Ⓓ Lyme disease

Ⓔ hepatitis A

4

Diseases usually spread via the faecal-oral route include

Ⓐ poliomyelitis

Ⓑ cholera

Ⓒ hepatitis E

Ⓓ hepatitis B

Ⓔ salmonellosis

5

Schedules of immunisation in the UK should include

Ⓐ *Haemophilus influenzae* type B at the age of 3 years

Ⓑ polio vaccine on three occasions during the first year of life

Ⓒ mumps, measles and rubella at the age of 6 months

Ⓓ diphtheria, tetanus and pertussis at 2, 3 and 4 months

Ⓔ diphtheria, tetanus and polio vaccination in the first year of school

6

Contraindications to active immunisation include

Ⓐ atopic disposition

Ⓑ HIV infection if live vaccines are required

Ⓒ pregnancy if live vaccines are required

Ⓓ chronic cardiac or respiratory failure

Ⓔ recent passive immunisation if live vaccines are required

7

Live viruses are usually used for active immunisation against

Ⓐ poliomyelitis

Ⓑ pertussis

Ⓒ typhoid fever

Ⓓ mumps, measles and rubella

Ⓔ hepatitis B

8

Indications for passive immunisation with human immunoglobulin include prevention of

Ⓐ hepatitis A and B

Ⓑ tetanus

Ⓒ rabies

Ⓓ meningococcaemia

Ⓔ chickenpox

9

Notification is a statutory obligation in the following infections

Ⓐ food poisoning
Ⓑ leptospirosis
Ⓒ viral hepatitis
Ⓓ meningococcaemia
Ⓔ measles and rubella

10

The infections listed below are associated with the following types of rash

Ⓐ anthrax—ulcerating nodules (chancres)
Ⓑ leptospirosis— haemorrhagic rash
Ⓒ toxocariasis—urticaria
Ⓓ herpes simplex—vesicular rash
Ⓔ rickettsial infection—erythema nodosum

11

The following are frequent causes of fever imported into the UK

Ⓐ malaria
Ⓑ hepatitis A
Ⓒ tuberculosis
Ⓓ brucellosis
Ⓔ pneumonia

12

With regard to travellers' diarrhoea

Ⓐ no causative organism is identified in 65% of patients
Ⓑ most attacks require drug treatment
Ⓒ antidiarrhoeal agents are particularly useful in children
Ⓓ ciprofloxacin is a useful first choice antibiotic
Ⓔ doxycycline prophylaxis is advised for all travellers to sub-Saharan Africa

13

Noteworthy factors in the assessment of pyrexia of unknown origin include

Ⓐ history of travel abroad
Ⓑ occupational history
Ⓒ leisure activities
Ⓓ recent drug therapy
Ⓔ contact with animals and pets

14

In the classification of HIV infection

Ⓐ group A = acute seroconversion simulating glandular fever
Ⓑ group B = persistent generalised lymphadenopathy
Ⓒ group C = constitutional symptoms and oral candidosis
Ⓓ group A1/B1/C1 all have absolute CD4 count >500/mm^3
Ⓔ group B = asymptomatic infection

15

Presenting features of HIV infection include

Ⓐ hairy leucoplakia
Ⓑ atypical pneumonia
Ⓒ thrombocytopenic purpura
Ⓓ pulmonary tuberculosis
Ⓔ candidiasis and cryptosporidiosis

16

HIV infection is associated with

Ⓐ an RNA retrovirus
Ⓑ transmission via drug abusers more often than by sexual transmission in the UK
Ⓒ absence of involvement of B lymphocytes
Ⓓ disordered suppressor rather than helper T lymphocytes
Ⓔ a better prognosis in the presence of Kaposi's sarcoma

17

In HIV infection

Ⓐ 80% of vertically transmitted infections are transplacental
Ⓑ a child born to an infected mother has a 90% chance of acquiring HIV
Ⓒ transmission can occur via breast milk
Ⓓ risk of fetal transmission is unaffected by pre-partum antiviral agents
Ⓔ vertical transmission is the major mode of transmission world-wide

18

HIV 2 infection is

Ⓐ typically more severe and aggressive than HIV 1 infection

Ⓑ a less common cause of disease than HIV 1

Ⓒ the predominant serotype in Europe

Ⓓ less easily transmitted vertically than HIV 1

Ⓔ identifiable as five distinct viral subtypes

19

In the diagnosis of HIV infection

Ⓐ ELISA testing has a low false negative rate

Ⓑ seroconversion invariably occurs in under 4 weeks

Ⓒ antibody detection tests are particularly helpful in neonates

Ⓓ the virus can be cultured from peripheral blood lymphocytes

Ⓔ serial testing is necessary to confirm infection in some individuals

20

In the treatment of HIV infection

Ⓐ all useful drugs work via inhibition of reverse transcriptase

Ⓑ reverse transcriptase inhibitors prevent replication in infected cells

Ⓒ reverse transcriptase inhibitors prevent spread of infectious virus into uninfected cells

Ⓓ drug-resistant strains of virus have not been recognised

Ⓔ monotherapy is preferred

21

Following an occupational needlestick injury with HIV-infected blood

Ⓐ the risk of HIV transmission is 30%

Ⓑ zidovudine reduces the risk of seroconversion by around 8%

Ⓒ infection is more likely if the patient has advanced disease

Ⓓ zidovudine should be started 12–24 hours after inoculation

Ⓔ zidovudine should be taken for 4 weeks after injury

22

In a patient with AIDS, cryptococcal meningitis is

Ⓐ the commonest cause of meningitis

Ⓑ characterised by abrupt onset of the classical features of a bacterial meningitis

Ⓒ diagnosed by Indian ink stain of cerebrospinal fluid (CSF)

Ⓓ typically associated with a normal cerebral CT scan

Ⓔ typically associated with a high CSF polymorph count

23

Cryptosporidiosis in an HIV-positive patient is

Ⓐ an AIDS defining diagnosis if chronic

Ⓑ likely to present with painless profuse diarrhoea

Ⓒ likely to resolve spontaneously

Ⓓ preventable by the use of boiled tap water

Ⓔ likely to respond well to anti-parasitic drug therapy

24

***Pneumocystis carinii* infection in an HIV-positive patient is**

Ⓐ the commonest cause of respiratory infection in African patients

Ⓑ characterised by copious sputum production

Ⓒ characterised by widespread fine pulmonary crackles

Ⓓ more likely to occur when the CD4 count is $< 200/mm^3$

Ⓔ excluded by the finding of a normal chest X-ray

25

In a schoolchild with measles

Ⓐ infection is due to a single-stranded RNA paramyxovirus

Ⓑ rhinorrhoea and conjunctivitis occur at the onset

Ⓒ Koplik's spots appear at the same time as the skin rash

Ⓓ the skin rash typically desquamates as it disappears

Ⓔ infectivity is confined to the prodromal phase

26

In patients with rubella infection

Ⓐ the RNA virus spreads by the faecal-oral route

Ⓑ the transient polyarthritis is more marked in children than in adults

Ⓒ infectivity is present for 7 days before and after the rash

Ⓓ suboccipital lymphadenopathy with a macular rash behind the ears is typical

Ⓔ the risk of serious fetal damage is < 5% after the 16th week of pregnancy

27

Typical complications of rubella include

Ⓐ an 80% risk of fetal damage within the first 6 weeks of pregnancy

Ⓑ post-viral encephalitis

Ⓒ gastroenteritis and acute appendicitis

Ⓓ polyarthritis

Ⓔ pericarditis

28

The characteristic features of mumps include

Ⓐ infection with an RNA paramyxovirus by airborne spread

Ⓑ high infectivity for 3 weeks after the onset of parotitis

Ⓒ presentation with an acute lymphocytic meningitis

Ⓓ abdominal pain attributable to mesenteric adenitis

Ⓔ orchitis which is usually bilateral and predominantly occurs prepubertally

29

The features of herpes simplex (HS) virus infections include

Ⓐ recurrent genital ulcers

Ⓑ acute gingivostomatitis

Ⓒ encephalitis

Ⓓ shingles

Ⓔ paronychia

30

The following statements about glandular fever are true

Ⓐ infection is usually attributable to the Epstein–Barr virus (EBV)

Ⓑ presentation is with fever, headache and abdominal pain

Ⓒ sore throat suggest cytomegalovirus rather than EBV infection

Ⓓ meningoencephalitis and hepatitis are recognised complications

Ⓔ severe oro-pharyngeal swelling requires prednisolone therapy

31

The clinical features of chickenpox include

Ⓐ infection due to varicella zoster virus from airborne spread

Ⓑ high infectivity until 7 days after the last crop of vesicles

Ⓒ clinical response to acyclovir therapy in the immunocompromised

Ⓓ palatal rash appears before involvement of the trunk then face

Ⓔ constitutional symptoms are particularly severe in children

32

Recognised complications of chickenpox include

Ⓐ pneumonia, particularly in children rather than adults

Ⓑ proliferative glomerulonephritis

Ⓒ acute pancreatitis

Ⓓ encephalitis with cerebellar involvement

Ⓔ myocarditis

33

The characteristic features of rabies include

Ⓐ a rhabdovirus infection transmitted in animal saliva

Ⓑ an incubation period of 4–8 days

Ⓒ a poor prognosis if symptoms develop

Ⓓ encephalitis or ascending paralysis

Ⓔ active and passive vaccination are useful in prevention and therapy

34

The clinical features of Lassa fever include

Ⓐ travel to South America

Ⓑ transmission via mosquito

Ⓒ no useful response to any antiviral agent

Ⓓ liver failure

Ⓔ incubation period 3–6 weeks

35

The clinical features of yellow fever include

Ⓐ a togavirus infection transmitted by mosquitoes

Ⓑ an incubation period of 3–6 weeks

Ⓒ peripheral blood leucocytosis in contrast to viral hepatitis

Ⓓ fever, headache and severe myalgia with bone pains

Ⓔ response to tribavirin drug therapy

36

Characteristics of the influenza virus include

Ⓐ restriction to human infection

Ⓑ low level of antigenic shift

Ⓒ transmission in respiratory secretions

Ⓓ incubation period 5–7 days

Ⓔ infection complicated by Reye's syndrome

37

Features of the respiratory syncytial virus include

Ⓐ childhood respiratory infection is uncommon but severe

Ⓑ infection is best diagnosed by serology

Ⓒ infants are protected via maternally acquired antibody

Ⓓ infection may be complicated by bronchiolitis

Ⓔ cough is characteristically absent during respiratory infection

38

Coxsackie viruses

Ⓐ are enteroviruses

Ⓑ cause hand, foot and mouth disease

Ⓒ cause chest pain

Ⓓ are a cause of aseptic meningitis

Ⓔ are detectable by the polymerase chain reaction in infected body fluids

39

Clinical features of dengue include

Ⓐ mosquito-borne infection with an incubation period of 5–6 days

Ⓑ continuous or saddleback fever

Ⓒ rigors, headache, photophobia and backache

Ⓓ morbilliform rash and cervical lymphadenopathy

Ⓔ protection by vaccination every 10 years in endemic areas

40

Diseases attributable to chlamydial infection include

Ⓐ psittacosis

Ⓑ epidemic typhus

Ⓒ trachoma

Ⓓ lymphogranuloma venereum

Ⓔ Q fever

41

In trachoma

A blepharospasm is a common presenting feature

B upper eyelid follicular conjunctivitis is typical

C acute ophthalmia neonatorum is a recognised presentation

D tetracycline eye drops are indicated

E blindness is usually due to cataracts

42

The typical features of psittacosis include

A an incubation period of 2 weeks

B constitutional upset with fever, headache and myalgia

C pulmonary infiltrates on chest X-ray not apparent clinically

D birds surviving the disease are no longer infectious

E prompt resolution with sulphonamide therapy

43

Diseases attributable to mycoplasmal infection include

A haemolytic anaemia

B pelvic inflammatory disease

C pneumonia

D myocarditis

E urethritis and prostatitis

44

The typical clinical features of typhus fevers include

A rickettsial infection from arthropods

B parasitisation of the endothelium of small blood vessels

C fever, headache and back pain and cutaneous haemorrhages

D mortality over 90%

E response to chloramphenicol or tetracycline therapy

45

Features consistent with the diagnosis of Q fever include

A exposure to sheep, cattle and unpasteurised milk

B an incubation period of 1–2 weeks

C pneumonia in the absence of fever, headache or myalgia

D blood culture-negative endocarditis

E prompt clinical response to sulphonamide therapy

46

The clinical features of Lyme disease include

A infection with the tick-borne spirochaete *Borrelia burgdorferi*

B an expanding erythematous rash (erythema chronicum migrans)

C cranial nerve palsies

D asymmetrical large joint recurrent oligoarthritis

E response to tetracycline or penicillin therapy

47

The clinical features of relapsing fevers include

A infection with borrelial spirochaetes

B an incubation period of 1–3 months

C rigors, headache, mental confusion and jaundice

D hepatosplenomegaly and thrombocytopenic purpura

E response to erythromycin or tetracycline therapy

48

The typical features of leptospirosis include

A incubation period of 1–3 months

B exposure risk in abattoirs, farms and inland waterways

C fever, severe myalgia, headache and conjunctival suffusion

D meningitis in *L. icterohaemorrhagiae* rather than *L. canicola* infection

E myocarditis, hepatitis and acute renal failure

49
Sexually-transmissible viral diseases include
Ⓐ cytomegalovirus
Ⓑ hepatitis A, B and C
Ⓒ papovavirus
Ⓓ herpes simplex
Ⓔ molluscum contagiosum

50
The following statements about syphilis are true
Ⓐ Infection is usually caused by *Treponema pertenue*
Ⓑ Untreated, infectivity is restricted to the first 2 months
Ⓒ The distinction between early and late syphilis is made at 2 years
Ⓓ The incubation period for primary syphilis is typically 2–4 weeks
Ⓔ Tertiary syphilis usually develops within one year of infection

51
The characteristic features of secondary syphilis include
Ⓐ fever and a macular rash occurring 8 weeks after the chancre
Ⓑ condylomata lata in warm moist areas appearing as flat papules
Ⓒ generalised lymphadenopathy and oro-genital mucous ulceration
Ⓓ cerebrospinal fluid pleocytosis is present in 90% indicating meningovascular disease
Ⓔ soft early diastolic murmur on cardiac auscultation

52
Characteristic features of late (tertiary and quaternary) syphilis include
Ⓐ negative specific treponemal antigen tests
Ⓑ destructive granulomas (gummas) in bones, joints and the liver
Ⓒ sensory ataxia
Ⓓ aneurysms of the ascending aorta
Ⓔ poor response of gummas to antibiotic therapy

53
The typical clinical features of gonorrhoea include
Ⓐ an incubation period of 2–3 weeks
Ⓑ anterior urethritis and cervicitis
Ⓒ right hypochondrial pain due to perihepatitis
Ⓓ pustular haemorrhagic rash and acute large joint arthritis
Ⓔ good response to ciprofloxacin therapy in penicillin allergy

54
Features suggestive of non-gonococcal urethritis include
Ⓐ urethral culture of *Chlamydia trachomatis*
Ⓑ urethral culture of *Ureaplasma urealyticum*
Ⓒ keratoderma and peripheral oligoarthritis
Ⓓ painless genital ulceration
Ⓔ good response to penicillin therapy

55
The typical features of lymphogranuloma venereum include
Ⓐ mononuclear cells exhibiting Donovan bodies within the lesion
Ⓑ transient genital ulceration 1–5 weeks after chlamydial infection
Ⓒ fever, weight loss and inguinal lymphadenopathy
Ⓓ proctitis and rectal stricture
Ⓔ response to tetracycline therapy

56
Recognised causes of genital ulcers include
Ⓐ herpes zoster
Ⓑ chancroid
Ⓒ primary syphilis
Ⓓ Behçet's syndrome
Ⓔ gonorrhoea

57

Anogenital herpes simplex is typically associated with

Ⓐ type 1 more often than type 2 herpes simplex infection

Ⓑ primary attacks more severe and prolonged than recurrent attacks

Ⓒ fever with painful genital ulceration and lymphadenopathy

Ⓓ sacral dermatomal pain and urinary retention

Ⓔ absence of clinical response to oral aciclovir

58

Scarlet fever is typically associated with

Ⓐ rigors, headache and acute pharyngitis or tonsillitis

Ⓑ generalised punctate erythema desquamating on resolution

Ⓒ group B rather than group A streptococcal infection

Ⓓ generalised rather than localised lymphadenopathy

Ⓔ a membranous adherent pharyngeal exudate

59

The typical features of erysipelas include

Ⓐ group A haemolytic streptococcal skin infection

Ⓑ absence of constitutional symptoms

Ⓒ well-defined area of cutaneous erythema and oedema

Ⓓ commoner in young rather than elderly patients

Ⓔ prompt response within 48 hours to benzylpenicillin

60

Staphylococcal infection is associated with

Ⓐ resistance to benzylpenicillin therapy

Ⓑ necrotising enterocolitis

Ⓒ bronchopneumonia

Ⓓ toxic shock syndrome

Ⓔ cellulitis

61

Clinical features suggesting toxic shock syndrome include

Ⓐ onset 24–48 hours after food ingestion

Ⓑ fever, myalgia, vomiting and diarrhoea

Ⓒ hypotension and hypovolaemia

Ⓓ prompt clinical response to benzylpenicillin

Ⓔ generalised erythema desquamating on resolution

62

In bacteraemic shock

Ⓐ endotoxin initiates disseminated intravascular coagulation

Ⓑ peripheral vascular resistance falls initially

Ⓒ acute circulatory failure is usually due to cardiac failure

Ⓓ leucocytosis and thrombocythaemia indicate a poor prognosis

Ⓔ antibiotic therapy should await bacteriological results

63

Diphtheria rather than streptococcal tonsillitis is suggested by

Ⓐ tender cervical lymphadenopathy

Ⓑ blood-stained nasal discharge and marked tachycardia

Ⓒ firm, adherent tonsillar exudate extending beyond the tonsils

Ⓓ paralysis of the soft palate, accommodation or ocular muscles

Ⓔ an incubation period of 2–4 days followed by marked fever

64

In the treatment of diphtheria

Ⓐ antitoxin should be avoided pending bacteriological confirmation

Ⓑ antitoxin-induced anaphylaxis is best treated with prednisolone

Ⓒ antitoxin-induced serum sickness produces intense bronchospasm

Ⓓ isolation is usually unnecessary

Ⓔ myocarditis typically results in permanent cardiac impairment

65

In whooping cough

Ⓐ the incubation period is 1–2 weeks

Ⓑ onset with rhinitis and conjunctivitis is characteristic

Ⓒ paroxysmal coughing bouts develop 2–3 weeks after exposure

Ⓓ *Bordetella pertussis* is best cultured from anterior nasal swabs

Ⓔ antibiotic therapy significantly reduces coughing bouts

66

The typical features of meningococcal infection include

Ⓐ airborne spread of infection

Ⓑ abrupt onset with headache, vomiting and meningism

Ⓒ acute circulatory failure and purpuric rash

Ⓓ isolation of serogroups A and C more commonly than group B

Ⓔ control of infection in contacts is best achieved by vaccination

67

Characteristic features of tetanus include

Ⓐ an incubation period of 2–3 days

Ⓑ muscular spasm typically starting in the masseters

Ⓒ convulsions associated with loss of consciousness

Ⓓ abdominal rigidity without pain or tenderness

Ⓔ bacteriological isolation of *Clostridium tetani* from the wound

68

In the treatment of tetanus

Ⓐ tetanus toxoid should be given intravenously as soon as possible

Ⓑ wound debridement should be undertaken prior to any other therapy

Ⓒ human antitetanus immunoglobulin should be given immediately

Ⓓ diazepam should be avoided because of the hazards of oversedation

Ⓔ penicillin or metronidazole therapy should be administered

69

The typical features of botulism include

Ⓐ ingestion of infected water 2–4 hours prior to symptom onset

Ⓑ onset with an afebrile gastroenteritis or postural hypotension

Ⓒ autonomic neuropathy induced by the cholinergic neurotoxin

Ⓓ ocular neuropathy and bulbar palsy developing over 3 days

Ⓔ dramatic clinical response to parenteral antitoxin

70

Clinical features of anthrax include

Ⓐ occupational exposure to animals and animal products

Ⓑ an incubation period of 1–3 weeks

Ⓒ a painless cutaneous papule with regional lymphadenopathy

Ⓓ gastroenteritis, meningitis or bronchopneumonia

Ⓔ multiple antibiotic resistance is common

71

Recognised features of brucellosis include

Ⓐ an incubation period of 3 months

Ⓑ fever, night sweats and back pain

Ⓒ hepatosplenomegaly and epididymoorchitis

Ⓓ oligoarthritis and spondylitis

Ⓔ peripheral blood neutrophil leucocytosis

72

The characteristic features of plague include

Ⓐ an incubation period of less than 7 days

Ⓑ transmission of *Yersinia pestis* in infected fish

Ⓒ predominantly pneumonic rather than bubonic presentation

Ⓓ rigors, severe headache and painful lymphadenopathy

Ⓔ absence of splenomegaly or hepatomegaly

73

The typical features of typhoid fever include

A faecal-oral spread of *Salmonella typhi* by food handlers

B an incubation period of 3–7 days

C onset with fever, headache, myalgia and septicaemia

D 'rose spots' on the trunk and splenomegaly 7–10 days after onset

E diarrhoea and abdominal pain and tenderness 10–14 days after onset

74

Recognised complications of typhoid fever include

A cholecystitis

B meningitis

C endocarditis

D osteomyelitis

E pneumonia

75

Paratyphoid fever rather than typhoid fever is suggested by

A onset with vomiting and diarrhoea

B an incubation period of 5–7 days

C absence of an erythematous macular rash

D the development of a reactive arthritis

E prominence of intestinal complications

76

In the diagnosis of the enteric fevers

A blood cultures are usually positive 2 weeks after onset

B stool cultures are usually positive within 7 days of onset

C peripheral blood neutrophil leucocytosis is typically marked

D the Widal reaction is typically positive within 7 days of onset

E persistent fever despite antibiotics indicates resistant organisms

77

Symptom patterns suggesting specific food poisoning include

A bloody diarrhoea after 12–48 hours—*Campylobacter jejuni*

B vomiting and abdominal pain after 3–6 hours—staphylococci

C vomiting and abdominal pain after 30–90 minutes—food allergy

D bloody diarrhoea after 24–48 hours—*Escherichia coli*

E vomiting and diarrhoea after 12–48 hours—salmonella

78

Bacillary dysentery in the UK

A is usually caused by *Shigella dysenteriae*

B has an incubation period of 1–7 days

C usually arises from contaminated water supplies

D is characterised by profuse watery diarrhoea

E should be treated with sulphonamide or tetracycline therapy

79

The characteristic features of cholera include

A the recent ingestion of contaminated water or shellfish

B an incubation period of 5–10 days

C sudden onset of profuse watery diarrhoea followed by vomiting

D acute circulatory failure developing within 12 hours of onset

E rapidly progressive metabolic alkalosis and dehydration

80
Antimicrobial therapy acts in the following ways
Ⓐ aminoglycosides disrupt bacterial protein synthesis

Ⓑ sulphonamides interrupt bacterial folate synthesis

Ⓒ penicillins disrupt bacterial protein synthesis

Ⓓ cephalosporins disrupt bacterial cell wall synthesis

Ⓔ tetracyclines disrupt bacterial protein synthesis

81
The antimicrobials listed below are contraindicated as follows
Ⓐ tetracyclines—in pregnancy

Ⓑ sulphonamides—in glucose 6 phosphate dehydrogenase deficiency

Ⓒ chloramphenicol—in neonatal infection

Ⓓ ampicillin—in infectious mononucleosis

Ⓔ cephalosporins—in the elderly

82
The following statements about penicillins are true
Ⓐ All penicillins are bactericidal

Ⓑ Like the cephalosporins, they contain a β-lactam ring

Ⓒ Clavulanic acid inhibits bacterial β-lactamase

Ⓓ They can safely be used in cephalosporin-allergic patients

Ⓔ They are best given intrathecally in bacterial meningitis

83
Tetracycline therapy is
Ⓐ bactericidal to sensitive bacteria

Ⓑ contraindicated in pregnancy

Ⓒ contraindicated in patients with renal failure

Ⓓ best given before meals

Ⓔ active against rickettsiae, mycoplasmas and chlamydiae

84
Aminoglycoside drug therapy
Ⓐ is ototoxic and nephrotoxic

Ⓑ should be avoided in patients requiring diuretic therapy

Ⓒ must be monitored using plasma drug concentrations

Ⓓ is effective against anaerobes and *Streptococcus faecalis*

Ⓔ is best avoided in patients with renal failure

85
Erythromycin is active against the following microorganisms
Ⓐ *Campylobacter jejuni*

Ⓑ *Escherichia coli*

Ⓒ *Legionella pneumophila*

Ⓓ *Mycoplasma pneumoniae*

Ⓔ *Clostridium welchii*

86
Chloramphenicol is active against the following microorganisms
Ⓐ *Haemophilus influenzae*

Ⓑ *Salmonella typhi*

Ⓒ *Klebsiella pneumoniae*

Ⓓ *Pseudomonas aeruginosa*

Ⓔ *Brucella abortus*

87
Ciprofloxacin is highly active against the following microorganisms
Ⓐ *Escherichia coli*

Ⓑ *Brucella abortus*

Ⓒ *Proteus mirabilis*

Ⓓ *Streptococcus pneumoniae*

Ⓔ *Bacteroides fragilis*

88

The following statements about antibiotic therapy are true

A Chloramphenicol therapy should be avoided in neonates

B Metronidazole is effective in giardiasis and amoebiasis

C Co-trimoxazole is effective in pneumocystis pneumonia

D Sodium fusidate is effective in staphylococcal osteomyelitis

E Ciprofloxacin is effective in syphilis

89

Indications for appropriate chemoprophylaxis include

A erythromycin in diphtheria contacts

B rifampicin in meningitis contacts

C penicillin following previous rheumatic fever

D rifampicin in susceptible tuberculosis contacts

E amoxycillin before dental surgery in patients with cardiac valve prostheses

90

Antiviral agents active against the following viruses include

A ganciclovir—cytomegalovirus

B amantadine—orthomyxovirus

C tribavirin—respiratory syncytial virus

D zidovudine—retrovirus

E famciclovir—herpes simplex and zoster virus

91

Characteristic features of leprosy include

A an incubation period of 2–5 years

B growth of the organism on Lowenstein–Jensen medium after 2–3 months

C spread of the tuberculoid form on prolonged patient contact

D spontaneous healing of the earliest macule

E a cell-mediated immune response in the lepromatous form

92

Typical features of tuberculoid leprosy include

A cell-mediated immune response around nerves and hair follicles

B absence of infectivity of affected patients

C palpable thickening of the peripheral nerves

D development of erythema nodosum leprosum

E persistently negative lepromin skin test

93

Typical features of lepromatous leprosy include

A absence of infectivity of affected patients

B unlike the tuberculoid form, organisms are scanty in number

C blood-borne spread from the dermis throughout the body

D strongly positive lepromin skin test

E anaesthetic hypopigmented skin macules and plaques

94

The following statements about the life cycle of plasmodia are true

A Sporozoites disappear from the blood within minutes of inoculation

B Merozoites re-entering red blood cells undergo both sexual and asexual development

C All plasmodia multiply in the liver then subsequently in red blood cells

D Dormant hypnozoites remain within the liver cells in all species

E Fertilisation of the gametocytes occurs in the human red blood cells

95
All species of plasmodia producing malaria in humans
Ⓐ are transmitted exclusively by anopheline mosquitoes
Ⓑ have a persistent exoerythrocytic phase often dormant for years
Ⓒ produce the initial symptoms on the release of red blood cell sporozoites
Ⓓ parasitise red blood cells and normoblasts in all stages of development
Ⓔ parasitise capillary endothelium throughout the body

96
Typical features of *Plasmodium falciparum* malaria include
Ⓐ febrile response more marked than in other forms of malaria
Ⓑ absence of intravascular haemolysis and splenomegaly
Ⓒ infected red blood cells causing capillary occlusion throughout the body
Ⓓ rarity of infection in haemoglobin S or C heterozygotes
Ⓔ longer incubation period of 3–4 weeks in non-immune subjects

97
Recognised clinical features of malaria include
Ⓐ absence of *P. vivax* infection in subjects lacking the Duffy blood group
Ⓑ asymptomatic *P. malariae* parasitaemia persisting for years
Ⓒ rarity of clinical relapses beyond two years
Ⓓ presentation with rigors, herpes simplex and haemolytic anaemia
Ⓔ flu-like symptoms, jaundice and hepatosplenomegaly in *P. falciparum*

98
The clinical features of amoebic dysentery typically include
Ⓐ an incubation period of 2–4 weeks
Ⓑ presentation with profuse watery diarrhoea
Ⓒ colonic mucosal involvement most marked in the rectum
Ⓓ characteristic appearances of the mucosa on sigmoidoscopy
Ⓔ *Entamoeba histolytica* cysts in the stool are pathognomonic of the disease

99
Recognised complications of amoebiasis include
Ⓐ severe intestinal haemorrhage
Ⓑ expectoration of amoebic pus from a liver abscess
Ⓒ cerebral abscess
Ⓓ amoebomas of the caecum, colon and rectum
Ⓔ genital and perineal ulceration from cutaneous amoebiasis

100
In the diagnosis and therapy of amoebiasis
Ⓐ amoebic liver abscesses usually reveal the presence of cysts
Ⓑ stool trophozoites are unlikely in the presence of blood or mucus
Ⓒ liver abscesses are best identified by ultrasound scanning
Ⓓ metronidazole therapy is effective in both liver and colonic disease
Ⓔ furamide therapy should also be given to eliminate colonic cyst

101
The characteristic features of giardiasis include
Ⓐ an incubation period of 2–3 days
Ⓑ infection transmitted by airborne droplet spread
Ⓒ predominant parasitisation of the duodenum and jejunum
Ⓓ presentation with watery diarrhoea and malabsorption
Ⓔ clinical response to metronidazole

102
Recognised features of toxoplasmosis include
Ⓐ infection derived from cats, pigs and sheep
Ⓑ asymptomatic infection is common in otherwise healthy subjects
Ⓒ congenital infection produces choroidoretinitis and cerebral palsy
Ⓓ glandular fever-like illness with peripheral blood monocytosis
Ⓔ pyrimethamine and sulphadiazine therapy is useful in AIDS

103
The typical features of African trypanosomiasis include
Ⓐ transmission of the parasite by the tsetse cattle fly
Ⓑ an incubation period of 2–3 weeks
Ⓒ onset with chancre-like skin lesion with local lymphadenopathy
Ⓓ generalised lymphadenopathy, hepatosplenomegaly and encephalitis
Ⓔ good prognosis given prompt pentamidine or suramin therapy

104
Typical features of American trypanosomiasis include
Ⓐ spread of the parasite by the reduviid bug of cats and dogs
Ⓑ Romaña's sign with eye closure due to a conjunctival infection
Ⓒ latent period of many years before onset of chronic disease
Ⓓ colonic and oesophageal dilatation due to neuropathy
Ⓔ response to nifurtimox therapy achieves cure rates of 90%

105
Typical features of visceral leishmaniasis (kala-azar) include
Ⓐ spread of *Leishmania donovani* by sandflies from dogs and rodents
Ⓑ an incubation period of 1–2 weeks
Ⓒ rigors with hepatomegaly but no splenomegaly
Ⓓ diagnosis confirmed on peripheral blood film
Ⓔ clinical response to pentavalent antimonials e g stibogluconate

106
Typical features of cutaneous leishmaniasis include
Ⓐ nasal and mouth mucosal ulcers
Ⓑ painful ulcers in the groins or axillae
Ⓒ marked splenomegaly and lymphadenopathy
Ⓓ ulcers which heal without scarring
Ⓔ negative leishmanin skin test

107
All forms of schistosomiasis are associated with
Ⓐ trematode helminths reproducing in freshwater snails
Ⓑ the passage of cercariae in the urine and/or stool
Ⓒ cercarial penetration of the skin or mucous membranes
Ⓓ progression to portal or pulmonary hypertension
Ⓔ eradication following praziquantel therapy

108
Typical features of *Schistosoma haematobium* infection include
Ⓐ disease confined to the urinary tract
Ⓑ presentation with painless haematuria
Ⓒ spontaneous resolution within a year of leaving endemic areas
Ⓓ involvement of the uterine cervix and seminal vesicles
Ⓔ an endemic disease in China and the Far East

109

Typical features of *Schistosoma mansoni* infection include

A an endemic disease in Egypt and East Africa

B abdominal pain with loose, blood-stained stools

C progression to jaundice and chronic liver failure

D paraplegia, cor pulmonale and bowel papillomata

E weight loss and malabsorption due to small bowel disease

110

Typical features of *Schistosoma japonicum* infection include

A parasitisation of rodents, domestic animals and man

B infestation follows the ingestion of raw fish and crustacea

C abdominal pain and diarrhoea due to ileal and colonic involvement

D epilepsy, hemiplegia, paraplegia and blindness

E morbidity and mortality rate less than that from the other species

111

Cestode infestation with *Taenia saginata* is associated with

A ingestion of undercooked pork

B abdominal pain and diarrhoea

C presentation with pruritus ani

D weight loss and malabsorption

E response to praziquantel therapy

112

***Echinococcus granulosus* infestation is usually associated with**

A contact with sheep, cattle and dogs

B acquisition of hydatid cysts in childhood

C cysts in the liver, brain and lungs

D absence of dissemination during liver aspiration

E prompt response to albendazole therapy if surgically inoperable

113

In infestation with the nematode *Enterobius vermicularis*

A adult threadworms occur in great numbers in the small bowel

B presentation with intense pruritus ani is typical

C identifiable ova are found on the perianal skin

D malabsorption usually develops following heavy infestations

E all family members should take piperazine or mebendazole therapy

114

In infestation with *Ascaris lumbricoides*

A the disease follows ingestion of food contaminated with larvae

B larval migration through the lungs produces pulmonary eosinophilia

C obstruction of the ileum, biliary and pancreatic ducts occurs

D malabsorption is the usual presentation

E levamisole in a single dose eradicates the disease

115

The typical features of strongyloidiasis include

A skin penetration with migration to the gut via the lungs

B larval penetration of the duodenal and jejunal mucosa

C abdominal pain, diarrhoea and malabsorption

D penetration of perianal skin producing a migrating linear weal

E systemic spread in the immunosuppressed, resulting in pneumonia

116

The clinical features of infection with *Toxocara canis* **include**

Ⓐ larval penetration of the gastric mucosa after contact with dogs

Ⓑ development of adult worms throughout the body tissues

Ⓒ hepatosplenomegaly and visual impairment

Ⓓ pulmonary and peripheral blood eosinophilia

Ⓔ effectively treated with diethylcarbamazine

117

Typical features of *Trichinella spiralis* **infestation include**

Ⓐ infection resulting from contact with the urine of rodents

Ⓑ larval migration from the small bowel to skeletal muscle

Ⓒ oedema of the eyelids with muscle pain and tenderness

Ⓓ acute myocarditis and encephalitis

Ⓔ response to corticosteroid and albendazole therapy

118

In infection with *Loa loa*

Ⓐ transmission of microfilaria is by the mosquito *Culex fatigans*

Ⓑ the incubation period is usually 1–2 weeks

Ⓒ intermittent Calabar swellings in the subdermis are typical

Ⓓ adult worms are visible traversing the eye beneath the conjunctiva

Ⓔ diethylcarbamazine therapy is curative

119

In onchocerciasis

Ⓐ larval infection is transmitted by the *Simulium* fly

Ⓑ worms mature over 2–4 weeks and persist for up to 1 year

Ⓒ cutaneous nodules and eosinophilia commonly develop

Ⓓ conjunctivitis, iritis and keratitis are characteristic

Ⓔ ivermectin is the drug therapy of choice

120

Children are no longer an infectious risk to others

Ⓐ 1 week after the last crop of chickenpox lesions

Ⓑ 5 days after the start of antibiotic therapy for scarlet fever

Ⓒ 1 week after the onset of a measles rash

Ⓓ 1 day after the onset of salivary gland swelling due to mumps

Ⓔ 1 week after the onset of a rubella rash

121

In patients with *Helicobacter pylori* **(HP) infection**

Ⓐ the diagnosis can be confirmed by decreased urease concentrations in the gastric mucosa

Ⓑ the presence of oesophagitis indicates the need for HP eradication therapy

Ⓒ HP eradication is enhanced by sustained elevation of gastric pH

Ⓓ amoxycillin plus metronidazole therapy is more effective than amoxycillin alone

Ⓔ HP eradication reduces recurrence rates of both duodenal and gastric ulcers

122

The typical features of *Yersinia* **infections include**

Ⓐ water-borne infection

Ⓑ exudative pharyngitis and enterocolitis

Ⓒ acute ileitis and mesenteric adenitis

Ⓓ erythema nodosum and reactive arthritis

Ⓔ clinical response to benzylpenicillin

DISEASES OF THE CARDIOVASCULAR SYSTEM

3

ANSWERS PAGE 172

1

The pain of myocardial ischaemia

Ⓐ is typically induced by exercise and relieved by rest

Ⓑ radiates to the neck and jaw but not the teeth

Ⓒ rarely lasts longer than 10 seconds after resting

Ⓓ is easily distinguished from oesophageal pain

Ⓔ invariably worsens as exercise continues

2

Syncope

Ⓐ followed by facial flushing suggests a tachyarrhythmia

Ⓑ without warning suggests a vaso-vagal episode

Ⓒ on exercise is a typical feature of mitral regurgitation

Ⓓ is the commonest cause of falls among elderly patients

Ⓔ is a recognised presenting feature of pulmonary embolism

3

Recognised features of severe cardiac failure include

Ⓐ tiredness

Ⓑ weight loss

Ⓒ epigastric pain

Ⓓ nocturia

Ⓔ nocturnal cough

4

In the normal human heart

Ⓐ the atrioventricular (AV) node is usually supplied by the left circumflex coronary artery

Ⓑ β_1-adrenoreceptors mediate chronotropic responses

Ⓒ pulmonary artery systolic pressure normally varies between 90 and 140 mmHg

Ⓓ the annulus fibrosus aids conduction of impulses from the atria to the ventricles

Ⓔ cardiac output is the product of heart rate and ventricular end-diastolic volume

5

In the normal electrocardiogram

Ⓐ the PR interval is measured from the end of the P wave to the beginning of the R wave

Ⓑ each small square represents 40 milliseconds at a standard paper speed of 25 mm/sec

Ⓒ the heart rate is 75 per minute if the R-R interval measures 4 cm

Ⓓ R waves become progressively larger from leads V_1–V_6

Ⓔ the P wave represents sinoatrial node depolarisation

6

The pulse characteristics listed below are typical features of the following disorders

Ⓐ pulsus bisferiens—combined mitral stenosis and regurgitation

Ⓑ pulsus paradoxus—aortic regurgitation

Ⓒ collapsing pulse—severe anaemia

Ⓓ pulsus alternans—extrasystoles every alternate beat

Ⓔ slow rising pulse—mitral stenosis

7

The following statements about the jugular venous pressure (JVP) are true

Ⓐ the external jugular vein is a reliable guide to right atrial pressure

Ⓑ the JVP is conventionally measured from the suprasternal notch

Ⓒ the normal JVP, unlike the blood pressure, does not rise with anxiety

Ⓓ the normal JVP does not rise on abdominal compression

Ⓔ the normal JVP falls during inspiration

8

The abnormalities of the jugular venous pulse listed below are associated with the following disorders

Ⓐ *cannon waves*—pulmonary hypertension

Ⓑ giant *a* waves—tricuspid stenosis

Ⓒ *v* waves—tricuspid regurgitation

Ⓓ inspiratory rise in jugular venous pressure—pericardial tamponade

Ⓔ absent *a* waves—atrioventricular dissociation

9

With regard to cardiovascular physiology

Ⓐ cardiac output is the product of heart rate and stroke volume

Ⓑ coronary blood vessels are innervated only by the parasympathetic nerves

Ⓒ intracoronary acetylcholine provokes vasoconstriction if atheroma is present

Ⓓ an atheromatous coronary lesion restricts blood flow during exercise if greater than 40%

Ⓔ bradykinin is an endogenous vasodilator

10

The auscultatory findings listed below are associated with the following phenomena

Ⓐ third heart sound—opening of mitral valve

Ⓑ varying intensity of first heart sound—atrioventricular dissociation

Ⓒ soft first heart sound—mitral stenosis

Ⓓ reversed splitting of second heart sound—left bundle branch block

Ⓔ fourth heart sound—atrial fibrillation

11

The following statements about the measurement of the blood pressure (BP) are true

Ⓐ An arm cuff smaller than recommended lowers BP recordings

Ⓑ Appearance of the first Korotkov sound denotes systolic pressure

Ⓒ Muffling of the sound denotes phase V diastolic pressure

Ⓓ Inter-observer variation is less with phase IV than with phase V

Ⓔ Resting BP should be recorded as random BP recordings do not correlate with morbidity

12

In the normal electrocardiogram (ECG)

Ⓐ depolarisation proceeds from epicardium to endocardium

Ⓑ depolarisation away from the positive electrode produces a positive deflection

Ⓒ depolarisation of the interventricular septum is recorded by the Q wave in V_5 + V_6

Ⓓ the AVR lead = right arm positive with respect to the other limb leads

Ⓔ voltage amplitudes vary with the thickness of cardiac muscle

13

Features that suggest a ventricular rather than supraventricular tachycardia include

Ⓐ a ventricular rate > 160/minute

Ⓑ termination of the arrhythmia with carotid sinus pressure

Ⓒ variable intensity of the first heart sound

Ⓓ the presence of cardiac failure

Ⓔ QRS complexes < 0.14 sec in duration on ECG

14
In the investigation of patients with suspected heart disease
Ⓐ the normal upper limit for the cardiothoracic ratio (CTR) on chest X-ray is 0.75

Ⓑ a negative exercise ECG excludes the diagnosis of ischaemic heart disease

Ⓒ a 'step-up' in oxygen saturation at cardiac catheterisation suggests an intracardiac shunt

Ⓓ Doppler echocardiography reliably assesses pressure gradients between cardiac chambers

Ⓔ radionuclide blood pool scanning accurately quantifies left ventricular function

15
The following statements about cardiac rhythms are true
Ⓐ Cardiac rate falls with inspiration in autonomic neuropathy

Ⓑ Re-entry tachyarrhythmias arise from anomalous atrioventricular conduction

Ⓒ Sinus bradycardia < 60/min is a normal occurrence during sleep

Ⓓ Sinus arrest is defined on ECG by P waves which do not elicit QRS complexes

Ⓔ Episodes of both bradycardias and tachycardias suggest the sick sinus syndrome

16
In a patient with a recurrent AV nodal re-entry tachycardia
Ⓐ adenosine is the prophylactic therapy of first choice

Ⓑ the cardiac rate is often 160–220 beats per minute

Ⓒ polyuria after a prolonged episode is characteristic

Ⓓ symptoms are invariably present during episodes

Ⓔ transient bundle branch block on ECG indicates coexistent myocardial ischaemia

17
Typical features of the Wolff–Parkinson–White (WPW) syndrome include
Ⓐ tachyarrhythmias resulting from re-entry phenomenon

Ⓑ ventricular pre-excitation via an accessory AV pathway

Ⓒ atrial fibrillation with a ventricular response of > 160/min

Ⓓ ECG between bouts showing prolonged PR interval with narrow QRS complexes

Ⓔ useful therapeutic response to verapamil or digoxin

18
Atrial tachycardia with AV block is typically associated with
Ⓐ an irregularly irregular pulse

Ⓑ slowing of the atrial rate on carotid sinus massage

Ⓒ presence of P waves identical to those found during sinus rhythm

Ⓓ digoxin toxicity and intracellular potassium depletion

Ⓔ bizarre broad QRS complexes on ECG

19
Atrial fibrillation (AF) is
Ⓐ present in 10% of the elderly population over the age of 75 years

Ⓑ usually readily converted to permanent sinus rhythm using DC cardioversion

Ⓒ associated with an annual stroke risk of 5% if structural heart disease is present

Ⓓ a common presenting feature of the sick sinus syndrome

Ⓔ usually associated with a ventricular rate < 100 /min even before therapy is introduced

20
In patients with atrial fibrillation (AF)

Ⓐ aspirin therapy alone does not reduce the risk of stroke

Ⓑ the radial pulse is typically irregularly irregular

Ⓒ the response in cardiac output to exercise is reduced due to the absence of atrial systole

Ⓓ elective direct current (DC) cardioversion is contraindicated during anticoagulant therapy

Ⓔ alcohol abuse should be considered as a likely cause

21
Ventricular ectopic beats

Ⓐ produce a clinically detectable reduction in stroke volume

Ⓑ which are symptomatic usually indicate underlying heart disease

Ⓒ secondary to cardiac disease typically disappear on exercise

Ⓓ are likely to be escape beats when there is underlying bradycardia

Ⓔ following acute myocardial infarction indicate the need for antiarrhythmic treatment

22
In ventricular tachycardia (VT)

Ⓐ underlying cardiac disease is usually present

Ⓑ amiodarone is useful in the prevention of recurrent episodes

Ⓒ a shortened QT interval on ECG predisposes to recurrent episodes

Ⓓ carotid sinus massage usually slows the cardiac rate transiently

Ⓔ complicated by acute cardiac failure, cardioversion should be avoided

23
In ventricular fibrillation

Ⓐ the radial pulse is extremely rapid and thready

Ⓑ which is unresponsive to treatment, profound hypokalaemia should be suspected

Ⓒ ECG confirmation is vital before DC shock is administered

Ⓓ cardioversion should be synchronised with the R wave on ECG

Ⓔ immediate lignocaine therapy avoids the need for cardioversion

24
In cardiopulmonary resuscitation

Ⓐ a sharp blow to the praecordium helps restore sinus rhythm

Ⓑ asystole is the commonest finding on ECG

Ⓒ a normal ECG suggests profound hypovolaemia

Ⓓ if cardioversion fails, intracardiac adrenaline should be given

Ⓔ the compression to ventilation ratio should be 5:1

25
In the management of cardiac arrhythmias

Ⓐ moderation of alcohol consumption should be advised

Ⓑ symptoms are a reliable guide to the efficacy of drug treatment

Ⓒ endocardial pacing should be considered for refractory paroxysmal tachycardias

Ⓓ combination drug therapy is often better than monotherapy

Ⓔ treatment of the causative disease is of no proven benefit

26
Digoxin
Ⓐ shortens the refractory period of conducting tissue
Ⓑ usually converts atrial flutter to sinus rhythm
Ⓒ acts primarily on cell membrane ionic pumps
Ⓓ effects are potentiated by hyperkalaemia
Ⓔ is a recognised cause of ventricular arrhythmias

27
The cardiac drugs listed below are associated with the following adverse effects
Ⓐ digoxin—acute confusional state
Ⓑ verapamil—constipation
Ⓒ amiodarone—photosensitivity
Ⓓ propafenone—corneal microdeposits
Ⓔ lignocaine—convulsions

28
In the classification of anti-arrhythmic drugs, the following statements are true
Ⓐ class I agents inhibit the fast sodium channel
Ⓑ class II agents are ß-adrenoreceptor antagonists
Ⓒ class III agents prolong the action potential
Ⓓ class IV agents inhibit the slow calcium channel
Ⓔ many antiarrhythmic agents have actions in more than one class

29
In echocardiography
Ⓐ endocarditis can be reliably excluded by transthoracic echocardiography (TTE)
Ⓑ transoesophageal echocardiography (TOE) is used to evaluate prosthetic mitral valve dysfunction
Ⓒ normal Doppler-derived intracardiac flow velocities are around 1 cm/sec
Ⓓ intracardiac clot cannot be distinguished from normal endocardial tissue
Ⓔ the pressure gradient between two cardiac chambers approximates to four times the square of blood flow velocity between the chambers squared ($P = 4 \times V^2$)

30
Amiodarone therapy
Ⓐ prolongs the plateau phase of the action potential
Ⓑ potentiates the effect of warfarin
Ⓒ is useful in the prevention of ventricular but not supraventricular tachycardia
Ⓓ should be withdrawn if corneal deposits occur
Ⓔ has a significant negative inotropic action

31
The following statements about atrioventricular block are true
Ⓐ first degree block produces a soft first heart sound
Ⓑ the PR interval is fixed in Mobitz type I second-degree block
Ⓒ decreasing PR intervals suggests Wenckebach's phenomenon
Ⓓ irregular cannon waves in the jugular venous pressure suggest complete heart block
Ⓔ the QRS complex in complete heart block is always broad and bizarre

32
Absolute indications for permanent endocardial pacing include
A asymptomatic congenital complete heart block

B asymptomatic Mobitz type I second-degree heart block

C Adams–Stokes attacks in the elderly

D complete heart block due to rheumatic mitral valve disease

E symptomatic second degree heart block following acute inferior myocardial infarction

33
The following statements about bundle branch block (BBB) are true
A Right BBB is most often the result of left ventricular hypertrophy

B Right BBB produces right axis deviation with a QRS > 0.12 sec on ECG

C Right BBB produces fixed splitting of the second heart sound

D Left BBB produces reversed splitting of the second heart sound

E Left posterior hemiblock produces left axis deviation on ECG

34
In a patient with central chest pain at rest
A intrascapular radiation suggests the possibility of aortic dissection

B postural variation in pain suggests the possibility of pericarditis

C chest wall tenderness is a typical feature of Tietze's syndrome

D relief of pain by nitrates excludes an oesophageal cause

E features of autonomic disturbance are specific to cardiac pain

35
In pericardial tamponade
A electrical alternans is a recognised ECG feature

B the systemic arterial pressure falls dramatically on inspiration

C the jugular venous pulse falls dramatically on inspiration

D an effusion > 250 ml must be present before detrimental haemodynamic effects ensue

E the chest X-ray is invariably abnormal

36
In a patient with cardiogenic shock due to acute myocardial infarction
A the absence of pulmonary oedema suggests right ventricular infarction

B the central venous pressure is the best index of left ventricular filling pressure

C dopamine in low dose increases renal blood flow

D high flow, high concentration oxygen is indicated

E colloid infusion is indicated if oliguria and pulmonary oedema develop

37
In the treatment of cardiac failure associated with acute pulmonary oedema
A controlled oxygen therapy should be restricted to 28% oxygen in patients who smoke

B morphine reduces angor animi and dyspnoea

C frusemide therapy given intravenously reduces preload and afterload

D nitrates should be avoided if the systolic blood pressure < 140 mmHg

E ACE inhibitors decrease the afterload but increase the preload

38

The following are recognised complications of heart failure

Ⓐ hyponatraemia

Ⓑ hypoalbuminaemia

Ⓒ impaired liver function tests

Ⓓ anaemia

Ⓔ sudden death

39

With regard to angiotensin-converting enzyme (ACE) inhibitors

Ⓐ ACE inhibitors reduce the conversion of angiotensinogen to angiotensin I

Ⓑ enalapril is a pro-drug

Ⓒ cough is a less common side-effect of ACE inhibitors than angiotensin II antagonists

Ⓓ first dose hypotension occurs less commonly in patients pretreated with diuretics

Ⓔ concurrent use of non-steroidal anti-inflammatory therapy increases the likelihood of severe renal dysfunction

40

In chronic biventricular cardiac failure

Ⓐ angiotensin II contributes to renal salt and water retention

Ⓑ excess ADH is the major cause of oedema

Ⓒ hyponatraemia usually indicates total body sodium depletion

Ⓓ cardiac sympathetic neural activity is markedly diminished

Ⓔ atrial natriuretic peptide is released

41

In the management of chronic heart failure

Ⓐ ACE inhibitor therapy reduces subsequent hospitalisation rates

Ⓑ coagulation is impaired and thromboembolic risk therefore declines

Ⓒ drug suppression of ventricular arrhythmia improves prognosis

Ⓓ ß-adrenoreceptor antagonists (ß-blockers) should always be avoided

Ⓔ digoxin is only of benefit if atrial fibrillation coexists

42

The diagnosis of rheumatic fever in a patient with an elevated ASO (antistreptolysin O) titre is confirmed by

Ⓐ fever with an elevated erythrocyte sedimentation rate

Ⓑ arthralgia and a previous history of rheumatic fever

Ⓒ chorea and a prolonged PR interval on ECG

Ⓓ erythema nodosum and arthritis

Ⓔ rheumatic nodules and pancarditis

43

In patients with significant mitral stenosis

Ⓐ the mitral valve orifice is reduced from 5 cm^2 to about 1 cm^2

Ⓑ a history of rheumatic fever or chorea is elicited in over 90% of patients

Ⓒ left atrial enlargement cannot be detected on the chest X-ray

Ⓓ the risk of systemic emboli is trivial in sinus rhythm

Ⓔ mitral balloon valvuloplasty is not advisable if there is also significant mitral regurgitation

44

Expected findings in a patient with significant mitral stenosis include

- **A** a soft early diastolic murmur
- **B** a quiet first sound and absence of an opening snap
- **C** left parasternal heave suggesting pulmonary hypertension
- **D** a displaced apex beat
- **E** the opening snap occurring just before the second heart sound

45

Recognised features of chronic mitral regurgitation include

- **A** soft first heart sound and loud third heart sound
- **B** presentation with signs of right ventricular failure
- **C** the severity of regurgitation is increased by afterload reduction
- **D** a pansystolic murmur and hyperdynamic displaced apex beat
- **E** atrial fibrillation requiring anticoagulation

46

Disorders typically producing the sudden onset of symptomatic mitral regurgitation include

- **A** Marfan's syndrome
- **B** acute myocardial infarction
- **C** acute rheumatic fever
- **D** infective endocarditis
- **E** diphtheria

47

Clinical features suggesting severe aortic stenosis include

- **A** late systolic ejection click
- **B** pulsus bisferiens
- **C** heaving, displaced apex beat
- **D** syncope associated with angina
- **E** loud second heart sound

48

Disorders associated with aortic regurgitation include

- **A** ankylosing spondylitis
- **B** Marfan's syndrome
- **C** syphilitic aortitis
- **D** persistent ductus arteriosus
- **E** Takayasu's disease

49

In a patient with aortic regurgitation in normal sinus rhythm

- **A** a mid-diastolic murmur is usually due to concomitant mitral stenosis
- **B** a systolic murmur is often due to coexistent aortic stenosis
- **C** a left parasternal heave and displaced apex beat are expected findings
- **D** systemic diastolic arterial pressure is usually low
- **E** a short early diastolic murmur suggests mild regurgitation

50

The following statements about tricuspid valve disease are true

- **A** Murmurs are best heard in mid-sternum at the end of expiration
- **B** Ascites occurs with tricuspid regurgitation but not stenosis
- **C** Tricuspid stenosis produces cannon waves in the jugular venous pressure
- **D** Both stenosis and regurgitation produce systolic hepatic pulsation
- **E** Endocarditis suggests the possibility of intravenous drug abuse

51

The typical features of congenital pulmonary stenosis include

- **A** breathlessness and central cyanosis
- **B** giant *a* waves in the jugular venous pressure
- **C** loud second heart sound preceded by an ejection systolic click
- **D** left parasternal heave and systolic thrill
- **E** enlargement of the pulmonary artery visible on chest X-ray

52
In infective endocarditis
Ⓐ streptococci and staphylococci account for over 80% of cases
Ⓑ left heart valves are more frequently involved than right heart valves
Ⓒ normal cardiac valves are not affected
Ⓓ glomerulonephritis usually occurs due to immune complex disease
Ⓔ a normal echocardiogram excludes the diagnosis

53
In the management of infective endocarditis
Ⓐ blood cultures are best obtained when the fever peaks
Ⓑ antibiotic therapy should be delayed pending bacteriological confirmation
Ⓒ parenteral antibiotic therapy should be continued for at least 4 months
Ⓓ persistent fever suggests the possibility of an allergy to antibiotic therapy
Ⓔ cardiac surgery should be considered if cardiac failure develops

54
The risks of developing clinical evidence of coronary artery disease are
Ⓐ increased by exogenous oestrogen use in postmenopausal females
Ⓑ diminished by stopping smoking
Ⓒ reduced by the moderate consumption of alcohol
Ⓓ increased in hyperfibrinogenaemia
Ⓔ increased by hypercholesterolaemia but not hypertriglyceridaemia

55
In the investigation of suspected angina pectoris
Ⓐ the resting ECG is usually abnormal
Ⓑ exercise-induced elevation in blood pressure indicates significant ischaemia
Ⓒ a normal ECG during exercise excludes angina pectoris
Ⓓ coronary angiography is only indicated if an exercise tolerance test (ETT) is abnormal
Ⓔ physical examination is of no clinical value

56
In the treatment of patients with angina pectoris
Ⓐ aspirin reduces the frequency of anginal attacks
Ⓑ glyceryl trinitrate is equally effective when swallowed as when taken sublingually
Ⓒ calcium antagonists may cause peripheral oedema
Ⓓ tissue levels of nitrates must be consistently high for maximum therapeutic effect
Ⓔ ß-blockers are more effective than other anti-anginal agents

57
In the management of angina pectoris
Ⓐ coronary angioplasty improves symptoms and subsequent mortality
Ⓑ coronary angioplasty should not be performed on stenotic coronary grafts
Ⓒ 90% of patients undergoing coronary artery grafting are pain free 5 years post-operation
Ⓓ coronary artery grafts improve prognosis in patients with stenosis of the left main coronary artery
Ⓔ the natural history of coronary artery disease is of progressively severe pain

58
Unstable angina is
- **A** invariably preceded by a history of effort angina
- **B** associated with progression to myocardial infarction in 15% of cases
- **C** due to plaque rupture, thrombosis or coronary artery spasm
- **D** an indication for immediate exercise testing to assess prognosis
- **E** best managed by emergency coronary artery bypass surgery

59
The clinical features of acute myocardial infarction include
- **A** nausea and vomiting
- **B** breathlessness and angor animi
- **C** hypotension and peripheral cyanosis
- **D** sinus tachycardia or sinus bradycardia
- **E** absence of any symptoms or physical signs

60
Findings consistent with an acute anterior myocardial infarction include
- **A** hypertension and raised jugular venous pressure
- **B** rumbling low-pitched diastolic murmur at the cardiac apex
- **C** ST elevation > 2 mm in leads II, III and AVF on ECG
- **D** gallop rhythm and soft first heart sound
- **E** an increased serum gamma-glutamyl transferase activity > 300 i.u./L

61
Drug therapies which improve the long-term prognosis after myocardial infarction include
- **A** aspirin
- **B** nitrates
- **C** calcium antagonists
- **D** ACE inhibitors
- **E** ß-blockers

62
Coronary artery thrombolysis with streptokinase therapy is
- **A** of no proven benefit to patients over the age of 75 years
- **B** more beneficial in patients with ST depression than ST elevation
- **C** relatively contraindicated in patients with uncontrolled hypertension
- **D** best avoided in patients with chest pain without elevation of serum creatine kinase activity
- **E** more likely to cause anaphylactic shock than therapy with tissue plasminogen activator

63
In the treatment of acute myocardial infarction
- **A** aspirin given within 6 hours of onset reduces the mortality
- **B** streptokinase therapy reduces infarct size and mortality by > 25%
- **C** diamorphine is better given intravenously than by any other route
- **D** immediate calcium channel blocker therapy reduces the early mortality rate
- **E** mobilisation should be deferred until cardiac enzymes normalise

64
In the treatment of arrhythmias following acute myocardial infarction
- **A** atropine should be given for all sinus bradycardias
- **B** frequent ventricular ectopics usually require lignocaine therapy
- **C** complete heart block in inferior infarcts usually requires endocardial pacing
- **D** lignocaine therapy should be given before cardioversion for ventricular fibrillation
- **E** cardioversion is indicated for all tachyarrhythmias inducing acute circulatory collapse

65
The following statements about the prognosis of acute myocardial infarction are true
Ⓐ 50% of all deaths occur within the first 24 hours
Ⓑ stress and social isolation adversely affect the prognosis
Ⓒ the 5-year survival is 75% for those who leave hospital
Ⓓ late mortality is determined by the extent of myocardial damage
Ⓔ survivors of ventricular fibrillation (VF) have a worse prognosis if VF occurs within the first 6–12 hours after the onset of symptoms rather than 6–12 days later

66
The following statements about systemic hypertension are true
Ⓐ Casual blood pressure (BP) recordings correlate poorly with life expectancy
Ⓑ Systolic hypertension alone is of little prognostic value
Ⓒ Most patients have a normal plasma renin concentration
Ⓓ 15% of the adult UK population have essential hypertension
Ⓔ 15% of hypertensives have hypertension secondary to other disorders

67
Recognised causes of secondary hypertension include
Ⓐ persistent ductus arteriosus
Ⓑ primary hyperaldosteronism
Ⓒ acromegaly
Ⓓ oestrogen-containing oral contraceptives
Ⓔ thyrotoxicosis

68
In a patient with systemic hypertension, the findings listed below suggest the following diagnoses
Ⓐ symmetrical small joint polyarthritis—hyperparathyroidism
Ⓑ radio-femoral delay in the pulses—renovascular disease
Ⓒ left ventricular failure—phaeochromocytoma
Ⓓ epigastric bruit—coarctation of the aorta
Ⓔ palpably enlarged kidneys—renovascular disease

69
Complications of systemic hypertension include
Ⓐ retinal microaneurysms
Ⓑ dissecting aneurysm of the ascending aorta
Ⓒ renal artery stenosis
Ⓓ lacunar strokes of the internal capsule
Ⓔ subdural haemorrhage

70
In the investigation of systemic hypertension
Ⓐ hyperkalaemic metabolic acidosis indicates hyperaldosteronism
Ⓑ excretion urography is useful in the diagnosis of renal artery stenosis
Ⓒ normal urinary 5-HIAA excretion makes the diagnosis of phaeochromocytoma unlikely
Ⓓ urine analysis for blood, protein and glucose is essential
Ⓔ the commonest cause of electrolyte abnormalities is diuretic treatment

71
Accelerated phase or malignant hypertension is suggested by hypertension and
Ⓐ a loud second heart sound
Ⓑ a heaving apex beat
Ⓒ headache
Ⓓ retinal soft exudates or haemorrhages
Ⓔ renal or cardiac failure

72

In the emergency treatment of accelerated hypertension

Ⓐ the aim is to lower the systolic blood pressure to normal within 60 minutes
Ⓑ intravenous sodium nitroprusside is usually necessary to control the severe hypertension
Ⓒ parenteral therapy is preferable to oral therapy
Ⓓ vasodilator therapy to reduce the afterload should be used
Ⓔ ACE inhibitors are indicated if renal artery stenosis is suspected

73

In the treatment of mild to moderate systemic hypertension

Ⓐ treatment has more effect on the risk of stroke than the risk of coronary heart disease
Ⓑ weight reduction is more important to prognosis than stopping smoking
Ⓒ treatment is less likely to be of benefit if cardiac or renal disease are present
Ⓓ there are no proven benefits of therapy in patients aged over 70 years
Ⓔ moderation of alcohol consumption is likely to improve blood pressure control

74

Important explanations for hypertension refractory to medical therapy include

Ⓐ poor compliance with drug therapy
Ⓑ inadequate drug therapy
Ⓒ phaeochromocytoma
Ⓓ primary hyperaldosteronism
Ⓔ renal artery stenosis

75

In the drug treatment of hypertension

Ⓐ thiazides exert their maximal effect after 1 week of treatment
Ⓑ lipid-soluble ß-blockers are less likely to cause neuropsychiatric complications
Ⓒ ACE inhibitors may cause hyperkalaemia
Ⓓ thiazides may cause hypouricaemia
Ⓔ ß-blockers may increase plasma cholesterol

76

The murmurs listed below are typical features of the following valvular heart disorders

Ⓐ low-pitched pansystolic murmur loudest at the right sternal edge—tricuspid regurgitation
Ⓑ apical late systolic murmur—mitral valve prolapse
Ⓒ mid-diastolic murmur at left sternal edge—pulmonary regurgitation
Ⓓ mid-diastolic murmur at the apex—mitral stenosis
Ⓔ systolic and diastolic murmur at left sternal edge—patent ductus arteriosus

77

With regard to ischaemic (coronary) heart disease

Ⓐ 25% of the male population of the UK die from this disease
Ⓑ the primary event in unstable angina is coronary artery spasm
Ⓒ 70% of cases of sudden death are attributable to this disease
Ⓓ 70% of occluded vessels undergo spontaneous revascularisation
Ⓔ 50% of all deaths occur in patients over the age of 75 years

78

With regard to anti-anginal drugs

Ⓐ nitrates dilate the venous and arterial vessels
Ⓑ non-selective ß-adrenoreceptor antagonists cause coronary vasodilatation
Ⓒ nifedipine is likely to cause a bradycardia
Ⓓ the usefulness of potassium channel-blockers is limited by tolerance
Ⓔ long acting nitrates have been proven to be the most effective first line therapy

79
In unstable angina
Ⓐ nitrates should only be used intravenously
Ⓑ heparin should only be given intravenously
Ⓒ an increased serum troponin T concentration suggests an acute myocardial infarction
Ⓓ left main stem disease should not be managed by percutaneous balloon angioplasty
Ⓔ if beta-blockers are contraindicated, nifedipine is the calcium antagonist of choice

80
Dilated (congestive) cardiomyopathy is
Ⓐ usually idiopathic
Ⓑ associated with pathognomic ECG changes
Ⓒ a recognised complication of cytotoxic chemotherapy
Ⓓ associated with chronic alcohol abuse
Ⓔ caused by Coxsackie A infection

81
The clinical features of restrictive (obliterative) cardiomyopathy include
Ⓐ a presentation which mimics that of constrictive pericarditis
Ⓑ primarily characterised by impaired diastolic function
Ⓒ association with primary or secondary amyloidosis
Ⓓ complication of conditions inducing a marked peripheral blood eosinophilia
Ⓔ gross cardiomegaly on chest X-ray

82
Clinical features compatible with idiopathic dilated cardiomyopathy include
Ⓐ absence of a previous history of angina or myocardial infarction
Ⓑ deep Q waves in anterior ECG leads
Ⓒ biventricular dilatation with an ejection fraction < 20%
Ⓓ dyskinetic segment of left ventricle on echocardiography
Ⓔ functional mitral regurgitation

83
Clinical features compatible with hypertrophic cardiomyopathy include
Ⓐ family history of sudden death
Ⓑ angina pectoris and exertional syncope
Ⓒ jerky pulse and heaving apex beat
Ⓓ murmurs suggesting both aortic stenosis and mitral regurgitation
Ⓔ soft or absent second heart sound

84
Typical features of acute pericarditis include
Ⓐ chest pain identical to that of myocardial infarction
Ⓑ a friction rub that is best heard in the axilla in mid-expiration
Ⓒ ST elevation on the ECG with upward concavity
Ⓓ elevation of the serum creatine kinase
Ⓔ ECG changes that are only seen in the chest leads

85
In a 20-year-old woman with acute pericarditis, the following disorders should be excluded
Ⓐ Hodgkin's disease
Ⓑ systemic lupus erythematosus
Ⓒ Coxsackie A virus infection
Ⓓ acute rheumatic fever
Ⓔ rubella virus infection

86

The typical features of constrictive pericarditis include

Ⓐ severe breathlessness

Ⓑ a normal chest X-ray

Ⓒ a previous history of tuberculosis

Ⓓ tachycardia and a loud third heart sound

Ⓔ marked elevation of the jugular venous pressure with a steep *x* and *y* descent

87

Central cyanosis in infancy is an expected finding in the following congenital heart diseases

Ⓐ persistent ductus arteriosus

Ⓑ transposition of the great arteries

Ⓒ coarctation of the aorta

Ⓓ Fallot's tetralogy

Ⓔ atrial septal defect

88

The following statements about persistent ductus arteriosus are true

Ⓐ Blood usually passes from the pulmonary artery to the aorta

Ⓑ The onset of heart failure usually occurs in early infancy

Ⓒ A systolic murmur around the scapulae is typical

Ⓓ Shunt reversal is indicated by cyanosis of the lower limbs

Ⓔ Prophylactic antibiotic therapy to prevent endocarditis is indicated

89

Typical clinical features of coarctation of the aorta include

Ⓐ an association with a bicuspid aortic valve

Ⓑ cardiac failure developing in male adolescents

Ⓒ palpable collateral arteries around the scapulae

Ⓓ rib notching on chest X-ray associated with weak femoral pulses

Ⓔ ECG showing right ventricular hypertrophy

90

In atrial septal defect

Ⓐ the lesion is usually of secundum type

Ⓑ the initial shunt is right to left

Ⓒ splitting of the second heart sound increases in expiration

Ⓓ the ECG typically shows right bundle branch block

Ⓔ surgery should be deferred until shunt reversal occurs

91

In small ventricular septal defects

Ⓐ the murmur is confined to late systole

Ⓑ the heart is usually enlarged

Ⓒ there is a risk of infective endocarditis

Ⓓ surgical repair before adolesence is usually indicated

Ⓔ most patients are asymptomatic

92

In right-to-left shunt reversals of congenital heart disease (Eisenmenger's syndrome)

Ⓐ pulmonary arterial hypertension is usually present

Ⓑ closure of the underlying lesion produces symptomatic relief

Ⓒ the chest X-ray is typically normal

Ⓓ central cyanosis and finger clubbing are often present

Ⓔ physical signs of the underlying lesion persist unchanged

93

In Fallot's tetralogy

Ⓐ pulmonary and aortic stenosis are combined with a ventricular septal defect

Ⓑ both finger clubbing and central cyanosis are present at birth

Ⓒ the second heart sound is loud and widely split on inspiration

Ⓓ the chest X-ray and ECG are typically normal

Ⓔ cyanotic spells occur due to episodes of dysrhythmia

94
Cardiovascular changes in normal pregnancy include
Ⓐ an increase in cardiac output of 150% by 12 weeks
Ⓑ tachycardia, elevated jugular venous pressure and third heart sound
Ⓒ reduction in systemic diastolic pressure
Ⓓ pulmonary systolic murmur
Ⓔ increased blood coagulability

95
After a myocardial infarction (MI)
Ⓐ car driving should not resume for at least 12 weeks
Ⓑ a total plasma cholesterol of 5.8 mmol/L does not require drug treatment
Ⓒ dietary treatment of hypercholesterolaemia is effective in most patients
Ⓓ exercise testing can usually be undertaken safely 4 weeks post-MI
Ⓔ ACE inhibitors confer a prognostic benefit in patients with symptomatic heart failure

96
The following features suggest that mitral valvuloplasty rather than mitral valve replacement would be the preferred treatment option in patients with mitral stenosis
Ⓐ a loud first heart sound and opening snap
Ⓑ moderate mitral regurgitation
Ⓒ pulmonary hypertension
Ⓓ left atrial thrombus
Ⓔ severe inoperable coronary artery disease

97
In intermittent claudication due to atherosclerosis
Ⓐ pain is typically relieved by rest and elevation of the leg
Ⓑ secondary ischaemic ulcers are usually painless
Ⓒ pedal pulses are often still palpable
Ⓓ exercise which causes pain should be avoided
Ⓔ the risk of progression is lessened by warfarin

98
Recognised causes of Raynaud's phenomenon include
Ⓐ ß-blocker therapy
Ⓑ cryoglobulinaemia
Ⓒ progressive systemic sclerosis
Ⓓ vibration trauma
Ⓔ giant cell arteritis

99
The risk of dissecting aortic aneurysm is increased in
Ⓐ Marfan's syndrome
Ⓑ coarctation of the aorta
Ⓒ pregnancy
Ⓓ calcific aortic stenosis
Ⓔ syphilitic aortitis

100
Characteristic features of dissecting aortic aneurysm include
Ⓐ haemopericardium
Ⓑ acute paraparesis
Ⓒ interscapular back pain
Ⓓ early diastolic murmur
Ⓔ pleural effusion

4 DISEASES OF THE RESPIRATORY SYSTEM

ANSWERS PAGE 184

1
Finger clubbing is a typical finding in
Ⓐ chronic bronchitis
Ⓑ bronchiectasis
Ⓒ primary biliary cirrhosis
Ⓓ cryptogenic fibrosing alveolitis
Ⓔ ventricular septal defect

2
Typical chest findings in a large right pleural effusion include
Ⓐ normal chest expansion
Ⓑ dull percussion note
Ⓒ absent breath sounds
Ⓓ vocal resonance decreased
Ⓔ pleural friction rub

3
Typical chest findings in right lower lobe consolidation include
Ⓐ decreased chest expansion
Ⓑ dull percussion note
Ⓒ decreased breath sounds
Ⓓ increased vocal resonance
Ⓔ rhonchi and crepitations

4
Typical chest findings in right lower lobe collapse include
Ⓐ decreased chest expansion
Ⓑ stony dull percussion note
Ⓒ bronchial breath sounds
Ⓓ decreased vocal resonance
Ⓔ crepitations

5
In the normal adult
Ⓐ the transverse fissure separates the right middle lobe from the right lower lobe
Ⓑ the left main bronchus is more vertical than the right
Ⓒ the left upper lobe lies anterior to the left lower lobe
Ⓓ the oblique fissure extends from the thoracic vertebral level T3
Ⓔ pulmonary surfactant is secreted by type I pneumocytes

6
An increase in ventilatory rate is associated with
Ⓐ lactic acidosis
Ⓑ respiratory alkalosis
Ⓒ exercise
Ⓓ fever
Ⓔ decrease in arterial $PaCO_2$

7
In the normal resting adult
Ⓐ pulmonary ventilation is 10 litres per minute
Ⓑ alveolar ventilation is 5 litres per minute
Ⓒ pulmonary blood flow is 10 litres per minute
Ⓓ the PaO_2 is 11–13 kPa and $PaCO_2$ is 4.8–6.0 kPa
Ⓔ pulmonary blood flow is higher at the lung base

8

In the central control of breathing

Ⓐ fever reduces the sensitivity of the respiratory centre

Ⓑ only central chemoreceptors are sensitive to arterial PCO_2

Ⓒ peripheral chemoreceptors are sensitive only to arterial PO_2

Ⓓ chronic alveolar hypoventilation decreases sensitivity to arterial PCO_2

Ⓔ chest wall and pulmonary stretch receptors stimulate ventilation during exercise

9

Alveolar hypoventilation is typically associated with

Ⓐ pulmonary embolism

Ⓑ severe chest wall deformity

Ⓒ salicylate intoxication

Ⓓ pulmonary fibrosis

Ⓔ severe chronic bronchitis

10

The following statements about pulmonary function tests are true

Ⓐ over 80% of vital capacity can normally be expelled in 1 second

Ⓑ the transfer factor is measured using inspired oxygen

Ⓒ residual volume is increased in chronic bronchitis and emphysema

Ⓓ the forced expiratory volume (FEV)/forced vital capacity (FVC) ratio is usually normal in ankylosing spondylitis

Ⓔ peak expiratory flow rates accurately reflect the severity of restrictive lung disorders

11

In a patient with severe acute breathlessness:

Ⓐ a normal arterial PaO_2 invariably suggests psychogenic hyperventilation

Ⓑ pulsus paradoxus is pathognomic of acute asthma

Ⓒ a normal chest X-ray excludes pulmonary embolism

Ⓓ the extremities are typically cool and sweaty in left ventricular failure

Ⓔ left bundle branch block is strongly suggestive of pulmonary embolism

12

The following are recognised causes of haemoptysis

Ⓐ tuberculosis

Ⓑ chronic obstructive pulmonary disease

Ⓒ bronchiectasis

Ⓓ Goodpasture's syndrome

Ⓔ mitral stenosis

13

The following disorders characteristically produce type I respiratory failure

Ⓐ kyphoscoliosis

Ⓑ Guillain–Barré polyneuropathy

Ⓒ adult (acute) respiratory distress syndrome (ARDS)

Ⓓ extrinsic allergic alveolitis

Ⓔ inhaled foreign body in a major airway

14

The following disorders characteristically produce type II respiratory failure

Ⓐ heroin overdose

Ⓑ poliomyelitis

Ⓒ pulmonary embolism

Ⓓ cryptogenic fibrosing alveolitis

Ⓔ bronchial asthma

15

The following statements about oxygen therapy are true

Ⓐ at sea level, the pressure of oxygen in inspired air is 20 kPa

Ⓑ chronic domiciliary oxygen therapy is indicated only when PaO_2 is < 6 kPa

Ⓒ dissolved oxygen contributes to tissue oxygenation in anaemia

Ⓓ oxygen toxicity in adults can produce retrolental fibroplasia

Ⓔ central cyanosis unresponsive to 100% oxygen indicates right-to-left shunting of > 20%

16

In the treatment of chronic bronchitis associated with type II respiratory failure

Ⓐ oxygen should be given so that the inspired oxygen content should be at least 40%

Ⓑ nebulised doxapram improves small airways obstruction

Ⓒ cough disturbing sleep should be treated with pholcodine

Ⓓ corticosteroid therapy is usually contraindicated

Ⓔ respiratory support should be considered if pH falls below 7.26

17

The following respiratory disorders are indications for heart-lung transplantation

Ⓐ bronchial adenocarcinoma

Ⓑ cystic fibrosis

Ⓒ cryptogenic pulmonary fibrosis

Ⓓ primary pulmonary hypertension

Ⓔ hepatopulmonary syndrome

18

The respiratory disorders listed below are commonly due to the following viral infections

Ⓐ laryngotracheobronchitis (croup)— Coxsackie A virus

Ⓑ epiglottitis—rhinoviruses

Ⓒ bronchiolitis—respiratory syncytial virus

Ⓓ viral pneumonia—enteroviruses

Ⓔ pharyngoconjunctival fever—echoviruses

19

Typical clinical features of acute tracheobronchitis include

Ⓐ an irritating unproductive cough at onset

Ⓑ superinfection with *Staphylococcus aureus*

Ⓒ retrosternal chest pain

Ⓓ pyrexia and neutrophil leucocytosis

Ⓔ crepitations rather than rhonchi on auscultation

20

Characteristic features of pneumococcal pneumonia include

Ⓐ sudden onset of rigors and pleuritic pain

Ⓑ peak frequency in childhood and old age

Ⓒ lobar collapse and diminished breath sounds

Ⓓ bacteraemia and neutrophil leucocytosis

Ⓔ herpes labialis

21

Recognised complications of pneumococcal pneumonia include

Ⓐ bronchial carcinoma

Ⓑ pericarditis

Ⓒ peripheral circulatory failure

Ⓓ pleural effusion and empyema

Ⓔ subphrenic abscess

22

The following features suggest a poor prognosis in pneumonia

Ⓐ diastolic blood pressure of 50 mmHg

Ⓑ confusion

Ⓒ respiratory rate of 20 breaths per minute

Ⓓ blood urea of 9 mmol/l

Ⓔ white cell count of 3000 x 10^9/L

23

Typical features of staphylococcal pneumonia include

Ⓐ an illness clinically indistinguishable from pneumococcal pneumonia

Ⓑ multiple lung abscesses appearing as thin-walled cysts

Ⓒ association with influenza A infection

Ⓓ staphylococcal sepsis elsewhere in the body

Ⓔ penicillin resistance

24

Typical features of klebsiella pneumonia include

Ⓐ upper lobe collapse on chest X-ray
Ⓑ severe systemic disturbance and high mortality
Ⓒ copious chocolate-coloured sputum
Ⓓ organisms resistant to chloramphenicol and gentamicin
Ⓔ occurrence in previously healthy individuals

25

Recognised features of mycoplasmal pneumonia include

Ⓐ institutional outbreaks in young adults
Ⓑ haemolytic anaemia and cold agglutinins in the serum
Ⓒ fever and malaise preceding respiratory symptoms by several days
Ⓓ inconspicuous physical signs in the chest
Ⓔ response to tetracycline or erythromycin therapy

26

Typical features of legionella pneumonia include

Ⓐ oro-faecal spread of infection
Ⓑ vomiting and diarrhoea
Ⓒ hyponatraemia and confusion
Ⓓ inconspicuous physical signs in the chest
Ⓔ response to rifampicin and/or erythromycin therapy

27

A non-pneumococcal pneumonia should be suspected if the clinical features include

Ⓐ respiratory symptoms preceding systemic upset by several days
Ⓑ chest signs less dramatic than the chest X-ray appearances
Ⓒ the development of a pleural effusion
Ⓓ the absence of a neutrophil leucocytosis
Ⓔ palpable splenomegaly and proteinuria

28

Pneumonia in the immunocompromised is best treated with the following drug regimes

Ⓐ *Pneumocystis carinii*—co-trimoxazole
Ⓑ *Pseudomonas aeruginosa*—azlocillin or ciprofloxacin
Ⓒ cytomegalovirus—ganciclovir
Ⓓ herpes simplex—acyclovir
Ⓔ respiratory syncytial virus—tribavirin

29

The following statements about aspiration pneumonias are true

Ⓐ bronchiectasis is a recognised complication
Ⓑ chest X-ray abnormalities are typically bilateral
Ⓒ lobar collapse predisposes to the development of lung abscess
Ⓓ systemic upset is usually marked
Ⓔ adult respiratory distress syndrome may be a complication

30

The clinical features of suppurative pneumonia and lung abscess include

Ⓐ prior pulmonary infarction
Ⓑ the presence of an inhaled foreign body
Ⓒ rigors and pleuritic chest pain
Ⓓ bronchial breathing if there is an underlying bronchial carcinoma
Ⓔ radiological features of cavitation

31

Post-primary tuberculosis in the UK is associated with

Ⓐ occurrence in childhood rather than old age
Ⓑ an increased prevalence in diabetic patients
Ⓒ human rather than bovine strains of mycobacteria
Ⓓ alcohol abuse and malnutrition
Ⓔ airborne reinfection rather than reactivation of infection

32
Typical features of primary tuberculosis include

Ⓐ a sustained pyrexial illness
Ⓑ caseation within the regional lymph nodes
Ⓒ bilateral hilar lymphadenopathy on chest X-ray
Ⓓ erythema nodosum
Ⓔ pleural effusion with a negative tuberculin skin test

33
Recognised features of miliary tuberculosis include

Ⓐ severe systemic upset with fever in childhood
Ⓑ blood dyscrasias and hepatosplenomegaly
Ⓒ normal chest X-ray and negative tuberculin test
Ⓓ inconspicuous physical signs in the chest
Ⓔ characteristic granulomata on liver and bone biopsy

34
Typical features of post-primary tuberculosis include

Ⓐ purulent sputum negative for tuberculosis on microscopy
Ⓑ bilateral upper lobe opacities on chest X-ray
Ⓒ conspicuous physical signs in the chest
Ⓓ haematogenous dissemination in most cases
Ⓔ cavitation of pulmonary lesions

35
Recognised complications of post-primary tuberculosis include

Ⓐ aspergilloma
Ⓑ amyloidosis
Ⓒ miliary tuberculosis
Ⓓ bronchiectasis
Ⓔ paraplegia

36
The following statements about tuberculin tine testing are true

Ⓐ False positives are common in sarcoidosis and acute exanthemata
Ⓑ the skin reaction is best assessed 3 days after inoculation
Ⓒ tuberculin-positive family contacts do not require BCG vaccination
Ⓓ grade 3 and 4 reactions are characterised by four discrete papules
Ⓔ tuberculin-positive children are immune to tuberculosis

37
In the treatment of post-primary pulmonary tuberculosis

Ⓐ combination drug therapy is always indicated
Ⓑ sputum remains infectious for at least 4 weeks after the onset of therapy
Ⓒ at least 12 months daily therapy is required for 100% effectiveness
Ⓓ isoniazid and pyrazinamide do not cross the blood–brain barrier
Ⓔ treatment failure is invariably due to multiple drug resistance

38
Recognised adverse reactions to anti-tuberculous drugs include

Ⓐ streptomycin—renal failure
Ⓑ isoniazid—hypothyroidism
Ⓒ rifampicin—optic neuritis
Ⓓ pyrazinamide—hepatitis
Ⓔ ethambutol—vestibular neuronitis

39
Prophylactic antituberculosis drug therapy is indicated in the following tuberculin-positive subjects

Ⓐ insulin-dependent diabetics
Ⓑ patients receiving long-term immunosuppressant drug
Ⓒ HIV antibody-positive subjects
Ⓓ children aged < 3 years who have not had BCG immunisation
Ⓔ adults who have recently become tuberculin-positive

40

Pulmonary infection with *Aspergillus fumigatus* is a recognised cause of the following

Ⓐ bullous emphysema

Ⓑ mycetoma

Ⓒ necrotising pneumonitis

Ⓓ bronchopulmonary eosinophilia

Ⓔ extrinsic allergic alveolitis

41

Typical features of early-onset bronchial asthma include

Ⓐ individuals are usually atopic

Ⓑ a single allergen is often identifiable

Ⓒ paroxysmal expiratory wheeze and dyspnoea

Ⓓ a strong family history of allergic disorders

Ⓔ *Aspergillus fumigatus* is usually present in the sputum

42

Typical features of late-onset bronchial asthma include

Ⓐ invariable history of cigarette smoking

Ⓑ multiple allergens are often identifiable

Ⓒ exposure to aspirin and certain chemicals induce attacks

Ⓓ asthma is more often chronic than episodic

Ⓔ serum IgE concentrations are often normal

43

Features indicative of severe acute asthma include

Ⓐ pulse rate = 120 per minute

Ⓑ peak expiratory flow rate (PEFR) = < 70% of expected

Ⓒ pulsus paradoxus = 30 mmHg

Ⓓ arterial PaO_2 = 10 kPa

Ⓔ arterial $PaCO_2$ = 6 kPa

44

The initial management of severe acute asthma should include

Ⓐ 24% oxygen delivered by a controlled flow mask

Ⓑ salbutamol 5 mg by inhalation

Ⓒ ampicillin 500 mg orally and cromoglycate 10 mg by inhalation

Ⓓ hydrocortisone 200 mg i.v. and prednisolone 40 mg orally

Ⓔ arterial blood gas analysis and chest X-ray

45

Typical features of asthma include

Ⓐ eosinophilic bronchial infiltrate

Ⓑ increased airway macrophages

Ⓒ goblet cell hyperplasia

Ⓓ epithelial shedding

Ⓔ subendothelial fibrosis

46

In the diagnosis of asthma

Ⓐ only increases in FEV_1 of > 15% following bronchodilators are likely to be significant

Ⓑ a peripheral blood eosinophilia is diagnostic

Ⓒ if doubt exists the methacholine bronchial provocation test should be carried out

Ⓓ the chest X-ray is usually unhelpful between attacks

Ⓔ arterial blood gas analysis is usually unhelpful between attacks

47

In the management of chronic persistent asthma

Ⓐ inhaled β_2-agonist use more than once per day is an indication for inhaled steroid therapy

Ⓑ cromoglycate therapy is often useful as an alternative to inhaled steroids in adults

Ⓒ patients taking high doses of inhaled steroids should use a spacer device

Ⓓ leucotriene antagonists are valuable substitutes for inhaled steroids

Ⓔ anticholinergic agents should be avoided

48
The sleep apnoea syndrome is associated with
Ⓐ obesity
Ⓑ an increased risk of road traffic accidents
Ⓒ nocturnal restlessness apparent to the patient
Ⓓ a good response to inhaled bronchodilator therapy administered at bedtime
Ⓔ acromegaly

49
The typical features of asthmatic pulmonary eosinophilia include
Ⓐ immediate hypersensitivity and immune complex reactions
Ⓑ positive skin and serum tests for *Aspergillus fumigatus*
Ⓒ isolation of *Aspergillus clavatus* in the sputum
Ⓓ recurrent upper lobe collapse
Ⓔ chronic asthma and bronchiectasis

50
Mediastinal opacification on the chest X-ray is a typical feature of
Ⓐ thymoma
Ⓑ retrosternal goitre
Ⓒ Pancoast tumour
Ⓓ hiatus hernia
Ⓔ neurofibroma

51
In a patient with hoarseness
Ⓐ a bovine cough suggests a functional cause
Ⓑ stridor suggests bilateral cord paralysis
Ⓒ inhaled corticosteroids are often beneficial
Ⓓ the finding of a left hilar mass is likely to explain the symptom
Ⓔ Teflon injection of the paralysed vocal cord aids functional improvement

52
Characteristic features of pulmonary eosinophilia include
Ⓐ an association with ascariasis and microfilariasis
Ⓑ eosinophilic pneumonia without peripheral blood eosinophilia
Ⓒ prominent asthmatic features
Ⓓ induction by exposure to sulphonamide drugs
Ⓔ opacities on chest X-ray

53
Clinical features compatible with a diagnosis of extrinsic allergic alveolitis include
Ⓐ expiratory rhonchi and sputum eosinophilia
Ⓑ dry cough, dyspnoea and pyrexia
Ⓒ end-inspiratory crepitations
Ⓓ FEV_1/FVC ratio of 50%
Ⓔ positive serum precipitin tests

54
In chronic obstructive pulmonary disease
Ⓐ FEV_1 declines by 50 ml per year in patients who continue to smoke
Ⓑ FEV_1 is typically < 80% of the predicted value
Ⓒ FEV_1/FVC ratio is typically < 50% of the predicted value
Ⓓ significant reversibility is defined as at least a 200 ml or 15% increase in FEV_1
Ⓔ total lung capacity (TLC) and residual volume (RV) are typically reduced

55
In the management of chronic obstructive pulmonary disease
Ⓐ influenza immunisation should only be offered once
Ⓑ long-term antibiotic treatment decreases the frequency of exacerbations
Ⓒ inhaled steroids are of no value
Ⓓ supplemental oxygen during air travel is necessary if the resting PaO_2 < 9 kPa
Ⓔ long term controlled oxygen therapy improves symptoms but not the prognosis

56
Typical findings in severe chronic obstructive pulmonary disease during inspiration include
Ⓐ elevation of the jugular venous pressure during inspiration
Ⓑ tracheal descent
Ⓒ indrawing of the intercostal muscles
Ⓓ contraction of the scalene muscles
Ⓔ widespread rhonchi

57
Typical chest X-ray findings in chronic obstructive pulmonary disease include
Ⓐ prominent pulmonary arteries at the hila
Ⓑ low flat diaphragms
Ⓒ prominent peripheral vascular markings
Ⓓ upper lobe pulmonary venous congestion
Ⓔ Kerley B lines and cardiomegaly

58
Recognised causes of bronchiectasis include
Ⓐ primary hypogammaglobulinaemia
Ⓑ an inhaled foreign body
Ⓒ cystic fibrosis
Ⓓ asthmatic pulmonary eosinophilia
Ⓔ sarcoidosis

59
Typical clinical features of bronchiectasis include
Ⓐ chronic cough with scanty sputum volumes
Ⓑ recurrent pleurisy
Ⓒ haemoptysis
Ⓓ empyema thoracis
Ⓔ crepitations on auscultation

60
Cystic fibrosis is associated with
Ⓐ an incidence of 1 in 2500 live births
Ⓑ a decreased sweat sodium concentration
Ⓒ male infertility
Ⓓ abnormal lung function at birth
Ⓔ recurring pneumococcal pulmonary infections

61
In the treatment of bronchiectasis
Ⓐ postural drainage is best undertaken twice daily
Ⓑ failure of medical therapy is a clear indication for surgery
Ⓒ antibiotic therapy is indicated if sputum purulence persists
Ⓓ thoracic CT is advisable before surgery is undertaken
Ⓔ pulmonary emphysema is a contraindication to surgery

62
The following statements about bronchial obstruction are true
Ⓐ lobar emphysema develops in the lung distal to a partial obstruction
Ⓑ mediastinal displacement is invariably towards the affected side
Ⓒ infection is inevitable especially in partial obstruction
Ⓓ a collapsed right middle lobe is best detected radiologically
Ⓔ inhaled foreign bodies usually lodge in the left main bronchus

63
Typical features of bronchial adenoma include
Ⓐ occurrence in elderly females
Ⓑ carcinoid syndrome if liver metastases are present
Ⓒ recurrent haemoptysis
Ⓓ lobar emphysema
Ⓔ recurrent pneumonia

64
Bronchial carcinoma
Ⓐ accounts for 10% of all male deaths from cancer
Ⓑ typically presents with massive haemoptysis
Ⓒ histology reveals adenocarcinoma in 50% of patients
Ⓓ is associated with asbestos exposure
Ⓔ is 40 times more common in smokers than in non-smokers

65
Bronchial carcinoma is
A surgically resectable in approximately 40% of cases
B reliably excluded by the finding of a normal chest X-ray
C associated with a 50% 5-year survival after surgical resection
D only reliably diagnosable by bronchoscopy
E usually small-cell in origin if associated with finger clubbing

66
Non-metastatic manifestations of bronchial carcinoma include
A cerebellar degeneration
B myasthenia
C gynaecomastia
D polyneuropathy
E dermatomyositis

67
Typical presentations of small-cell bronchial carcinoma include
A nephrotic syndrome
B inappropriate antidiuretic hormone (ADH) secretion
C ectopic adrenocorticotropic hormone (ACTH) secretion
D ectopic parathyroid hormone secretion
E hypertrophic pulmonary osteoarthropathy

68
The following are contraindications to surgical resection in bronchial carcinoma
A distant metastases
B malignant pleural effusion
C $FEV_1 < 0.8$ litres
D ipsilateral mediastinal lymphadenopathy
E oesophageal involvement

69
Typical features of cryptogenic fibrosing alveolitis include
A hypercapnic respiratory failure
B positive antinuclear and rheumatoid factors
C finger clubbing
D recurrent wheeze and haemoptysis
E increased neutrophil and eosinophil count in bronchial washings

70
In coal worker's pneumoconiosis
A the disease usually progresses despite avoidance of coal dust
B certification for compensation depends upon the clinical features
C upper lobe opacities suggest progressive massive fibrosis
D accompanying chronic bronchitis is not due to coal dust exposure
E confirmatory physical findings are often present

71
Typical findings in silicosis include
A chest X-ray abnormalities similar to those found in coal workers
B 'egg-shell' calcification of the hilar lymph nodes
C progression of the disease arrested when dust exposure ceases
D fibrotic peripheral nodules in patients with rheumatoid disease
E occupational history of coal, tin and mineral mining

72
The following statements about asbestos-related disease are true
A pleural plaques usually progress to become mesotheliomas
B benign pleural effusions are not blood-stained
C finger clubbing and basal crepitations suggest pulmonary asbestosis
D the FEV_1/FVC ratio is typically decreased
E mesothelioma can only be reliably diagnosed at thoracotomy

73

Occupational exposure to the following substances produces an extrinsic allergic alveolitis

Ⓐ cotton dust—bagassosis
Ⓑ mouldy hay—farmer's lung
Ⓒ tin dioxide—siderosis
Ⓓ avian protein—bird fancier's lung
Ⓔ mouldy barley—bysinnosis

74

The following statements about sarcoidosis are true

Ⓐ pulmonary lesions typically cavitate
Ⓑ the tuberculin tine test is usually positive
Ⓒ erythema marginatum is a characteristic finding
Ⓓ spontaneous resolution is unusual
Ⓔ hypercalcaemia suggests skeletal involvement

75

Typical features of subacute sarcoidosis include

Ⓐ hilar lymphadenopathy on chest X-ray
Ⓑ cranial neuropathies
Ⓒ conjunctivitis
Ⓓ erosive polyarthritis
Ⓔ swollen parotid glands

76

A pleural effusion with a protein content of 50 g/L would be compatible with

Ⓐ congestive cardiac failure (CCF)
Ⓑ pulmonary infarction
Ⓒ subphrenic abscess
Ⓓ pneumonia
Ⓔ nephrotic syndrome

77

In a patient with a symptomatic pleural effusion

Ⓐ physical signs in the chest are invariably present
Ⓑ pleural biopsy should be avoided given a protein content of 50 g/L
Ⓒ tuberculosis can be excluded if the chest X-ray is otherwise normal
Ⓓ lymphocytosis in the pleural fluid is pathognomonic of pleural tuberculosis
Ⓔ milky pleural fluid suggests thoracic duct obstruction

78

Typical features of an empyema thoracis include

Ⓐ bilateral effusions on chest X-ray
Ⓑ a fluid level on chest X-ray suggests a bronchopleural fistula
Ⓒ persistent pyrexia despite antibiotic therapy
Ⓓ recent abdominal surgery
Ⓔ bacteriological culture of the organism despite antibiotic therapy

79

The following statements about spontaneous pneumothorax are true

Ⓐ breathlessness and pleuritic chest pain are usually present
Ⓑ bronchial breathing is audible over the affected hemithorax
Ⓒ absent peripheral lung markings on chest X-ray suggests tension
Ⓓ surgical referral is required if there is a bronchopleural fistula
Ⓔ pleurodesis should be considered for recurrent pneumothoraces

80

The following are causes of an elevated hemidiaphragm

Ⓐ recurrent laryngeal nerve paralysis
Ⓑ surgical lobectomy
Ⓒ subphrenic abscess
Ⓓ severe pleuritic pain
Ⓔ chronic severe asthma

81

Clinical features characteristic of massive pulmonary embolism include

Ⓐ central and peripheral cyanosis

Ⓑ pleuritic chest pain and haemoptysis

Ⓒ breathlessness and syncope

Ⓓ tachycardia and elevated jugular venous pressure

Ⓔ Q waves in leads I, II and AVL on ECG

82

Recognised features of pulmonary infarction include

Ⓐ peripheral blood leucocytosis and fever

Ⓑ pleuropericardial friction rub

Ⓒ bloodstained pleural effusion

Ⓓ development of a lung abscess

Ⓔ ipsilateral elevation of the hemidiaphragm

83

In the treatment of acute pulmonary thromboembolism

Ⓐ streptokinase therapy should be given immediately

Ⓑ 24% oxygen therapy should correct hypoxaemia

Ⓒ diamorphine therapy should be avoided if the patient is severely hypoxic

Ⓓ heparin infusion should be given until warfarin therapy has become effective

Ⓔ warfarin therapy should be continued for 4 weeks

DISTURBANCES IN WATER, ELECTROLYTE AND ACID-BASE BALANCE

5

ANSWERS PAGE 193

1
In a normal 65 kg man, the following statements are true
A total body water is approximately 40 litres
B 70% of the total body water is intracellular
C 75% of extracellular water is intravascular
D sodium, bicarbonate and chloride ions are mainly intracellular
E potassium, magnesium, phosphate and sulphate ions are mainly extracellular

2
In a healthy man living in a temperate climate
A 500 ml of water per day are derived from metabolic processes
B water loss from the skin and lungs is about 250 ml per day
C obligatory urinary water loss is about 500 ml per day
D faecal water loss is about 750 ml per day
E urinary sodium losses should be < 10 mmol per day in response to sodium depletion

3
Within the normal kidney
A 33% of the filtered water is reabsorbed in the proximal tubules
B antidiuretic hormone (ADH) increases the water permeability of the distal tubules
C the glomerular filtrate contains about 200 mg protein per litre
D 33% of the filtered sodium is reabsorbed in the proximal tubules
E the juxtaglomerular apparatus comprises specialised cells of the efferent arterioles and proximal convoluted tubules

4
In the proximal convoluted tubules of the normal kidney
A 33% of filtered chloride is reabsorbed
B > 90% of filtered potassium is reabsorbed
C 65% of the filtered sodium is reabsorbed
D 99% of the filtered glucose is reabsorbed
E 10% of the filtered bicarbonate is reabsorbed

5
In the distal convoluted tubules of the normal kidney
A sodium ions are reabsorbed with chloride ions
B sodium ions are reabsorbed in exchange for potassium or hydrogen
C the active secretion of potassium is controlled by aldosterone
D passive water loss is controlled by the effects of antidiuretic hormone (ADH)
E two-thirds of the secreted hydrogen ions are excreted as ammonium

6
Typical causes of combined salt and water depletion include
A inadequate sodium intake
B chronic diuretic drug therapy
C uncontrolled diabetes mellitus
D primary hypoadrenalism
E acute pancreatitis

7
Typical causes of hyponatraemia include
A diabetes insipidus
B hepatocellular failure
C psychogenic polydipsia
D Cushing's syndrome
E diuretic drug therapy

8

In the treatment of moderately severe combined sodium and water depletion

A the pulse and blood pressure are reliable indices of the severity of losses

B 5% dextrose should be used to replace the extracellular fluid volume losses

C 2–4 litres of isotonic saline should be given in the first 12 hours of therapy

D potassium and hydrogen ion balance are often disturbed

E 1.26% sodium bicarbonate should be given parenterally if metabolic acidosis is present and there is evidence of preexisting renal disease

9

Primary water depletion is a recognised complication of

A primary hyperparathyroidism

B toxic confusional states

C oesophageal carcinoma

D lithium therapy

E acute pancreatitis

10

Expected features of severe primary water depletion include

A urine osmolality of 300 mosmol/kg

B plasma sodium of 130 mmol/L

C marked thirst and oliguria

D hypotension and peripheral circulatory failure

E muscle weakness and a 'doughy' consistency of skin tissue

11

In the treatment of moderately severe water depletion

A the use of isotonic sodium chloride should be avoided

B 8 litres of isotonic dextrose should be given within the first 12 hours

C the urine volume reliably indicates the volume of fluid required

D the use of hypotonic fluids is contraindicated because of the risk of cerebral oedema

E the finding of peripheral circulatory failure suggests that there is also significant sodium depletion

12

The following statements about potassium balance are true

A 85% of the daily potassium intake is excreted in the urine

B intracellular potassium ion concentrations are about 140 mmol/L

C cellular uptake of potassium is enhanced by adrenaline and insulin

D bicarbonate ions impair cellular uptake of potassium

E the normal dietary potassium intake is about 2–3 g (50–80 mmol) per day

13

Recognised causes of potassium depletion include

A metabolic alkalosis

B cardiac failure

C corticosteroid treatment

D renal tubular acidosis

E amiloride diuretic therapy

14

The clinical features of severe potassium depletion include

A polyuria due to renal tubular dysfunction

B muscle weakness, paraesthesiae and depressed tendon reflexes

C flattening of the T wave, ST depression and U waves on ECG

D abdominal distension and paralytic ileus

E sinus bradycardia and decreased digoxin sensitivity

15
Hyperkalaemia is a recognised finding in
Ⓐ severe untreated diabetic ketoacidosis
Ⓑ primary hypoadrenalism
Ⓒ rhabdomyolysis
Ⓓ prostaglandin inhibitor therapy in renal impairment
Ⓔ angiotensin-converting enzyme (ACE) inhibitor therapy

16
Clinical features of hyperkalaemia include
Ⓐ tall peaked T waves and ST depression on ECG
Ⓑ asystole and ventricular fibrillation
Ⓒ peripheral paraesthesiae
Ⓓ widening of the QRS and conduction defects on ECG
Ⓔ symptoms and signs indistinguishable from those induced by hypokalaemia

17
The emergency treatment of severe hyperkalaemia should include
Ⓐ dietary restriction of coffee and fruit juices
Ⓑ parenteral dextrose and glucagon therapy
Ⓒ parenteral calcium gluconate therapy
Ⓓ restoration of sodium and water balance
Ⓔ calcium resonium orally and/or rectally

18
Recognised causes of hypophosphataemia include
Ⓐ primary hyperparathyroidism
Ⓑ secondary hyperparathyroidism
Ⓒ malnutrition
Ⓓ corticosteroid-induced osteoporosis
Ⓔ peritoneal dialysis

19
Magnesium deficiency is
Ⓐ a cause of confusion, depression and epilepsy
Ⓑ usually due to prolonged vomiting and diarrhoea
Ⓒ Found in uncontrolled diabetes mellitus and alcoholism
Ⓓ Found in primary hyperparathyroidism and hyperaldosteronism
Ⓔ best treated with oral magnesium sulphate

20
The renal excretion of water is dependent on
Ⓐ the glomerular filtration rate
Ⓑ the proximal tubular reabsorption of solute
Ⓒ solute concentrations in the thick ascending limb of the loop of Henle
Ⓓ the plasma concentration of antidiuretic hormone arginine vasopressin (AVP)
Ⓔ the integrity of the distal convoluted tubules

21
Expected findings in acute water intoxication include
Ⓐ serum sodium concentration < 130 mmol/L
Ⓑ urinary osmolality 290 mosm/kg
Ⓒ nausea, headache and confusion
Ⓓ prompt response to 1 litre of normal sodium chloride
Ⓔ clinical evidence of increased extracellular fluid (ECF) volume

22

In a patient with hyponatraemia and a serum sodium of 110–120 mmol/L

Ⓐ 2–3 litres of isotonic sodium chloride should be given over 24 hours

Ⓑ water intake should be restricted to 1.5 litres per day

Ⓒ the finding of an increased urine osmolality suggests inappropriate excess antidiuretic hormone (ADH) secretion

Ⓓ frusemide therapy should be administered if there is evidence of fluid overload

Ⓔ associated with chronic liver failure, the urinary osmolality is usually reduced

23

Dilutional hyponatraemia due to inappropriate antidiuretic hormone (ADH) secretion is associated with the following

Ⓐ abdominal surgery

Ⓑ meningoencephalitis

Ⓒ hypothyroidism

Ⓓ morphine and phenothiazine therapy

Ⓔ pulmonary tuberculosis

24

Sodium and water retention should be expected following drug therapy with

Ⓐ amiloride

Ⓑ naproxen

Ⓒ oestrogen

Ⓓ thyroxine

Ⓔ captopril

25

The following statements about diuretic therapy are true

Ⓐ frusemide reduces sodium reabsorption in the proximal tubules

Ⓑ thiazides aggravate hyperglycaemia and hyperuricaemia

Ⓒ triamterene antagonises aldosterone in the distal tubules

Ⓓ amiloride is contraindicated in oliguric renal failure

Ⓔ bumetanide produces hyponatraemia even when oedema is still present

26

The following statements about hydrogen ion balance are true

Ⓐ $[H^+]$ = dissociation constant $(K) \times [HCO_2] / [HCO_3^-]$

Ⓑ The normal plasma hydrogen ion concentration is 36–44 nmol/L

Ⓒ The plasma bicarbonate concentration is predominantly regulated by the renal tubules

Ⓓ Phosphates and sulphates are excreted principally in the bile

Ⓔ Carbon dioxide is principally transported in the blood as carbaminohaemoglobin

27

The following statements about acid-base regulation in healthy subjects are true

Ⓐ the blood pH is calculated from the measured arterial $PaCO_2$

Ⓑ $H^+ + HCO_3^- \Leftrightarrow H_2CO_3 \Leftrightarrow H_2O + CO_2$

Ⓒ the normal anion gap = Plasma $(Na^+ + K^+) - (Cl^- + HCO_3^-) < 15$ mmol/L

Ⓓ the blood $PaCO_2$ correlates closely with alveolar $PaCO_2$

Ⓔ the normal plasma bicarbonate concentration is 36–44 mmol/L

28

Metabolic acidosis induced by the following disorders is typically associated with an increased

Ⓐ plasma bicarbonate concentration in lactic acidosis

Ⓑ anion gap in starvation acidosis

Ⓒ blood $PaCO_2$ in diabetic ketoacidosis

Ⓓ plasma chloride concentration in proximal (type II) renal tubular acidosis

Ⓔ red cell carbonic acid production during acetazolamide therapy

29

Metabolic acidosis would be an expected finding in

Ⓐ chronic alveolar hyperventilation

Ⓑ acute insulin deficiency

Ⓒ acute inflammatory polyneuropathy (Guillain–Barré syndrome)

Ⓓ failure of distal renal tubular hydrogen ion secretion

Ⓔ fulminant liver failure

30

In a patient breathing room air, these arterial blood gases would be compatible with the diagnoses listed below: PaO_2 7.4 kPa, $PaCO_2$ 5.6 kPa, Hydrogen ion 78 nmol/L

Ⓐ prolonged frusemide therapy in chronic cardiac failure

Ⓑ chronic bronchitis with type II respiratory failure (ventilatory failure)

Ⓒ immediately following resuscitation from a cardiac arrest

Ⓓ chronic bronchitic patient in acute renal failure

Ⓔ prolonged vomiting due to pyloric stenosis

6 DISEASES OF THE KIDNEY AND URINARY SYSTEM

ANSWERS PAGE 197

1
The following statements about renal physiology in health are correct
Ⓐ each kidney comprises approximately 1 000 000 nephrons
Ⓑ the kidneys receive approximately 5% of the cardiac output
Ⓒ variations in the calibre of afferent and efferent arterioles control the filtration pressure
Ⓓ the glomerular capillaries are supplied by the afferent arterioles
Ⓔ the blood supply of the medulla arises from efferent arterioles

2
The kidney produces the following substances
Ⓐ erythropoietin
Ⓑ 25-hydroxycholecalciferol
Ⓒ prostaglandins PGE_2 and PGI_2
Ⓓ angiotensin-converting enzyme
Ⓔ aldosterone

3
Causes of polyuria include
Ⓐ chronic hyperglycaemia
Ⓑ lithium toxicity
Ⓒ adrenocorticotrophic hormone (ACTH) deficiency
Ⓓ Addison's disease
Ⓔ hypercalcaemia

4
Urinary protein excretion
Ⓐ in Bence Jones proteinuria is readily detectable by stick tests
Ⓑ > 3.5 g/day is invariably due to glomerular disease
Ⓒ is greater in the night than during the day
Ⓓ comprising myoglobin produces a positive labstix test for blood
Ⓔ in early diabetic nephropathy typically comprises albumin predominantly

5
Proteinuria in excess of 3.5 g per day is a typical feature of
Ⓐ cardiac failure
Ⓑ polycystic renal disease
Ⓒ renal amyloidosis
Ⓓ minimal change nephropathy
Ⓔ chronic pyelonephritis

6
Microscopic haematuria would be an expected finding in
Ⓐ urinary tract infection
Ⓑ renal papillary necrosis
Ⓒ membranous glomerulonephritis
Ⓓ infective endocarditis
Ⓔ renal infarction

7

In the investigation of renal disease

Ⓐ a random urinary pH of 4 suggests renal tubular acidosis (RTA)

Ⓑ creatinine clearance is calculated from the ratio of the urinary and plasma concentrations

Ⓒ urinary albumin/creatinine ratio of 1 mg/mmol indicates glomerular disease

Ⓓ a urinary protein/creatinine ratio of 50 mg/mmol indicates glomerular disease

Ⓔ renal biopsy is mandatory in chronic renal failure

8

Typical features of the acute glomerulonephritis syndrome include

Ⓐ bilateral renal angle pain and tenderness

Ⓑ hypertension and periorbital facial oedema

Ⓒ oliguria < 800 ml and haematuria

Ⓓ highly selective proteinuria

Ⓔ history of allergy with oedema of the lips

9

Typical features of the nephrotic syndrome include

Ⓐ bilateral renal angle pain

Ⓑ generalised oedema and pleural effusions

Ⓒ hypoalbuminaemia and proteinuria > 3.5 g /day

Ⓓ hypertension and polyuria

Ⓔ urinary sodium concentration > 20 mmol/L

10

Focal segmental glomerulonephritis would be an expected feature of

Ⓐ acute pyelonephritis

Ⓑ acute hepatitis B virus infection

Ⓒ microscopic polyarteritis nodosa

Ⓓ acute IgA nephropathy

Ⓔ renal amyloidosis

11

Typical features of acute post-infectious glomerulonephritis include

Ⓐ subendothelial immune deposits on the glomerular basement membrane

Ⓑ bacterial rather than viral infections

Ⓒ diffuse glomerular involvement

Ⓓ recurrent haemoptyses

Ⓔ a poor prognosis when the disease occurs in childhood

12

Typical features of acute post-infectious glomerulonephritis include

Ⓐ hypertension

Ⓑ impaired renal tubular function

Ⓒ hypocomplementaemia

Ⓓ oliguria

Ⓔ microscopic haematuria

13

IgA nephropathy is characterised by

Ⓐ recurrent macroscopic haematuria

Ⓑ onset 4–6 weeks after a respiratory tract infection

Ⓒ nephrotic syndrome in 20% of patients

Ⓓ progression to chronic renal failure in 10% of patients

Ⓔ mesangial cell proliferation on renal biopsy

14

Typical features of mesangiocapillary glomerulonephritis (MCGN) include

Ⓐ presentation with the nephrotic syndrome

Ⓑ hypertension and renal impairment at presentation

Ⓒ associated with partial lipodystrophy

Ⓓ progression to chronic renal failure

Ⓔ elevated complement levels

15

Glomerulonephritis associated with decreased serum complement concentrations is characteristic of

Ⓐ bacterial endocarditis
Ⓑ systemic lupus erythematosus
Ⓒ cryoglobulinaemia
Ⓓ mesangiocapillary glomerulonephritis
Ⓔ post-infectious glomerulonephritis

16

The typical features of Goodpasture's disease include

Ⓐ circulating antiglomerular basement membrane antibodies
Ⓑ crescentic nephritis
Ⓒ presentation with acute renal failure
Ⓓ haemoptysis and pulmonary infiltrates on chest X-ray
Ⓔ association with HLA-DR15

17

The characteristic features of membranous glomerulonephritis include

Ⓐ absence of glomerular or mesangial cell proliferation histologically
Ⓑ presentation with a nephrotic syndrome
Ⓒ progression to renal failure in one-third of patients
Ⓓ spontaneous remission occurs in one-third of patients
Ⓔ treatment with immunosuppression is useful in the majority

18

Typical causes of rapidly progressive glomerulonephritis include

Ⓐ post-infectious glomerulonephritis
Ⓑ systemic vasculitis
Ⓒ Goodpasture's disease
Ⓓ IgA nephropathy
Ⓔ membranous glomerulonephritis

19

Characteristic features of minimal change nephropathy are

Ⓐ occurrence in adults usually follows an acute infection
Ⓑ marked mesangial cell proliferation on renal biopsy
Ⓒ nephrotic syndrome with unselective proteinuria
Ⓓ hypertension and microscopic haematuria
Ⓔ progression to chronic failure in patients not responding to corticosteroid therapy

20

In the treatment of minimal change nephropathy

Ⓐ therapy should be deferred pending renal biopsy in childhood
Ⓑ diuretics should be avoided to minimise the risk of renal impairment
Ⓒ following remission, more than one-third of patients relapse within 3 years
Ⓓ immunosuppressant therapy is indicated for frequent relapses
Ⓔ impaired renal function commonly develops in the long term

21

Characteristic features of renal tubular acidosis (RTA) include

Ⓐ normal anion gap
Ⓑ hyperchloraemic acidosis
Ⓒ inappropriately high urinary pH > 5.4
Ⓓ decreased glomerular filtration rate (GFR)
Ⓔ normocytic normochromic anaemia

22

Recognised causes of distal type 1 renal tubular acidosis (RTA) include

Ⓐ lithium therapy
Ⓑ hyperparathyroidism
Ⓒ Sjögren's syndrome
Ⓓ chronic renal transplant rejection
Ⓔ chronic pyelonephritis

23
Typical features of acute interstitial nephritis (AIN) include
Ⓐ skin rashes, arthralgia and fever
Ⓑ peripheral blood eosinophilia
Ⓒ renal biopsy evidence of an eosinophilic interstitial nephritis
Ⓓ renal impairment typically follows withdrawal of the drug
Ⓔ onset following antibiotic or anti-inflammatory drug therapy

24
Causes of acute interstitial nephritis include
Ⓐ penicillin therapy
Ⓑ naproxen therapy
Ⓒ tuberculosis
Ⓓ myeloma
Ⓔ cytomegalovirus

25
Causes of chronic interstitial nephritis include
Ⓐ Sjögren's syndrome
Ⓑ Wilson's disease
Ⓒ sickle-cell nephropathy
Ⓓ chronic transplant rejection
Ⓔ analgesic abuse

26
The following findings would support a diagnosis of pre-renal rather than established acute renal failure
Ⓐ oliguria < 700 ml per day
Ⓑ urine/plasma urea ratio > 10:1
Ⓒ a urinary osmolality > 600 mosm/kg
Ⓓ a urinary sodium concentration < 20 mmol/L
Ⓔ hypertension rather than hypotension

27
The typical features of lower urinary tract infections (UTIs) include
Ⓐ rigors, loin pain and renal impairment
Ⓑ suprapubic pain, dysuria and haematuria
Ⓒ progression to acute pyelonephritis if untreated
Ⓓ midstream urine culture producing *Escherichia coli* > 100 000 /ml
Ⓔ the drug of choice for the majority is ciprofloxacin

28
The typical features of acute pyelonephritis in adults include
Ⓐ normal anatomy of the urinary tract
Ⓑ vomiting, rigors and renal angle tenderness
Ⓒ renal angle pain is usually bilateral
Ⓓ evidence of reflux on isotope renography
Ⓔ loin pain and fullness in the flank

29
During pregnancy
Ⓐ asymptomatic bacteriuria is present in 50% of pregnant women
Ⓑ ureteric atonia predisposes to the onset of acute pyelonephritis
Ⓒ treatment of asymptomatic bacteriuria prevents symptom onset
Ⓓ intravenous urography is mandatory if acute pyelonephritis ensues
Ⓔ trimethoprim is the treatment of choice in acute cystitis

30
Chronic pyelonephritis is
Ⓐ a recognised association of nephrocalcinosis
Ⓑ usually symptomatic from the onset of the condition
Ⓒ associated with a poorer prognosis in paraplegic or diabetic patients
Ⓓ likely to present with renal impairment only after the age of 60 years
Ⓔ a recognised cause of chronic sodium depletion

31

Chronic pyelonephritis in adults

Ⓐ accounts for the majority of patients with chronic renal failure (CRF) in the UK

Ⓑ is usually attributable to vesicoureteric reflux in childhood

Ⓒ has pathognomic histopathological features on renal biopsy

Ⓓ is usually associated with demonstrable ureteric reflux

Ⓔ producing hypotension should be treated with oral sodium salts

32

Complications of chronic renal failure include

Ⓐ macrocytic anaemia

Ⓑ peripheral neuropathy

Ⓒ bone pain

Ⓓ pericarditis

Ⓔ metabolic alkalosis

33

Typical biochemical features of chronic renal failure include

Ⓐ impaired urinary concentrating ability

Ⓑ hypophosphataemia

Ⓒ hypercalcaemia

Ⓓ metabolic acidosis

Ⓔ proteinuria > 3.5 g/day

34

Ureteric obstruction

Ⓐ predisposes to stone formation

Ⓑ is a recognised complication of cervical carcinoma

Ⓒ unlike bladder-neck obstruction, seldom causes haematuria

Ⓓ at the pelvi-ureteric junction in childhood is usually congenital

Ⓔ is typically pain-free if the onset is gradual

35

Disorders predisposing to renal stone formation include

Ⓐ urinary tract infection

Ⓑ prolonged immobilisation

Ⓒ hypoparathyroidism

Ⓓ renal tubular acidosis

Ⓔ sarcoidosis

36

In the treatment of renal calculi

Ⓐ anuria indicates the need for urgent surgical intervention

Ⓑ the urine should be alkalinised if the stone is radio-opaque

Ⓒ bendrofluazide increases urinary calcium excretion

Ⓓ allopurinol increases urinary urate excretion in gouty patients

Ⓔ renal pelvic stones require removal at open surgery

37

The clinical features of adult polycystic renal disease include

Ⓐ an autosomal recessive mode of inheritance

Ⓑ cystic disease of the liver and pancreas

Ⓒ renal angle pain and haematuria

Ⓓ aortic and mitral regurgitation

Ⓔ aneurysms of the circle of Willis

38

The features of Alport's syndrome include

Ⓐ an autosomal dominant mode of inheritance

Ⓑ degeneration of the glomerular basement membrane

Ⓒ mutation of genes encoding type IV collagen

Ⓓ association with progressive chronic renal failure

Ⓔ association with high-tone deafness

39
Recognised features of renal carcinoma include
A persistent fever
B bone metastases
C haematuria
D polycythaemia
E serum alpha-fetoprotein in high titre

40
Tumour metabolites associated with renal carcinoma are responsible for
A hypertension
B abnormalities of liver function values
C neuromyopathy
D hypercalcaemia
E hyperglycaemia

41
Typical features of bladder carcinoma include
A squamous cell rather than transitional cell in origin
B presentation with urinary frequency and nocturia
C unresponsive to radiotherapy
D early metastatic spread to the liver and lungs
E association with exposure to dyes and tobacco consumption

42
Typical features of prostatic carcinoma include
A slowly progressive obstructive uropathy
B presentation with urinary frequency and nocturia
C preservation of the normal anatomy on digital rectal examination
D local spread along the lumbosacral nerve plexus
E osteolytic rather than osteosclerotic bone metastases

43
The typical features of benign prostatic hypertrophy include
A peak incidence in the age-group 40–60 years
B acute urinary retention and haematuria
C increased plasma testosterone concentration
D normal serum prostatic acid phosphatase concentration
E asymmetrical prostatic enlargement on rectal examination

44
Characteristic features of testicular tumours include
A testicular pain in seminoma of the testis
B secretion of alpha-fetoprotein and chorionic gonadotrophin by teratomas
C absence of distant metastases
D peak incidence after the age of 60 years
E seminomas are both radio- and chemosensitive

7 DIABETES MELLITUS, AND NUTRITIONAL AND METABOLIC DISORDERS

ANSWERS PAGE 202

1
The following statements about diabetes mellitus in the UK are true
A the prevalence is approximately 1–2%
B the disorder is more common in nulliparous than multiparous women
C type 1 diabetes (IDDM) is typically inherited as an autosomal dominant trait
D type 2 diabetes (NIDDM) increases in prevalence with advancing age
E hyperglycaemia occurs only after 25% reduction in islet cell mass

2
Type 1 insulin-dependent diabetes mellitus (IDDM) is associated with
A 'insulitis'—T lymphocyte infiltrate of the islets of Langerhans
B cows milk feeding of infants < 3 months old
C serum islet cell antibodies in > 80% of newly-diagnosed patients
D 35% concordance rates in monozygotic twins
E possession of HLA antigens DR3 and DR4

3
The following statements about type 2 diabetes mellitus (NIDDM) are true
A there is clear evidence of disordered autoimmunity in most patients with NIDDM
B monozygotic twins show almost 100% concordance for NIDDM
C patients with NIDDM typically exhibit hypersensitivity to insulin
D obesity predisposes to NIDDM in genetically-susceptible individuals
E insulin secretion in response to amino acids is normal in NIDDM

4
Secondary diabetes mellitus is associated with
A thiazide diuretic therapy
B haemochromatosis
C primary hyperaldosteronism
D pancreatic carcinoma
E thyrotoxicosis

5
The physiological effects of insulin include
A increased glycolysis
B decreased glycogenolysis
C increased lipolysis
D increased gluconeogenesis
E increased protein catabolism

6
In decompensated diabetes mellitus
A thirst results from the increased osmolality of glomerular filtrate
B hyperpnoea is the result of acidosis due to increased lactic and ketoacid production
C negative nitrogen balance results from the increased protein catabolism
D lipolysis increases as a result of relative insulin deficiency
E insulin deficiency inhibits the peripheral utilisation of ketoacids

7
In the diagnosis of diabetes mellitus
Ⓐ glycated haemoglobin (HbA$_{1c}$) is a sensitive screening test
Ⓑ absence of glycosuria excludes diabetes
Ⓒ glycosuria is usually due to reduced renal threshhold in young patients
Ⓓ 2% of patients have significant diabetic complications at presentation
Ⓔ plasma glucose concentrations are 15% higher than whole blood levels

8
The oral glucose tolerance test is
Ⓐ diabetic if the 2 hour plasma glucose > 11.1 mmol/L
Ⓑ diabetic if the fasting plasma glucose > 7.8 mmol/L
Ⓒ undertaken following 3 days of dietary carbohydrate restriction
Ⓓ best administered using 75 g of glucose in 250 ml of water
Ⓔ diabetic if any plasma glucose exceeds 12 mmol/L

9
Typical presentations of diabetes mellitus include
Ⓐ weight loss and nocturia
Ⓑ balanitis or pruritus vulvae
Ⓒ epigastric pain and vomiting
Ⓓ limb pains with absent ankle reflexes
Ⓔ asymptomatic glycosuria in the elderly

10
In the dietary management of diabetes mellitus
Ⓐ 90% of patients also require hypoglycaemic drug therapy
Ⓑ carbohydrate intakes should be 50–55% of total calorie intake
Ⓒ ice-cream and chocolates should never be consumed
Ⓓ fat intakes should not exceed 35% of total calorie intake
Ⓔ in obese patients, calorie intake should not exceed 600 kcal/day

11
Sulphonylurea drug therapy in diabetes mellitus
Ⓐ causes more weight gain when given with biguanide therapy
Ⓑ increases hepatic gluconeogenesis
Ⓒ decreases the number of peripheral insulin receptors
Ⓓ decreases hepatic glycogenolysis
Ⓔ causes alcohol-induced flushing as a dominantly-inherited trait

12
Biguanide drug therapy in diabetes mellitus
Ⓐ is more likely to cause weight loss than weight gain
Ⓑ increases plasma immunoreactive insulin concentration
Ⓒ decreases pancreatic glucagon release
Ⓓ inhibits hepatic glycogenolysis
Ⓔ causes troublesome constipation

13
The following statements about insulin therapy are true
Ⓐ The duration of action of unmodified insulins = 6 hours
Ⓑ The duration of action of depot insulins = 12 hours +
Ⓒ Obese individuals tend to require lower total doses
Ⓓ The standard UK solution strength = 100 iu/ml
Ⓔ Human insulins are less potent than animal-derived insulins

14

In the management of a newly-diagnosed 20-year-old diabetic

Ⓐ insulin-induced hypoglycaemia should be experienced as part patient education

Ⓑ insulin requirements during the first 8 weeks often decrease

Ⓒ insulin should normally be administered once daily initially

Ⓓ glycated haemoglobin (HbA$_{1c}$) concentrations should be monitored weekly

Ⓔ 6-hourly urine testing is recommended during pregnancy

15

Typical symptoms of hypoglycaemia in diabetic patients include

Ⓐ feelings of faintness and hunger

Ⓑ tremor, palpitation and dizziness

Ⓒ headache, diplopia and confusion

Ⓓ abnormal behaviour despite plasma glucose consistently > 5 mmol/L

Ⓔ nocturnal sweating, nightmares and convulsions

16

In the treatment of severe hypoglycaemia in a diabetic patient

Ⓐ 50 ml 50% glucose should be given intravenously

Ⓑ glucagon should be avoided if the episode was due to sulphonylurea therapy

Ⓒ an alternative explanation is likely if the patient is taking metformin therapy alone

Ⓓ recovery is invariably complete within 1 hour of therapy

Ⓔ hospital admission is usually unnecessary if due to chlorpropamide therapy

17

Factors predisposing to frequent hypoglycaemic episodes in a diabetic patient include

Ⓐ delayed meals

Ⓑ unusual exercise

Ⓒ excessive alcohol intake

Ⓓ development of hypoadrenalism

Ⓔ errors in drug administration

18

In a comatose diabetic patient, clinical features suggesting hypoglycaemia rather than ketoacidosis include

Ⓐ systemic hypotension

Ⓑ brisk tendon reflexes

Ⓒ air hunger

Ⓓ moist skin and tongue

Ⓔ abdominal pain

19

In a typical diabetic patient attending the diabetic follow-up clinic, the following features should be included in the routine assessment

Ⓐ blood pressure

Ⓑ lower limb peripheral pulses

Ⓒ body weight

Ⓓ urinalysis

Ⓔ visual acuity and fundoscopy

20

The typical clinical features of diabetic ketoacidosis include

Ⓐ abdominal pain and air hunger

Ⓑ rapid, weak pulse and hypotension

Ⓒ profuse sweating and oliguria

Ⓓ vomiting and constipation

Ⓔ coma with extensor plantar responses

21
Expected findings in severe diabetic ketoacidosis include
Ⓐ water deficit of 5–10 litres
Ⓑ both sodium and potassium deficits of > 400 mmol
Ⓒ arterial blood gas analysis PaO_2 7 kPa, $PaCO_2$ 7 kPa and pH = 7.20
Ⓓ decreased serum potassium concentration at presentation
Ⓔ peripheral blood leucocytosis

22
In the management of diabetic keto-acidosis
Ⓐ intracellular water deficit is best restored using half-strength saline (0.45% saline)
Ⓑ potassium should be given even before checking the serum potassium concentration
Ⓒ bicarbonate infusion is often only necessary in renal failure
Ⓓ 5% dextrose solution should be avoided unless hypoglycaemia supervenes
Ⓔ peripheral circulatory failure requires rapid volume replacement initially

23
In the long-term management of diabetes
Ⓐ retinal neovascularisation should resolve with better glycaemic control
Ⓑ microaneurysms are usually only visible with fluorescein angiography
Ⓒ visual symptoms correlate well with the severity of retinal disease
Ⓓ microalbuminuria suggests renal tubular dysfunction
Ⓔ the development of an autonomic neuropathy confers an increased risk of sudden death

24
In the management of diabetes mellitus during pregnancy
Ⓐ there is an increased perinatal mortality rate
Ⓑ the baby is usually smaller than expected from gestational age
Ⓒ delivery should be undertaken by Caesarian section at week 36
Ⓓ mild diabetes responds well to sulphonylurea and diet therapy
Ⓔ glucose intolerance usually decreases throughout pregnancy

25
In the management of diabetics requiring elective surgery
Ⓐ patients should stop sulphonylureas 24 hours prior to surgery
Ⓑ usual insulin should be given preoperatively to prevent ketoacidosis
Ⓒ patients with NIDDM require insulin cover for major surgery
Ⓓ those undergoing cardiopulmonary bypass have lower insulin needs
Ⓔ 10% dextrose and insulin infusion is the optimal perioperative method of control

26
The clinical features of the metabolic syndrome (syndrome X) include
Ⓐ hyperuricaemia
Ⓑ hypertension
Ⓒ central obesity
Ⓓ hyperinsulinaemia
Ⓔ hypertriglyceridaemia

27
The clinical features of diabetic retinopathy include
Ⓐ arteriolar spasm with arteriovenous nipping
Ⓑ venous dilatation and increased venous tortuosity
Ⓒ soft and hard exudates
Ⓓ 'dot' and 'blot' retinal haemorrhages
Ⓔ microaneurysms

28
The complications of malnutrition are the result of
Ⓐ impaired haematopoiesis
Ⓑ impaired cellular responses to infection
Ⓒ impaired humoral responses to infection
Ⓓ impaired tissue healing
Ⓔ mucosal cell atrophy

29
The daily essential nutrient requirements in man include
Ⓐ 1–2mg vitamins D, K, and B_{12}
Ⓑ 1 kg water
Ⓒ 50 g protein
Ⓓ 50 mg vitamin C
Ⓔ 10 mg calcium and phosphate

30
The following statements about adult dietary energy sources are true
Ⓐ Carbohydrates have a calorific value of 4 kcal/g
Ⓑ Fats have a calorific value of 5 kcal/g
Ⓒ 1 litre of whisky (40% alcohol) contains about 1000 calories
Ⓓ Linoleic and linolenic acids are both essential fatty acids
Ⓔ Proteins provide 4 kcal/g and all nine essential amino acids

31
A healthy daily diet for a slim, active man should include
Ⓐ 1700 kcal (8.4 MJ)
Ⓑ 50 g of carbohydrate
Ⓒ 15 mg of both iron and zinc
Ⓓ 60 g of protein of good biological value
Ⓔ 50 mg of folic acid

32
Clinical features of protein-energy malnutrition in adults include
Ⓐ a body mass index (BMI) of between 18 and 20
Ⓑ oedema in the absence of hypoalbuminaemia
Ⓒ nocturia, cold intolerance and diarrhoea
Ⓓ skin depigmentation, hair loss and covert infection
Ⓔ cerebral atrophy and sinus tachycardia

33
Expected laboratory findings in protein-energy malnutrition in adults include
Ⓐ decreased plasma free fatty acid (FFA) concentrations
Ⓑ increased plasma cortisol and reverse T3 concentrations
Ⓒ impaired delayed skin sensitivity to tuberculin
Ⓓ decreased plasma insulin, glucose and T3 concentrations
Ⓔ decreased urinary osmolality and creatinine excretion

34
The following statements about protein-energy malnutrition (PEM) in children are true
Ⓐ kwashiorkor is a combined protein and calorie deficiency state
Ⓑ nutritional marasmus occurs in isolated total calorie deficiency
Ⓒ nutritional dwarfism is usually associated with a body mass index (BMI) of < 16
Ⓓ there is an increased susceptibility to all types of infection
Ⓔ premature weaning and childhood illnesses predispose to protein-energy malnutrition

35
The clinical features of protein-energy malnutrition include
A marked muscle wasting and abdominal distension in marasmus
B weight loss more than growth retardation in marasmus
C hepatic steatosis and hypoproteinaemic oedema in kwashiorkor
D desquamative dermatosis, stomatitis and anorexia in marasmus
E associated zinc deficiency in kwashiorkor

36
In the treatment of severe protein-energy malnutrition
A mortality rates of about 20% occur even in hospitalised patients
B correction of fluid and electrolyte balance is vital
C calorie and protein intake restoration worsens the oedema
D fatty liver leads to cirrhosis if calorie intakes remain poor
E mortality rates would be greatly reduced by rehydration, breast feeding and immunisation

37
The following statements about calcium balance in adult man are true
A total body calcium is about 1.2 kg of which 99% is in bone
B the UK recommended adult intake is 800 mg daily
C 70% of dietary calcium is excreted in the faeces
D dietary phytates and oxalates enhance calcium absorption
E the serum calcium is a sensitive index of total body calcium

38
The following statements about iron balance in a healthy young adult female are true
A the healthy daily diet should provide 15 mg of iron
B 60% of dietary inorganic iron is absorbed
C organic iron is better absorbed than inorganic iron
D daily iron losses of 1 mg results from desquamated cells
E 500 ml of blood contains 25 µg of iron

39
The following statements about deficiency states are true
A iodine deficiency produces goitre and thyrotoxicosis
B soft drinking water contains more fluoride than hard waters
C zinc deficiency produces dermatitis, hair loss and diarrhoea
D copper deficiency in children produces anaemia and poor growth
E phosphate deficiency occurs in neonates fed on cow's milk

40
Vitamin A is
A a fat-soluble vitamin
B present as retinol in carrots and certain green vegetables
C the treatment of choice in xerophthalmia and keratomalacia
D recommended in minimum dietary requirements of 50 mg daily for adults
E present in high concentrations in fish liver oils

41
Vitamin D
Ⓐ is present in high concentrations in dairy products
Ⓑ is non-essential in the diet given adequate sunlight exposure
Ⓒ like vitamin A is stored mainly in the liver
Ⓓ is converted from cholecalciferol to 1,25 dihydroxycholecalciferol
Ⓔ enhances calcium absorption by the induction of specific enterocyte transport proteins

42
Vitamin K is
Ⓐ a fat-soluble vitamin found in leafy vegetables
Ⓑ synthesised in the liver by the conversion of vitamin K_2
Ⓒ vital for the synthesis of clotting factors 2, 7, 9, 10
Ⓓ often deficient in neonates due to the absence of normal gut flora
Ⓔ absorbed by an active process which is inhibited by warfarin therapy

43
Vitamin C deficiency
Ⓐ impairs wound healing due to defective collagen synthesis
Ⓑ would develop within 4 months given a daily intake of 5 mg
Ⓒ produces bleeding gums in edentulous individuals
Ⓓ produces perifollicular haemorrhages and 'corkscrew' hairs
Ⓔ in childhood produces anaemia and bone and joint pains

44
In thiamin deficiency
Ⓐ anaerobic glycolysis is impaired resulting in lactic acidosis
Ⓑ the diet is deficient in green vegetables and dairy products
Ⓒ sudden death results from low output cardiac failure
Ⓓ peripheral neuropathy results in marked muscle wasting
Ⓔ Wernicke's encephalopathy is usually suggested by ataxia and nystagmus

45
Deficiency of the B vitamins listed below is associated with the following disorders
Ⓐ niacin—pellagra
Ⓑ pyridoxine—isoniazid-induced peripheral neuropathy
Ⓒ pyridoxine—haemolytic anaemia
Ⓓ riboflavin—angular stomatitis
Ⓔ riboflavin—cheilosis

46
The following statements about vitamin B_{12} and folic acid are true
Ⓐ The serum vitamin B_{12} level is lower in vegetarians than in omnivores
Ⓑ Both vitamin B_{12} and folate are essential for DNA synthesis
Ⓒ A daily intake of 1–2 µg of vitamin B_{12} is recommended
Ⓓ A daily intake of 1–2 mg of folic acid is recommended
Ⓔ Deficiency of either vitamin produces a peripheral blood macrocytosis and pancytopenia

47
In the nutritional support of hospital patients

Ⓐ vitamin K deficiency is associated with antibiotic use

Ⓑ enteral feeding aids healing in inflammatory bowel disease

Ⓒ 2.5 L of 10% dextrose provides 1000 kcal

Ⓓ solutions of up to 20% dextrose can safely be given by peripheral vein

Ⓔ the use of dextrose alone as a calorie source produces muscle wasting

48
In the assessment of nutritional deficiency in hospital patients

Ⓐ nutritional supplementation is not required until clinical signs are apparent

Ⓑ 1 kg of weight loss approximates to 6000 kcal of energy

Ⓒ plasma albumin is a reliable index of visceral protein depletion

Ⓓ elevated serum methyl malonate suggests vitamin B_{12} deficiency

Ⓔ lymphocytosis suggests protein depletion

49
Characteristic findings in simple obesity in adults include

Ⓐ a body mass index > 30

Ⓑ increased plasma cortisol and insulin concentrations

Ⓒ a family history of obesity of similar degree and distribution

Ⓓ onset in females at the menarche, in pregnancy or menopause

Ⓔ basal metabolic rates and thermic responses to food are similar to lean subjects

50
Recognised associations of obesity include

Ⓐ hyperuricaemia

Ⓑ depression

Ⓒ gallstones

Ⓓ type 2 diabetes mellitus

Ⓔ hyperlipidaemia

51
Drug therapies known to increase appetite and body weight include

Ⓐ oral contraceptives

Ⓑ chlorpromazine

Ⓒ amitriptyline

Ⓓ fluoxetine

Ⓔ glipizide

52
Ideal weight reducing diets in the treatment of moderate obesity should

Ⓐ provide no more than 600 kcal (2.5 MJ)

Ⓑ achieve a theoretical weight loss of at least 2 kg per week

Ⓒ aim to achieve a weight loss of 10%

Ⓓ maintain nitrogen balance given a daily intake of 25 g protein

Ⓔ reduce carbohydrate intake much more than total fat intake

53
The following statements about the management of obesity are correct

Ⓐ the risk of obesity in males is increased if the waist circumference > 37 inches (94 cm)

Ⓑ jogging for 20 minutes five times per week will expend an additional 900 kcal per week

Ⓒ effective calorie restriction usually produces symptomatic ketosis

Ⓓ the calorie content of 200 ml of wine or 500 ml of beer = 150 kcal

Ⓔ drug therapy to suppress the appetite or induce satiety is of proven long-term efficacy

54
The benefits of a sustained 10% weight reduction in the obese include

Ⓐ fall in the blood pressure of 10 mmHg (systolic) and 20 mmHg (diastolic)

Ⓑ reduction in total mortality of 20–25%

Ⓒ reduction in the risk of developing diabetes mellitus by > 50%

Ⓓ reduction in total cholesterol by 50%

Ⓔ improvement in the symptoms of angina pectoris by 10%

55

The functions of the main lipoproteins include

Ⓐ chylomicrons transport mainly cholesterol

Ⓑ very low density lipoprotein (VLDL) transports endogenous triglycerides

Ⓒ low density lipoprotein (LDL) transports cholesterol

Ⓓ high density lipoprotein (HDL) transports cholesterol from the peripheral tissues to the liver

Ⓔ low density lipoprotein is important for the excretion of cholesterol and is cardioprotective

56

In the classification of hyperlipidaemias, the following findings are typical

Ⓐ chylomicronaemia in types I and V

Ⓑ hypertriglyceridaemia in types III, IV and V

Ⓒ hypercholesterolaemia in types II, III and IV

Ⓓ tendon xanthomata in type IIa hypercholesterolaemia

Ⓔ defective low density lipoprotein (LDL) catabolism and receptor binding in type V hyperlipidaemia

57

Common causes of secondary hyperlipidaemia include

Ⓐ chronic renal failure

Ⓑ diabetes mellitus

Ⓒ hyperthyroidism

Ⓓ alcohol abuse

Ⓔ oestrogen replacement therapy

58

The actions of the lipid-lowering drugs include

Ⓐ the statins inhibit HMG CoA reductase and reduce cholesterol synthesis

Ⓑ the statins increase plasma LDL and triglycerides

Ⓒ nicotinic acid increases lipolysis and lower HDL

Ⓓ fibrates increase VLDL lipolysis

Ⓔ colestipol diverts hepatic cholesterol synthesis into an increased bile acid production

59

In the treatment of hyperlipidaemia in patients aged < 60 years

Ⓐ dietary fat restriction reduces the plasma cholesterol by about 10%

Ⓑ lowering the plasma cholesterol is only of value if elevated > 6.5 mmol/L

Ⓒ drug therapy is usually necessary if the plasma cholesterol > 7.8 mmol/L

Ⓓ high plasma HDL/LDL ratios indicate the need for drug therapy

Ⓔ fibrates reduce cholesterol synthesis by inhibiting HMG CoA reductase

60

Spontaneous hypoglycaemia is

Ⓐ confirmed by a blood glucose concentration < 2.2 mmol/L

Ⓑ a recognised complication of acute alcoholic intoxication

Ⓒ best investigated using a 48-hour fast if unexplained

Ⓓ the cause of early dumping syndrome following partial gastrectomy

Ⓔ most obvious pre-prandially in patients with an insulinoma

61

Causes of spontaneous hypoglycaemia include

Ⓐ primary hepatoma

Ⓑ autoimmune insulin syndrome

Ⓒ hepatic failure

Ⓓ Addison's disease

Ⓔ pancreatic islet-cell tumour

62
In the classification of acute and non-acute porphyrias
Ⓐ delta-ALA synthetase activity is increased in all porphyrias

Ⓑ porphobilinogen deaminase activity is reduced in acute porphyrias

Ⓒ neuropsychiatric features are typical of the non-acute porphyrias

Ⓓ photosensitivity is typical of the acute porphyrias

Ⓔ variegate porphyria and coproporphyria are acute porphyrias

63
The typical features of acute intermittent porphyria include
Ⓐ increased porphobilinogen deaminase activity

Ⓑ the absence of clinical symptoms or signs

Ⓒ vomiting, constipation and abdominal pain

Ⓓ hypertension and tachycardia

Ⓔ exacerbation by diamorphine or chlorpromazine therapy

64
Disorders associated with amyloid deposition include
Ⓐ familial Mediterranean fever

Ⓑ multiple myeloma

Ⓒ type 1 diabetes mellitus

Ⓓ Alzheimer's disease

Ⓔ rheumatoid arthritis

8 ENDOCRINE DISEASE

ANSWERS PAGE 210

1

The hypothalamic releasing factors listed below stimulate the pituitary gland to secrete the following hormones
Ⓐ dopamine—prolactin
Ⓑ somatostatin—growth hormone
Ⓒ thyrotrophin releasing hormone (TRH)—TSH and prolactin
Ⓓ gonadotrophin releasing hormone (GnRH)—LH and FSH independently
Ⓔ corticotrophin releasing hormone (CRH)—ß-lipotrophic hormone (LPH) and ACTH

2

The following statements about pituitary tumours are true
Ⓐ chromophobe adenomas cause pressure effects but do not secrete pituitary hormones
Ⓑ diabetes insipidus usually indicates suprasellar extension
Ⓒ Cushing's disease is usually caused by acidophilic macroadenomas
Ⓓ acromegaly is most often associated with basophilic microadenomas
Ⓔ tumour enlargement with expansion of the pituitary fossa typically presents with headaches and/or a bitemporal upper quadrantanopia

3

Causes of hyperprolactinaemia include
Ⓐ oral contraceptive therapy
Ⓑ chlorpromazine therapy
Ⓒ primary hypothyroidism
Ⓓ hypoadrenalism
Ⓔ Cushing's disease

4

The clinical features of hyperprolactinaemia include
Ⓐ hypogonadism and galactorrhoea
Ⓑ infertility associated with secondary amenorrhoea
Ⓒ an increased likelihood of macroadenoma in males
Ⓓ bitemporal hemianopia associated with microadenomas
Ⓔ prompt response to dopamine agonist therapy

5

The clinical features of acromegaly include
Ⓐ arthropathy and myopathy
Ⓑ hypertension and impaired glucose tolerance
Ⓒ goitre and cardiomegaly
Ⓓ increased sweating and headache
Ⓔ skin atrophy and decreased sebum secretion

6

Typical results of investigations in a patient with acromegaly include
Ⓐ failure of the plasma growth hormone (GH) to rise during a glucose tolerance test (GTT)
Ⓑ decreased serum prolactin
Ⓒ increased serum insulin-like growth factor (IGF-1)
Ⓓ abnormality of the pituitary fossa on plain X-ray
Ⓔ tumour shrinkage in response to octreotide therapy

7

Typical features of anterior pituitary hormone deficiency in adults include

Ⓐ loss of growth hormone function before luteinising hormone

Ⓑ hypertension due to ACTH deficiency

Ⓒ skin pigmentation

Ⓓ myxoedema due to TSH defiency

Ⓔ dilutional hyponatraemia

8

Causes of hypopituitarism include

Ⓐ Kallmann's syndrome

Ⓑ craniopharyngioma

Ⓒ head injury

Ⓓ Sheehan's syndrome

Ⓔ sarcoidosis

9

Causes of diabetes insipidus include

Ⓐ congenital sex-linked recessive disorder

Ⓑ craniopharyngioma

Ⓒ DIDMOAD syndrome

Ⓓ severe hypocalcaemia

Ⓔ sarcoidosis

10

The typical features of cranial diabetes insipidus include

Ⓐ serum sodium concentration > 150 mmol/L with urine SG < 1.001

Ⓑ increased polyuria following corticosteroid therapy for hypopituitarism

Ⓒ onset following basal meningitis or hypothalamic trauma

Ⓓ decreased renal responsiveness to ADH following carbamazepine therapy

Ⓔ unlike psychogenic polydipsia, the response to ADH is invariably normal

11

Causes of nephrogenic diabetes insipidus include

Ⓐ lithium therapy

Ⓑ heavy metal poisoning

Ⓒ congenital sex-linked recessive disorder

Ⓓ chlorpropamide therapy

Ⓔ demeclocycline therapy

12

Causes of inappropriate ADH secretion include

Ⓐ meningitis

Ⓑ head injury

Ⓒ lobar pneumonia

Ⓓ small cell bronchial carcinoma

Ⓔ phenothiazine therapy

13

The insulin-induced hypoglycaemia stimulation test is

Ⓐ mandatory to confirm the diagnosis of hypopituitarism

Ⓑ best terminated as soon as the plasma glucose falls below 2.4 mmol/L

Ⓒ contraindicated in ischaemic heart disease and epilepsy

Ⓓ contraindicated in severe hypopituitarism

Ⓔ an unreliable test of hypothalamic function

14

In childhood growth hormone deficiency

Ⓐ panhypopituitarism is a typical finding

Ⓑ most patients have a craniopharyngioma

Ⓒ a genetic deficiency of growth hormone releasing factor is common

Ⓓ delayed bone development is a characteristic feature

Ⓔ treatment with human growth hormone produces precocious puberty

15

Causes of short stature in childhood include

Ⓐ Klinefelter's syndrome

Ⓑ Turner's syndrome

Ⓒ emotional deprivation

Ⓓ Cushing's syndrome

Ⓔ hyperthyroidism

16

The following statements about thyroid hormones are true

Ⓐ T_3 and T_4 are both stored in colloid vesicles as thyroglobulin

Ⓑ T_4 is metabolically more active than T_3

Ⓒ T_3 and T_4 are mainly bound to albumin in the serum

Ⓓ 85% of the circulating T_3 arises from extra-thyroidal T_4

Ⓔ conversion of T_4 to T_3 decreases in acute illness

17

The finding of reduced serum free T_4 and thyroid-stimulating hormone (TSH) concentrations is compatible with the following conditions

Ⓐ hypopituitarism

Ⓑ primary hypothyroidism

Ⓒ nephrotic syndrome

Ⓓ pneumonia

Ⓔ pregnancy

18

The following statements about thyrotoxicosis are true

Ⓐ most patients have Graves' disease

Ⓑ multinodular goitre is more common than uninodular goitre

Ⓒ amiodarone treatment should be considered as a possible cause

Ⓓ the thyroid gland is diffusely hyperactive in Graves' disease

Ⓔ there is an increased prevalence of HLA-DR3 in Graves' disease

19

The clinical features of thyrotoxicosis include

Ⓐ atrial fibrillation with a collapsing pulse

Ⓑ weight loss and oligomenorrhoea

Ⓒ peripheral neuropathy

Ⓓ proximal myopathy and exophthalmos

Ⓔ decreased insulin requirements in type 1 diabetes mellitus

20

In the treatment of thyrotoxicosis

Ⓐ propranolol should not be given in atrial fibrillation

Ⓑ carbimazole blocks the secretion of T_3 and T_4 by the thyroid

Ⓒ persistent suppression of the serum TSH is an indication for surgery

Ⓓ serum TSH receptor antibodies usually persist despite carbimazole

Ⓔ surgery is more likely to be necessary in young men than in women

21

Following ^{131}I radioiodine treatment for thyrotoxicosis

Ⓐ rising plasma TSH suggests disease recurrence

Ⓑ at least 50% of patients develop hypothyroidism within 7 years

Ⓒ relapse is common in patients with a solitary 'hot' nodule

Ⓓ a clinical effect should be expected within 4–12 weeks

Ⓔ 70% of patients require further radioiodine therapy

22

The following regimes would be appropriate in the management of a 30-year-old woman with severe thyrotoxic Graves' disease

Ⓐ carbimazole with ^{131}I radioiodine

Ⓑ potassium perchlorate with carbimazole

Ⓒ propranolol with carbimazole

Ⓓ subtotal thyroidectomy following thyrotoxic control

Ⓔ prednisolone with potassium iodide and propranolol

23

Complications of subtotal thyroidectomy for thyrotoxicosis include

Ⓐ transient hypothyroidism

Ⓑ recurrent laryngeal nerve palsy

Ⓒ hypoparathyroidism

Ⓓ recurrent thyrotoxicosis

Ⓔ thyroid carcinoma

24

In Graves' ophthalmopathy

Ⓐ diplopia is the most common presenting symptom

Ⓑ the patient is invariably thyrotoxic

Ⓒ serum eye muscle antibodies are pathognomonic

Ⓓ in 90% of patients the condition resolves spontaneously

Ⓔ hypothyroidism exacerbates the condition

25

The clinical features of primary hypothyroidism include

Ⓐ carpal tunnel syndrome and proximal myopathy

Ⓑ cold sensitivity and menorrhagia

Ⓒ deafness and dizziness

Ⓓ puffy eyelids and malar flush

Ⓔ absent ankle tendon reflexes

26

Biochemical findings in primary hypothyroidism include

Ⓐ decreased serum free T_4 and decreased serum TSH concentration

Ⓑ increased serum prolactin concentration

Ⓒ inappropriate ADH secretion

Ⓓ increased serum alkaline phosphatase concentration

Ⓔ increased serum cholesterol concentration

27

Clinical features of primary hypothyroidism in childhood include

Ⓐ malabsorption with diarrhoea

Ⓑ precocious puberty

Ⓒ retardation of growth and sexual development

Ⓓ epiphyseal dysgenesis on bone X-rays

Ⓔ permanent mental retardation

28

Causes of goitre include

Ⓐ acromegaly

Ⓑ lithium and amiodarone therapy

Ⓒ Hashimoto's thyroiditis

Ⓓ oral contraceptive therapy and pregnancy

Ⓔ Pendred's syndrome (thyroidal dyshormonogenesis)

29

The following statements about goitre are true

Ⓐ onset in later life favours a diagnosis of thyroid carcinoma

Ⓑ hypothyroidism favours a diagnosis of Hashimoto's thyroiditis

Ⓒ deafness in childhood suggests a diagnosis of dyshormonogenesis

Ⓓ thyroxine treatment for associated hypothyroidism causes goitre enlargement

Ⓔ serum thyroid antibodies favour a diagnosis of subacute thyroiditis

30

Typical features of de Quervain's (subacute) thyroiditis include

Ⓐ a large painless goitre

Ⓑ giant cells on histopathology

Ⓒ clinical signs of hyperthyroidism

Ⓓ an elevated ESR and serum thyroid antibodies

Ⓔ long-term hypothyroidism in most patients

31

The development of a simple colloid goitre is associated with

Ⓐ Coxsackie B viral infection

Ⓑ dietary iodine deficiency

Ⓒ excess dietary calcium intake

Ⓓ cranial irradiation

Ⓔ dietary goitrogens

32

Thyroid carcinoma of

Ⓐ lymphomatous type usually presents as a single 'hot' thyroid nodule

Ⓑ anaplastic type is usually cured by local radiotherapy

Ⓒ follicular type is best treated by ^{131}I radioiodine therapy alone

Ⓓ papillary type should be treated with total thyroidectomy

Ⓔ medullary type secretes calcitonin causing severe hypocalcaemia

33

The serum calcium concentration is typically increased in

Ⓐ hypoalbuminaemia

Ⓑ pyloric stenosis

Ⓒ carcinomatosis

Ⓓ hypoparathyroidism

Ⓔ chronic sarcoidosis

34

Typical clinical features of primary hyperparathyroidism include

Ⓐ recurrent acute pancreatitis and renal colic due to calculi

Ⓑ hyperplasia of all the parathyroid glands on histology

Ⓒ osteitis fibrosa on bone X-rays at presentation

Ⓓ the complications of pseudo-gout and hypertension

Ⓔ renal tubular acidosis and nephrogenic diabetes insipidus

35

Typical biochemical findings in primary hyperparathyroidism include

Ⓐ increased serum calcium and phosphate concentrations

Ⓑ decreased serum 1,25-dihydroxy-cholecalciferol concentration

Ⓒ hypercalciuria and hyperphosphaturia

Ⓓ increased serum alkaline phosphatase with bony involvement

Ⓔ increased serum calcium and PTH concentrations

36

Features of secondary hyperparathyroidism include

Ⓐ calcification of the basal ganglia

Ⓑ complication of chronic renal failure

Ⓒ parathyroid enlargement is often palpable

Ⓓ development of parathyroid adenomas

Ⓔ complication of gluten enteropathy

37

Causes of hypercalcaemia include

Ⓐ bone metastases

Ⓑ carcinomas secreting PTH-like peptides

Ⓒ severe Addison's disease

Ⓓ severe hypothyroidism

Ⓔ chronic sarcoidosis

38

The clinical features of hypoparathyroidism include

Ⓐ carpopedal and laryngeal spasm

Ⓑ fungal infection of the finger nails

Ⓒ abdominal pain and constipation

Ⓓ peripheral paraesthesiae and psychosis

Ⓔ cataracts and epilepsy

39

Causes of hypoparathyroidism include

Ⓐ autoimmune disease often also involving other endocrine glands

Ⓑ Di George syndrome with congenital thymic aplasia

Ⓒ subtotal thyroidectomy for thyrotoxicosis

Ⓓ medullary carcinoma of the thyroid gland

Ⓔ metastatic disease within the thyroid gland

40

The typical features of pseudohypoparathyroidism include

Ⓐ impaired coupling of adenyl cyclase with the renal PTH receptor

Ⓑ decreased serum PTH and calcitonin concentrations

Ⓒ decreased serum calcium and phosphate concentrations

Ⓓ family history of short stature and growth retardation

Ⓔ good response to parenteral PTH

41

Causes of tetany due to hypocalcaemia include

- **A** hyperventilation
- **B** pyloric stenosis
- **C** primary hyperaldosteronism
- **D** acute pancreatitis
- **E** gluten enteropathy

42

In the treatment of primary hypoparathyroidism

- **A** if tetany develops, 20 ml of 10% calcium gluconate should be given
- **B** if tetany is not relieved by calcium gluconate, give magnesium sulphate
- **C** calcitonin therapy prevents the onset of cataracts
- **D** oral 1-α-hydroxycholecalciferol restores calcium homeostasis
- **E** 5% carbon dioxide inhalation is required if tetany develops

43

The following statements about adrenal gland physiology are true

- **A** ACTH normally controls the adrenal secretion of aldosterone
- **B** ACTH increases adrenal androgen and cortisol secretion
- **C** the plasma cortisol concentration normally peaks in the evening
- **D** hyperglycaemia increases the rate of cortisol secretion
- **E** cortisol enhances gluconeogenesis and lipogenesis from amino acids

44

A cushingoid appearance would be an expected finding in

- **A** chronic alcohol abuse
- **B** pituitary macroadenomas
- **C** ACTH-secreting bronchial carcinoma
- **D** adrenocortical adenoma
- **E** fludrocortisone therapy

45

The typical clinical features of Cushing's syndrome include

- **A** generalised osteoporosis
- **B** systemic hypotension
- **C** hirsutism and amenorrhoea
- **D** proximal myopathy
- **E** hypoglycaemic episodes

46

Typical features of pituitary-dependent Cushing's disease include

- **A** enlargement of the pituitary fossa
- **B** amenorrhoea and depression
- **C** proximal myopathy and diabetes mellitus
- **D** suppression of plasma cortisol following dexamethasone
- **E** hypotension and hyperkalaemia

47

Expected findings in patients with benign adrenal adenomas include

- **A** preservation of the normal diurnal rhythm of cortisol secretion
- **B** plasma cortisol < 170 nmol/L 10 hours after 2 mg oral dexamethasone
- **C** increased free cortisol/creatinine ratios in early-morning urine
- **D** increased plasma dehydroepiandrosterone concentration
- **E** elevated ACTH at 0800 hours

48

Adverse effects of oral corticosteroid therapy include

- **A** peptic ulceration
- **B** hypertension
- **C** avascular bone necrosis
- **D** pseudogout
- **E** insomnia

49

In primary hyperaldosteronism (Conn's syndrome)

Ⓐ peripheral oedema is usually present

Ⓑ proximal myopathy is due to hypokalaemia

Ⓒ polyuria and polydipsia are characteristic

Ⓓ diabetes mellitus is often present

Ⓔ hypertension is associated with hyperreninaemia

50

Causes of primary adrenocortical insufficiency include

Ⓐ haemochromatosis

Ⓑ autoimmune adrenalitis

Ⓒ amyloidosis

Ⓓ sarcoidosis

Ⓔ tuberculosis

51

Typical features of primary adrenocortical insufficiency include

Ⓐ anorexia, weight loss and diarrhoea

Ⓑ pigmentation of scars from surgery preceding hypoadrenalism

Ⓒ vitiligo, weakness and hypotension

Ⓓ increased insulin requirements in diabetic patients

Ⓔ amenorrhoea and loss of body hair

52

Typical features of secondary adrenocortical insufficiency include

Ⓐ impaired gonadotrophin secretion usually precedes ACTH deficiency

Ⓑ impaired plasma cortisol response 30 minutes after ACTH stimulation

Ⓒ vitiligo and skin hyperpigmentation

Ⓓ hypotension and hyperkalaemia

Ⓔ preservation of the normal diurnal rhythm of cortisol secretion

53

In the treatment of primary adrenocortical insufficiency

Ⓐ oral hydrocortisone is the glucocorticoid of choice

Ⓑ fludrocortisone is usually unnecessary unless there is hyperkalaemia

Ⓒ the dose of cortisol should not be increased without medical advice

Ⓓ adrenal crisis requires intravenous crystalloids and hydrocortisone

Ⓔ typical maintenance therapy comprises at least 50 mg cortisol daily

54

Features of congenital adrenal hyperplasia include

Ⓐ 21-hydroxylase enzyme deficiency

Ⓑ decreased plasma cortisol and aldosterone concentrations

Ⓒ increased mortality in male infants

Ⓓ growth acceleration and precocious puberty

Ⓔ increased plasma 17-α-hydroxy-progesterone concentration

55

The typical features of phaeochromocytoma include

Ⓐ predominantly adrenaline rather than noradrenaline secretion

Ⓑ episodic nausea with sweating and marked skin pallor

Ⓒ underlying malignant tumour in the majority

Ⓓ presentation with hypertension and hypercalcaemia

Ⓔ control of symptoms following propranolol therapy alone

56

Causes of impotence include

Ⓐ pituitary microprolactinoma

Ⓑ psychological distress

Ⓒ peripheral vascular disease

Ⓓ diabetes mellitus

Ⓔ multiple sclerosis

57
In male infertility associated with oligospermia
Ⓐ increased plasma FSH concentrations suggest testicular dysfunction
Ⓑ testicular biopsy should be undertaken to exclude malignancy
Ⓒ testicular production of sperm may be normal
Ⓓ gonadotrophin therapy usually restores normal fertility
Ⓔ low plasma FSH concentrations suggest obstruction is the cause

58
Causes of gynaecomastia include
Ⓐ androgen deficiency and /or excessive oestrogen production
Ⓑ microprolactinoma or macroprolactinoma
Ⓒ cimetidine therapy
Ⓓ haemochromatosis
Ⓔ human chorionic gonadotrophin secreting tumour

59
Hypogonadotrophic hypogonadism is typically associated with
Ⓐ atrophy of the testicular interstitial (Leydig) cells
Ⓑ Klinefelter's syndrome (XXY)
Ⓒ isolated GnRH deficiency (Kallmann's syndrome)
Ⓓ haemochromatosis
Ⓔ hepatic cirrhosis

60
The clinical features of male hypogonadism include
Ⓐ total absence of pubic hair if prepubertal in onset
Ⓑ growth retardation if prepubertal in onset
Ⓒ atrophy of the external genitalia if postpubertal in onset
Ⓓ impairment of strength, libido and erectile function
Ⓔ sweating with hot flushes after postpubertal castration

61
Causes of hypergonadotrophic hypogonadism include
Ⓐ Klinefelter's syndrome
Ⓑ Turner's syndrome
Ⓒ autoimmune ovarian disease
Ⓓ leprosy
Ⓔ cryptorchidism

62
In cryptorchidism with inguinal testes in a child
Ⓐ the individual is usually otherwise normal
Ⓑ hypogonadotrophic hypogonadism should be excluded
Ⓒ the seminiferous tubules are typically normal
Ⓓ testicular interstitial cell function is usually normal
Ⓔ treatment with chorionic gonadotrophin or GnRH is contraindicated

63
Causes of primary amenorrhoea include
Ⓐ endometriosis
Ⓑ congenital adrenal hyperplasia
Ⓒ Turner's syndrome (XO)
Ⓓ gluten enteropathy
Ⓔ craniopharyngioma

64
Causes of secondary amenorrhoea include
Ⓐ pituitary microprolactinoma
Ⓑ anorexia nervosa
Ⓒ Cushing's syndrome
Ⓓ renal failure
Ⓔ Stein–Leventhal syndrome

65
The typical features of idiopathic premature menopause include
Ⓐ decreased plasma LH and FSH concentrations
Ⓑ hirsutism and clitoral hypertrophy
Ⓒ bone fractures due to osteomalacia
Ⓓ superficial dyspareunia and dysuria
Ⓔ age at onset 45–55 years

66
Causes of hirsutism include
- Ⓐ idiopathic familial hirsutism
- Ⓑ polycystic ovarian syndrome (PCO)
- Ⓒ Cushing's syndrome
- Ⓓ autoimmune polyglandular syndrome
- Ⓔ ovarian tumour

67
Features in type I multiple endocrine neoplasia (MEN) syndrome (Wermer's syndrome) include
- Ⓐ sex-linked mode of inheritance
- Ⓑ functioning pituitary adenomas
- Ⓒ medullary thyroid carcinoma
- Ⓓ gastrinoma
- Ⓔ insulinoma

68
Features in type II multiple endocrine neoplasia (MEN) syndrome (Sipple's syndrome) include
- Ⓐ recessive mode of inheritance
- Ⓑ primary hyperparathyroidism
- Ⓒ medullary thyroid carcinoma
- Ⓓ neurofibromata associated with phaeochromocytoma
- Ⓔ Wilm's nephroblastoma

DISEASES OF THE ALIMENTARY TRACT AND PANCREAS

9

ANSWERS PAGE 218

1
In the neuroendocrine control of the alimentary tract
Ⓐ mucosal secretion is mediated by neuropeptides
Ⓑ the initial release of gastrin occurs in response to gastric distension
Ⓒ sympathetic nerve fibres run in the splanchnic nerves
Ⓓ parasympathetic stimuli mediate the inhibition of secretin secretion
Ⓔ somatostatin induces the secretion of upper GI hormones

2
In the normal alimentary tract
Ⓐ mucosa-associated lymphoid tissue constitutes 25% of the total body lymphatic tissue
Ⓑ secretory IgA protects the gut from bacterial invasion
Ⓒ fat soluble drugs and vitamins enter the portal and systemic circulations via lymphatics
Ⓓ folic acid is chiefly absorbed in the terminal ileum
Ⓔ exocrine pancreatic secretion is controlled solely by hormonal factors

3
In the normal alimentary tract
Ⓐ small bowel contractile activity ceases during fasting
Ⓑ triglycerides are hydrolysed to monoglycerides by the effects of secretin
Ⓒ disaccharides are absorbed by an active process and metabolised in the liver
Ⓓ pancreatic trypsinogen is stimulated by the release of cholecystokinin
Ⓔ colonic motility is principally controlled by the hormone motilin

4
Causes of mouth ulcers include
Ⓐ gluten enteropathy
Ⓑ Crohn's disease
Ⓒ lichen planus
Ⓓ adverse drug reaction
Ⓔ herpes simplex

5
Causes of salivary gland enlargement include
Ⓐ alcoholic liver disease
Ⓑ Sjögren's syndrome
Ⓒ bacterial infection
Ⓓ sarcoidosis
Ⓔ measles

6
Recognised causes of dysphagia include
Ⓐ iron deficiency anaemia
Ⓑ pharyngeal pouch
Ⓒ Barrett's oesophagus
Ⓓ myasthenia gravis
Ⓔ achalasia

7
The following statements about pharyngeal pouch are true
Ⓐ Upper gastrointestinal endoscopy is the investigation of choice
Ⓑ Patients experience gurgling in the throat after swallowing
Ⓒ Presentation typically occurs in adolescence
Ⓓ Recurrent pneumonia is a recognised complication
Ⓔ Dysphagia is typically rapidly progressive

8
Typical features of oesophageal achalasia include
Ⓐ recurrent pneumonia
Ⓑ spasm of the lower oesophageal sphincter (LOS)
Ⓒ heartburn and acid reflux
Ⓓ predisposition to oesophageal carcinoma
Ⓔ symptomatic response to pneumatic balloon dilatation

9
In diffuse oesophageal spasm
Ⓐ Auerbach's plexus is normal
Ⓑ most patients are over the age of 60 at presentation
Ⓒ strong uncoordinated contractions occur unrelated to swallowing
Ⓓ dysphagia is most often due to an associated oesophagitis
Ⓔ acid lowering drug therapy typically reduces the frequency of chest pain

10
Gastro-oesophageal reflux disease is associated with the following factors
Ⓐ decreased intra-abdominal pressure
Ⓑ delayed gastric emptying
Ⓒ prolonged oesophageal transit time
Ⓓ increased lower oesophageal sphincter tone
Ⓔ presence of a hiatus hernia

11
Causes of oesophageal stricture include
Ⓐ gastro-oesophageal reflux disease
Ⓑ oesophageal carcinoma
Ⓒ bronchial carcinoma
Ⓓ prolonged nasogastric intubation
Ⓔ the presence of a sliding hiatus hernia

12
Oesophageal carcinoma in the UK is
Ⓐ associated with gluten enteropathy
Ⓑ more likely to be due to adenocarcinoma than squamous carcinoma
Ⓒ associated with Barret's oesophagus
Ⓓ more likely to arise in the upper third rather than the lower third of the oesophagus
Ⓔ associated with alcohol and tobacco consumption

13
Typical features of oesophageal carcinoma at presentation include
Ⓐ acid reflux and odynophagia
Ⓑ painless obstruction to the passage of a food bolus
Ⓒ nausea and weight loss
Ⓓ metastatic spread in the majority of patients
Ⓔ overall survival rates at 5 years of approximately 50%

14
Factors associated with chronic peptic ulcer disease include
Ⓐ oral contraceptive therapy
Ⓑ duodenogastric reflux
Ⓒ pernicious anaemia
Ⓓ *Helicobacter pylori*—associated gastritis
Ⓔ tobacco consumption

15
Typical features of peptic ulcer dyspepsia include
Ⓐ pain relieved by eating
Ⓑ well-localised pain relieved by vomiting
Ⓒ pain-free remissions lasting many weeks
Ⓓ nausea and epigastric pain lasting > 4 hours
Ⓔ nocturnal pain causing frequent night waking

16

***Helicobacter pylori* eradication is likely to benefit patients with**

Ⓐ non-ulcer dyspepsia

Ⓑ erosive oesophagitis

Ⓒ duodenal ulcer disease

Ⓓ gastric ulcer disease

Ⓔ gastric B-cell lymphoma

17

In the investigation and treatment of chronic dyspepsia

Ⓐ most patients aged < 45 years have an underlying peptic ulcer

Ⓑ 25% of duodenal ulcers relapse unless *H. pylori* has been eradicated

Ⓒ magnesium-containing antacids produce constipation

Ⓓ bismuth compounds should not be used for maintenance therapy

Ⓔ gastric ulcers associated with NSAID therapy are less likely to be associated with *H. pylori* gastritis than gastric ulcers occurring in patients not taking NSAIDs

18

Gastroduodenal haemorrhage in the UK is

Ⓐ more often due to peptic ulcer than to oesophageal varices

Ⓑ associated with a 5% mortality when due to chronic peptic ulceration

Ⓒ a recognised complication of severe head injury

Ⓓ best investigated by endoscopy within 24 hours of admission

Ⓔ significantly associated with anti-inflammatory drug therapy

19

Typical features of major acute gastroduodenal haemorrhage include

Ⓐ severe abdominal pain

Ⓑ angor animi and restlessness

Ⓒ syncope preceding other evidence of bleeding

Ⓓ elevated blood urea and creatinine concentrations

Ⓔ peripheral blood microcytosis

20

When acute gastroduodenal haemorrhage is suspected

Ⓐ a pulse rate > 100 /min is most likely to be due to anxiety

Ⓑ hypotension without a tachycardia suggests an alternative diagnosis

Ⓒ the absence of anaemia suggests the volume of blood loss is modest

Ⓓ nasogastric aspiration provides an accurate estimate of blood loss

Ⓔ endoscopy is best deferred pending blood volume replacement

21

In resuscitating a patient with an acute gastrointestinal bleed

Ⓐ oxygen should be administered if there are signs of hypovolaemia

Ⓑ transfusion requires whole blood rather than packed red cells

Ⓒ volume replacement with colloids is preferable to crystalloids

Ⓓ monitoring central venous pressure and/or urine output is advisable

Ⓔ surgical intervention should be considered if rebleeding occurs despite ulcer sclerotherapy

22

Perforation of a peptic ulcer is typically associated with

Ⓐ acute rather than chronic ulcers

Ⓑ duodenal more often than gastric ulcers

Ⓒ abdominal pain radiating to the shoulder tip

Ⓓ the absence of nausea and vomiting

Ⓔ symptomatic improvement several hours following onset

23

Characteristic features of gastric outlet obstruction include

Ⓐ metabolic acidosis

Ⓑ bile vomiting

Ⓒ urinary pH < 5

Ⓓ symptomatic relief after vomiting

Ⓔ absent gastric peristalsis

24
Typical features of a gastrinoma include
Ⓐ a small gastric tumour
Ⓑ hepatic metastases at presentation
Ⓒ parathyroid adenomas
Ⓓ constipation rather than diarrhoea
Ⓔ absent acid secretory response to pentagastrin stimulation

25
The pathological changes of acute gastritis are typically associated with
Ⓐ *Helicobacter pylori* infection
Ⓑ severe head injury
Ⓒ alcohol abuse
Ⓓ iron therapy
Ⓔ NSAID therapy

26
The pathological changes of chronic gastritis are typically associated with
Ⓐ *Helicobacter pylori* infection
Ⓑ pernicious anaemia
Ⓒ tuberculosis
Ⓓ post-partial gastrectomy
Ⓔ functional dyspepsia

27
Complications of partial gastrectomy include
Ⓐ early satiety
Ⓑ iron deficiency anaemia
Ⓒ weight loss
Ⓓ reactive hypoglycaemia
Ⓔ vomiting and diarrhoea soon after meals

28
The typical features of functional dyspepsia include
Ⓐ onset under the age of 45 years
Ⓑ nausea and bloating
Ⓒ weight loss and anaemia
Ⓓ constipation with pelletty stools
Ⓔ symptoms of anxiety and depression

29
Carcinoma of the stomach is associated with
Ⓐ adenomatous gastric polyps
Ⓑ chronic hypochlorhydria
Ⓒ *Helicobacter pylori* infection
Ⓓ Ménétrier's disease
Ⓔ alcohol and tobacco consumption

30
Typical features of gastric carcinoma in the UK include
Ⓐ progression to involve the duodenum
Ⓑ origin within a chronic peptic ulcer
Ⓒ overall 5-year survival rate of 50%
Ⓓ folate deficiency anaemia on presentation
Ⓔ supraclavicular lymphadenopathy

31
In gluten enteropathy (coeliac disease)
Ⓐ the typical age at onset is 11–19 years
Ⓑ there is a predisposition to gut lymphoma and carcinoma
Ⓒ the toxic agent is the polypeptide α-gliadin
Ⓓ gluten-free diets improve absorption but not the villous atrophy
Ⓔ serum antiendomysium IgA antibody titres are characteristically elevated

32
Causes of subtotal villous atrophy include
Ⓐ dermatitis herpetiformis
Ⓑ Whipple's disease
Ⓒ Zollinger–Ellison syndrome
Ⓓ hypogammaglobulinaemia
Ⓔ tropical sprue

33
Causes of small bowel bacterial overgrowth (blind loop syndrome) include
Ⓐ diabetic autonomic neuropathy
Ⓑ chronic hypochlorhydria
Ⓒ jejunal diverticulosis
Ⓓ progressive systemic sclerosis
Ⓔ enterocolic fistula

34

In the blind loop syndrome

Ⓐ the finding of 10^3 coliform organisms/ml in the duodenal aspirate is diagnostic

Ⓑ anaemia is typically due to folate deficiency

Ⓒ the finding of steatorrhoea suggests the problem is pancreatic in origin

Ⓓ the diagnosis is best confirmed using the SeHCAT absorption test

Ⓔ the absence of serum IgA raises the possibility of giardiasis

35

The clinical features of Whipple's disease include

Ⓐ predominance in elderly females

Ⓑ ankylosing spondylitis

Ⓒ pericarditis and myocarditis

Ⓓ meningitis and cranial nerve palsies

Ⓔ weight loss and diarrhoea

36

The diarrhoea associated with radiation enteritis is likely to be the result of

Ⓐ proctocolitis

Ⓑ bile salt malabsorption

Ⓒ enterocolic fistulas

Ⓓ small bowel strictures

Ⓔ giardiasis

37

Causes of protein-losing enteropathy include

Ⓐ Crohn's disease

Ⓑ radiation enteritis

Ⓒ intestinal lymphoma

Ⓓ Ménétrier's disease

Ⓔ intestinal lymphangiectasia

38

Ulcerative lesions of the small bowel are associated with the following disorders

Ⓐ NSAID therapy

Ⓑ yersiniosis

Ⓒ ulcerative colitis

Ⓓ enteric-coated potassium tablets

Ⓔ tropical sprue

39

The typical clinical features of abdominal tuberculosis include

Ⓐ involvement of the sigmoid colon

Ⓑ perianal fistulas

Ⓒ exudative ascites

Ⓓ granulomatous hepatitis

Ⓔ predominant symptoms of diarrhoea rather than abdominal pain

40

Clinical features suggesting the carcinoid syndrome include

Ⓐ facial blanching and sweating

Ⓑ constipation

Ⓒ intestinal ischaemia

Ⓓ granulomatous hepatitis

Ⓔ late occurrence of metastatic disease

41

Causes of acute pancreatitis include

Ⓐ measles

Ⓑ hypothermia

Ⓒ choledocholithiasis

Ⓓ azathioprine therapy

Ⓔ alcohol abuse

42

The following are characteristic of acute pancreatitis

Ⓐ abdominal guarding develops soon after the onset of pain

Ⓑ normal serum amylase concentration in the first 4 hours after onset

Ⓒ persistent serum hyperamylaseaemia suggests a developing pseudocyst

Ⓓ hypercalcaemia 5–7 days after onset

Ⓔ hyperactive loud bowel sounds

43

Adverse prognostic factors in acute pancreatitis include

Ⓐ arterial hypoxaemia with a $PaO_2 < 8$ kPa

Ⓑ leucopaenia with white blood cell count $< 5 \times 10^9$/L

Ⓒ serum albumin < 30 g/L and serum calcium < 2 mmol/L

Ⓓ hypoglycaemia < 2.3 mmol/L

Ⓔ blood urea > 16 mmol/L after rehydration

44
In the management of acute pancreatitis
A early laparotomy is advisable to exclude alternative diagnoses

B opiates should be avoided because of spasm of the sphincter of Oddi

C intravenous fluids are unnecessary in the absence of a tachycardia

D the urine output and PaO_2 should be monitored

E persistent elevation in the serum amylase suggests pancreatic duct obstruction

45
In the investigation of chronic pancreatic disease
A glucose tolerance is typically normal in pancreatic carcinoma

B duodenal ileus is a characteristic feature of chronic pancreatitis

C ultrasound scanning is more sensitive than CT scanning

D ERCP can reliably distinguish carcinoma from chronic pancreatitis

E pancreatic calcification suggests alcohol as the cause

46
Features consistent with the diagnosis of chronic pancreatitis include
A back pain persisting for days or weeks

B decreased vitamin B_{12} absorption

C increased sodium concentration in the sweat

D abdominal pain occurring 12–24 hours after alcohol intake

E pancreatic calcification on plain X-ray or ultrasound scan

47
Typical causes of chronic pancreatitis include
A annular pancreas

B alcoholism

C gallstones

D cystic fibrosis

E mumps

48
Typical complications of chronic pancreatitis include
A pancreatic pseudocyst formation

B obstructive jaundice

C portal vein thrombosis

D diabetes mellitus

E opiate drug dependence

49
Pancreas divisum
A occurs with a prevalence rate of about 1% in the normal population

B results in both acute and chronic pancreatitis

C represents a failure of fusion of the embryonic dorsal and ventral ducts

D progresses to produce gastric outlet obstruction

E is typically associated with malrotation of the foregut

50
Cystic fibrosis affecting the pancreas
A typically causes severe steatorrhoea

B results in impaired glucose tolerance

C is also associated with a predisposition to peptic ulceration

D limits survival beyond the childhood years

E causes widespread obstruction of the pancreatic ductules

51
The typical features of pancreatic carcinoma include
A adenocarcinomatous histology

B origin in the body of the pancreas in 60% of patients

C abdominal pain when arising in the ampulla of Vater

D back pain and weight loss indicate a poor prognosis

E presentation with painless jaundice

52

Characteristic features of ulcerative colitis include

Ⓐ invariable involvement of the rectal mucosa

Ⓑ segmental involvement of the colon and rectum

Ⓒ pseudopolyposis following healing of mucosal damage

Ⓓ inflammation extending from the mucosa to the serosa

Ⓔ enterocutaneous and enteroenteric fistulae

53

Ulcerative colitis (UC) differs from Crohn's colitis in that

Ⓐ UC occurs at any age

Ⓑ cessation of smoking is likely to reduce activity of Crohn's disease

Ⓒ toxic dilatation only occurs in ulcerative colitis

Ⓓ there is no association with aphthous mouth ulcers in UC (unlike Crohn's disease)

Ⓔ there is no involvement of the small bowel in UC

54

Recognised complications of ulcerative colitis include

Ⓐ pyoderma gangrenosum

Ⓑ pericholangitis

Ⓒ amyloidosis

Ⓓ colonic carcinoma

Ⓔ enteropathic arthritis

55

In the treatment of severe acute ulcerative colitis

Ⓐ antibiotic therapy is mandatory if the patient is febrile

Ⓑ antidiarrhoeal agents increase the risk of toxic dilatation

Ⓒ systemic corticosteroids induce a remission in the majority

Ⓓ hypoproteinaemia indicates the need for albumin infusion

Ⓔ failure of medical therapy indicates the need for surgery

56

In the maintenance treatment of ulcerative colitis

Ⓐ corticosteroid therapy should be given orally rather than rectally

Ⓑ aminosalicylate therapy reduces the risk of colonic carcinoma

Ⓒ azathioprine will reduce maintenance corticosteroid requirements

Ⓓ the development of renal impairment suggests aminosalicylate toxicity

Ⓔ aminosalicylate therapy is effective only if given by mouth

57

Characteristic features of Crohn's disease include

Ⓐ familial association with ulcerative colitis

Ⓑ onset after the age of 70 years

Ⓒ disease confined to the terminal ileum and colon

Ⓓ predisposition to biliary and renal calculi

Ⓔ giant cell granulomata on histopathology

58

The typical clinical features of Crohn's disease include

Ⓐ association with tobacco consumption

Ⓑ presentation with bloody diarrhoea

Ⓒ presentation with subacute intestinal obstruction

Ⓓ segmental involvement of the colon and rectum

Ⓔ inflammatory changes confined to the mucosa on histopathology

59

Recognised complications of Crohn's disease include

Ⓐ pernicious anaemia

Ⓑ erythema nodosum

Ⓒ enteropathic arthritis

Ⓓ aphthous mouth ulcers

Ⓔ small bowel lymphoma

60
In the treatment of ileo-caecal Crohn's disease

Ⓐ surgical bypass is preferable to limited gut resection

Ⓑ stopping smoking reduces the risk of symptomatic relapses

Ⓒ corticosteroid therapy is contraindicated in the acute phase

Ⓓ cholestyramine reduces the diarrhoea but increases steatorrhoea

Ⓔ aminosalicylate therapy reduces the risk of small bowel obstruction

61
Intestinal obstruction

Ⓐ of mechanical type is a complication of inguinal hernia

Ⓑ of paralytic type is a feature of peripheral circulatory failure

Ⓒ from peritonitis is typically mechanical in type

Ⓓ associated with strangulation is invariably mechanical in type

Ⓔ of paralytic type eventually progresses to a mechanical type

62
In patients with intestinal obstruction

Ⓐ vomiting is an invariable feature

Ⓑ the finding of an empty rectum usually excludes faecal impaction

Ⓒ hyperactive loud bowel sounds suggest mechanical obstruction

Ⓓ persisting diarrhoea excludes obstruction

Ⓔ abdominal tenderness suggests strangulation or peritonitis

63
The typical features of the irritable bowel syndrome include

Ⓐ nocturnal diarrhoea and weight loss

Ⓑ onset after the age of 45 years

Ⓒ history of abdominal pain in childhood

Ⓓ right iliac fossa pain and urinary frequency

Ⓔ abdominal distension, flatulence and pellety stools

64
The management of the irritable bowel syndrome should include

Ⓐ explanation and reassurance after a detailed clinical examination

Ⓑ barium enema and barium follow-through examinations in all patients

Ⓒ evaluation of social and emotional factors

Ⓓ referral for psychiatric assessment and therapy

Ⓔ dihydrocodeine for abdominal pain and diarrhoea

65
Typical features of colonic diverticulosis include

Ⓐ predominant involvement of the right hemicolon

Ⓑ predisposition to the development of colonic carcinoma

Ⓒ complications are more common in patients receiving NSAID therapy

Ⓓ reduction in the number of diverticula with a high-fibre diet

Ⓔ the absence of symptoms in the absence of complications

66
Typical features of colonic diverticulitis include

Ⓐ severe rectal bleeding

Ⓑ chronic iron deficiency anaemia

Ⓒ septicaemia and paralytic ileus

Ⓓ right iliac fossa pain

Ⓔ vesicocolic fistula

67
The typical features of acute small bowel ischaemia include

Ⓐ occlusion of the inferior mesenteric artery

Ⓑ the recent onset of atrial fibrillation

Ⓒ the sudden onset of abdominal pain, vomiting and diarrhoea

Ⓓ peripheral circulatory failure and signs of peritonitis

Ⓔ gaseous distension of the small bowel on plain abdominal X-rays

68

The typical features of acute ischaemic colitis include

Ⓐ rigors, abdominal pain and constipation

Ⓑ occlusion of the superior mesenteric artery (SMA)

Ⓒ profuse bloody diarrhoea and abdominal tenderness

Ⓓ mucosal oedema with 'thumb-printing' on barium enema radiology

Ⓔ resolution with the later development of a colonic stricture

69

Typical features of pseudomembranous colitis include

Ⓐ onset within 3 weeks of antibiotic therapy

Ⓑ normal appearance of the rectal mucosa

Ⓒ *Clostridium difficile* toxin in the stool

Ⓓ presentation with abdominal pain and diarrhoea

Ⓔ clinical relapse despite prompt treatment

70

In Hirschsprung's disease of the colon

Ⓐ there is a family history in 90% of cases

Ⓑ presentation typically occurs between the ages of 3 and 5 years

Ⓒ there is a segmental absence of the myenteric nerve plexus

Ⓓ the rectum is typically loaded on digital examination

Ⓔ the surgical treatment of choice is a defunctioning colostomy

71

The following statements about colonic polyps are true

Ⓐ 75% of polyps occur in the right hemicolon

Ⓑ The typical histology is that of tubular adenoma

Ⓒ Polyps > 2 cm in diameter are usually malignant

Ⓓ Intussusception is a recognised complication

Ⓔ Presentation with constipation is typical

72

Familial adenomatous polyposis is

Ⓐ inherited as an autosomal recessive trait

Ⓑ usually clinically apparent before the age of 10 years

Ⓒ likely to progress to carcinoma before the age of 40 years

Ⓓ associated with gastric and small bowel polyps

Ⓔ best treated with immunosuppressant therapy in patients aged < 20 years

73

The following statements about colonic carcinoma are true

Ⓐ it is the commonest of all gastrointestinal carcinomas

Ⓑ the majority of carcinomas arise in the right hemicolon

Ⓒ after resection, there is a recognised risk of a second carcinoma

Ⓓ Dukes' A classifies tumour extending to the serosa only

Ⓔ only a minority of rectal tumours are palpable per rectum

74

In colonic carcinoma

Ⓐ of the caecum, presentation with iron deficiency anaemia is typical

Ⓑ obstruction is typically an early event in carcinoma of the sigmoid

Ⓒ metastatic spread is to the lungs rather than the liver

Ⓓ concomitant multiple tumours are present in 20% of patients

Ⓔ rising serum carcinoembryonic antigen (CEA) levels post-resection suggest recurrent tumour

10 DISEASES OF THE LIVER AND BILIARY SYSTEM

ANSWERS PAGE 227

1
In the normal liver
A the space of Disse separates the hepatocytes from sinusoidal endothelium

B the hepatic artery supplies 50% of the total hepatic oxygen supply

C Kupffer cells are derived from blood monocytes

D Ito cells are responsible for the uptake and storage of vitamin D

E the right and left hemilivers are divided into 10 segments

2
Bilirubin is
A derived exclusively from the breakdown of haemoglobin

B bound in the unconjugated form to plasma ß-globulin

C conjugated in the microsomes of the hepatocytes

D reabsorbed in the small bowel as bilirubin diglucuronide

E normally excreted as stercobilinogen in the faeces and as urobilinogen in the urine

3
The concentration of conjugated bilirubin in the
A serum in haemolytic anaemia is typically increased

B urine of healthy subjects is typically undetectable

C serum normally constitutes most of the total serum bilirubin

D serum in Gilbert's syndrome is typically increased

E urine in viral hepatitis parallels that of urobilinogen

4
The serum alanine aminotransferase (ALT) concentration is
A derived from a microsomal enzyme specific to hepatocytes

B typically more than six times normal in alcoholic hepatitis

C usually normal in both obstructive and haemolytic jaundice

D likely to rise and fall in parallel with the serum bilirubin in viral hepatitis

E likely to increase in response to the intake of enzyme-inducing drugs

5
The serum alkaline phosphatase concentration is
A derived from the liver, bone, small bowel and placenta

B typically increased to more than six times normal in viral hepatitis

C derived mainly from hepatic sinusoidal and canalicular membranes

D of particular prognostic value in chronic liver disease

E increased more in extrahepatic than intrahepatic cholestasis

6
When monitoring serum liver function values in liver disease
A the albumin concentration falls rapidly in acute liver failure

B persistent hypergammaglobulinaemia indicates hepatocyte necrosis

C an increased IgA concentration is typical of alcoholic hepatitis

D the prothrombin time increases rapidly in severe acute hepatitis

E an increased IgG concentration suggests primary biliary cirrhosis

7

In the investigation of suspected liver disease

Ⓐ ultrasonography reliably distinguishes solid from cystic masses

Ⓑ ultrasonography reliably excludes liver disease

Ⓒ normal liver function values exclude significant liver disease

Ⓓ the mortality rate of percutaneous liver biopsy is about 5%

Ⓔ ascitic protein concentrations > 30 g/L are compatible with diagnosis of carcinomatosis

8

Drugs known to cause hepatic microsomal enzyme induction include

Ⓐ amoxycillin

Ⓑ carbamazepine

Ⓒ rifampicin

Ⓓ phenytoin

Ⓔ naproxen

9

Characteristic features of Gilbert's syndrome include

Ⓐ an autosomal recessive mode of inheritance

Ⓑ decreased hepatic glucuronyl transferase activity

Ⓒ unconjugated hyperbilirubinaemia < 100 μmol/L

Ⓓ serum bilirubin concentration increased by fasting

Ⓔ increased serum bile acid concentrations

10

Characteristic features of cholestatic jaundice include

Ⓐ dark green stools

Ⓑ dark brown urine

Ⓒ unconjugated hyperbilirubinaemia

Ⓓ serum alkaline phosphatase concentration increased > 2.5 normal

Ⓔ increased serum bile acid concentrations

11

Causes of extrahepatic cholestatic jaundice include

Ⓐ primary sclerosing cholangitis

Ⓑ primary biliary cirrhosis

Ⓒ cystic fibrosis

Ⓓ alcoholic cirrhosis

Ⓔ choledocholithiasis

12

The following features suggest extrahepatic cholestasis rather than viral hepatitis

Ⓐ a palpable gallbladder

Ⓑ right hypochondrial tenderness

Ⓒ serum alkaline phosphatase concentration > 2.5 times normal

Ⓓ pruritus and rigors

Ⓔ peripheral blood polymorph leucocytosis

13

The histopathological characteristics of acute hepatitis include

Ⓐ polymorph leucocyte infiltration of the lobules

Ⓑ sparing of the centrilobular areas

Ⓒ enlargement of the portal tracts

Ⓓ hepatocyte necrosis with deeply-stained acidophilic bodies

Ⓔ fatty infiltration

14

The typical histopathology of interface hepatitis includes

Ⓐ lymphocytic infiltration limited to the portal tracts

Ⓑ periportal hepatocytic damage with the formation of 'rosettes'

Ⓒ destruction of the lobular architecture

Ⓓ bridging of the portal tracts with fibrotic tissue

Ⓔ association with the recovery phase of hepatitis A infection

15
The typical causes of macrovesicular steatosis include
Ⓐ alcohol abuse
Ⓑ pregnancy
Ⓒ Reye's syndrome
Ⓓ starvation and malnutrition
Ⓔ diabetes mellitus

16
The typical features of type A viral hepatitis (HAV) include
Ⓐ picornavirus infection spread by the faecal-oral route
Ⓑ an incubation period of 3 months
Ⓒ a greater risk of acute liver failure in the young than in the old
Ⓓ right hypochondrial pain and tenderness
Ⓔ progression to cirrhosis if cholestasis is prolonged

17
The following statements about type A viral hepatitis are true
Ⓐ persistent viraemia produces the post-hepatitis syndrome
Ⓑ relapsing hepatitis usually indicates a poorer prognosis
Ⓒ the virus is not usually transmitted via infected blood
Ⓓ drug-induced acute hepatitis produces identical liver histology
Ⓔ travellers given immune serum globulin are protected for 3 months

18
Circulating hepatitis B surface antigen (HBsAg) is
Ⓐ detectable during the prodrome of acute type B hepatitis
Ⓑ a DNA viral particle transmissible in all body fluids
Ⓒ likely to persist in about 50% of adults following acute type B hepatitis
Ⓓ invariably present in a patient with jaundice attributable to type B hepatitis infection
Ⓔ commoner in asymptomatic subjects in the Western rather than the Eastern hemisphere

19
The typical features of type B viral hepatitis (HBV) include
Ⓐ an incubation period of 1 month
Ⓑ history of exposure to unsafe sex or drug abuse
Ⓒ prodromal illness with polyarthralgia
Ⓓ hepatitic illness more severe than with type A virus
Ⓔ absence of progression to chronic hepatitis

20
In hepatitis C (HCV)
Ⓐ a chronic carriage rate of > 50% is the rule
Ⓑ the infecting agent is an RNA flavivirus
Ⓒ the disease does not progress to chronic hepatitis
Ⓓ most patients experience the symptoms of acute hepatitis
Ⓔ the virus is responsible for 90% of all post-transfusion hepatitis

21
In hepatitis D (HDV)
Ⓐ the infective agent is a DNA virus
Ⓑ transmission is usually via the enteral route
Ⓒ replication of the virus requires the presence of type B virus
Ⓓ simultaneous infection with type B virus often produces severe hepatitis
Ⓔ pre-existing hepatitis B carriage predisposes to the progression to cirrhosis

22
In hepatitis E (HEV)
Ⓐ the infective agent is a calicivirus
Ⓑ the principal mode of transmission is via the faecal-oral route
Ⓒ the clinical illness resembles that of HAV infection
Ⓓ acute hepatitis is more likely to occur if infection is acquired in pregnancy
Ⓔ chronic infection does not occur

23
The typical features of acute hepatic failure include
Ⓐ onset within 8 weeks of the initial illness

Ⓑ hepatosplenomegaly and ascites

Ⓒ encephalopathy and fetor hepaticus

Ⓓ nausea, vomiting and renal failure

Ⓔ cerebral oedema without papilloedema

24
Typical liver function values in acute hepatic failure include
Ⓐ hypoalbuminaemia

Ⓑ hypoglycaemia

Ⓒ prolonged prothrombin time

Ⓓ serum alkaline phosphatase > three times normal

Ⓔ peripheral blood lymphocytosis

25
The management of acute liver failure includes
Ⓐ avoidance of dietary protein

Ⓑ acid-lowering drug therapy to prevent erosive gastritis

Ⓒ fresh frozen plasma to correct coagulation disorders

Ⓓ parenteral dextrose 10% to correct hypoglycaemia

Ⓔ parenteral mannitol 20% to control cerebral oedema

26
The clinical features of autoimmune hepatitis include
Ⓐ predominance of females aged 20–40 years

Ⓑ acute onset simulating viral hepatitis in 25% of patients

Ⓒ arthralgia, fever and amenorrhoea

Ⓓ spider telangiectasia and hepatosplenomegaly

Ⓔ cushingoid facies, hirsutism and acne

27
Hepatitis B chronic hepatitis differs from autoimmune hepatitis in that it
Ⓐ typically affects males over 30 years of age

Ⓑ often produces acute hepatic failure

Ⓒ is characterised by florid physical signs

Ⓓ typically progresses slowly without exacerbations

Ⓔ is less likely to be complicated by hepatoma

28
Diseases associated with autoimmune hepatitis include
Ⓐ autoimmune haemolytic anaemia

Ⓑ Hashimoto's thyroiditis

Ⓒ ulcerative colitis

Ⓓ nephrotic syndrome

Ⓔ rheumatoid arthritis

29
Eight weeks after the onset of hepatitis, the following serum tests strongly support a diagnosis of autoimmune hepatitis
Ⓐ antinuclear and smooth muscle antibodies in high titres

Ⓑ anti-LKM antibodies

Ⓒ hypoalbuminaemia with hypergammaglobulinaemia

Ⓓ decreased caeruloplasmin concentration

Ⓔ antimitochondrial antibodies in titres > 640

30
In the management of patients with autoimmune hepatitis
Ⓐ liver biopsy should be undertaken as soon as possible after the onset of the illness

Ⓑ remissions and relapses are characteristic

Ⓒ associated with autoantibodies, 50% of patients die within 5 years despite treatment

Ⓓ corticosteroid and azathioprine therapy are life-saving

Ⓔ interferon is of proven value in neonatally-acquired chronic type B viral hepatitis

31
The typical features of advanced hepatic cirrhosis include
Ⓐ progressive hepatomegaly
Ⓑ massive splenomegaly
Ⓒ peripheral blood macrocytosis
Ⓓ parotid gland enlargement
Ⓔ central cyanosis

32
Hepatic cirrhosis in adults in the UK is
Ⓐ cryptogenic in aetiology in 60% of patients
Ⓑ an early complication of severe acute type B viral hepatitis
Ⓒ a recognised complication of acute paracetamol poisoning
Ⓓ more likely if alcohol abuse is chronic rather than in episodic binges
Ⓔ a recognised complication of kwashiorkor

33
In patients with hepatic cirrhosis
Ⓐ central cyanosis responds well to oxygen therapy
Ⓑ increasing jaundice suggests progressive liver failure
Ⓒ the peripheral blood flow is typically reduced
Ⓓ the glomerular filtration rate is decreased
Ⓔ oesophageal varices indicate portal hypertension

34
Causes of hepatic cirrhosis include
Ⓐ haemochromatosis
Ⓑ Wilson's disease
Ⓒ macrovesicular steatosis complicating diabetes mellitus
Ⓓ hepatitis A infection
Ⓔ α_1-antitrypsin deficiency

35
Hepatic encephalopathy due to progressive liver failure is suggested by
Ⓐ dysarthria and chorea
Ⓑ focal neurological signs
Ⓒ yawning and hiccoughing
Ⓓ serum aminotransferase activity > 10 times normal
Ⓔ epilepsy and disorientation

36
Hepatic encephalopathy in cirrhosis is typically precipitated by
Ⓐ infection
Ⓑ hypokalaemia
Ⓒ abdominal surgery
Ⓓ gastrointestinal bleeding
Ⓔ lactulose therapy

37
In the management of hepatic cirrhosis with ascites
Ⓐ the dietary sodium intake should be restricted to 80 mmol/day
Ⓑ paracentesis and parenteral albumin replacement improves the survival rate
Ⓒ the daily calorie intake should be restricted to 1500 calories
Ⓓ diuretic therapy should achieve a weight loss of 2 kg/day
Ⓔ protein intake should be at least 60 g/day unless encephalopathy is suspected

38
The management of severe hepatic encephalopathy should include
Ⓐ withdrawal of dietary protein intake
Ⓑ sedatives to minimise neuropsychiatric symptoms
Ⓒ neomycin to reduce colonic bacterial flora
Ⓓ diuretic therapy with potassium supplementation
Ⓔ enteral or parenteral glucose 300 g/day

39

The hepatorenal syndrome in cirrhosis is characterised by

Ⓐ acute renal tubular necrosis

Ⓑ proteinuria and an abnormal urinary sediment

Ⓒ urinary sodium concentration < 10 mmol/L

Ⓓ urine/plasma osmolality ratio < 1.0

Ⓔ an elevated central venous pressure in most patients

40

Causes of portal hypertension include

Ⓐ alcoholic cirrhosis

Ⓑ myeloproliferative disease

Ⓒ hepatic schistosomiasis

Ⓓ neonatal umbilical sepsis

Ⓔ hepatic vein obstruction (Budd–Chiari syndrome)

41

Complications of portal hypertension include

Ⓐ variceal haemorrhage

Ⓑ congestive gastropathy

Ⓒ hepatorenal failure

Ⓓ hepatic encephalopathy

Ⓔ ascites

42

In the management of acute bleeding from oesophageal varices due to hepatic cirrhosis

Ⓐ the mortality rate of the first bleed is about 40%

Ⓑ variceal banding or sclerotherapy are contraindicated

Ⓒ somatostatin and vasopressin both reduce portal venous pressure

Ⓓ balloon tamponade is better deferred until endoscopic confirmation of bleeding varices

Ⓔ transjugular intrahepatic portasystemic stent shunting (TIPSS) is contraindicated in hepatic failure

43

Prevention of recurrent variceal bleeding is achievable using

Ⓐ somatostatin (octreotide) therapy

Ⓑ transjugular intrahepatic portasystemic stent shunting (TIPSS)

Ⓒ ß-adrenoreceptor antagonist treatment

Ⓓ variceal banding

Ⓔ sclerotherapy

44

Causes of ascites in the absence of intrahepatic liver disease include

Ⓐ congestive cardiac failure

Ⓑ nephrotic syndrome

Ⓒ peritoneal tuberculosis

Ⓓ lymphatic obstruction

Ⓔ Budd–Chiari syndrome

45

In primary biliary cirrhosis

Ⓐ middle-aged males are affected predominantly

Ⓑ pruritus is invariably accompanied by jaundice

Ⓒ osteomalacia and osteoporosis are often present

Ⓓ rigors and abdominal pain are a typical presentation

Ⓔ serum smooth muscle antibodies are present in high titres

46

The typical features of primary biliary cirrhosis include

Ⓐ xanthomata of the palmar creases and eyelids

Ⓑ poor prognosis even in asymptomatic patients

Ⓒ hepatomegaly preceding splenomegaly

Ⓓ dilated bile ducts on ultrasonography

Ⓔ improved survival rate with immunosuppressant therapy

47

The typical features of primary haemochromatosis include

Ⓐ association with HLA A3 in 75% of cases
Ⓑ male predominance
Ⓒ hepatic cirrhosis and diabetes mellitus
Ⓓ hypertrophic cardiomyopathy
Ⓔ grey skin pigmentation due to ferritin deposition

48

The typical features of Wilson's disease include

Ⓐ acute haemolytic anaemia
Ⓑ acute hepatitis and chronic hepatitis
Ⓒ parkinsonian syndrome and hepatic cirrhosis
Ⓓ osteomalacia and raised serum copper concentration
Ⓔ renal tubular acidosis and Kayser–Fleischer rings

49

The typical features of alcoholic liver disease include

Ⓐ macrovesicular steatosis
Ⓑ acute hepatitis and chronic hepatitis
Ⓒ hepatic cirrhosis
Ⓓ cholestatic jaundice
Ⓔ alcohol intake > 30 g per day for > 5 years

50

Indications for orthotopic liver transplantation in chronic liver failure include

Ⓐ serum bilirubin > 100 mmol/L
Ⓑ ascites or encephalopathy resistant to medical therapy
Ⓒ decompensated alcoholic cirrhosis in an abstinent patient
Ⓓ arterial hypoxaemia due to intrapulmonary shunting
Ⓔ presence of a hepatoma in a cirrhotic liver

51

Primary hepatocellular carcinoma is associated with

Ⓐ hepatic cirrhosis in 80% of patients in the UK
Ⓑ ingestion of aflatoxin-contaminated food in the tropics
Ⓒ haemochromatosis
Ⓓ hepatitis A virus infection
Ⓔ androgen and oestrogen ingestion

52

The typical features of hepatocellular carcinoma include

Ⓐ fever, weight loss and abdominal pain
Ⓑ ascites and intra-abdominal bleeding
Ⓒ venous hum over the liver
Ⓓ serum alpha-fetoprotein in high titre
Ⓔ surgically resectable disease in 50% of patients

53

Pyogenic liver abscess is a recognised complication of

Ⓐ ascending cholangitis
Ⓑ Crohn's disease
Ⓒ pancreatitis
Ⓓ septicaemia
Ⓔ subphrenic abscess

54

The typical features of pyogenic liver abscess include

Ⓐ obstructive jaundice and weight loss
Ⓑ tender hepatomegaly without splenomegaly
Ⓒ pleuritic pain and pleural effusion
Ⓓ multiple abscesses especially in ascending cholangitis
Ⓔ *Escherichia coli*, anaerobes and streptococci present in pus

55
The following statements about the biliary tract are true
🅐 the right and left hepatic ducts join to form the common bile duct
🅑 the normal common bile duct measures 25 mm in diameter
🅒 the bile and pancreatic ducts usually join the duodenum separately
🅓 the gallbladder is chiefly innervated by sympathetic nerves
🅔 1–2 litres of bile are secreted daily and concentrated 10-fold in the gallbladder

56
Gallstones are
🅐 more common in Africa and in India than in Europe
🅑 demonstrable in over 80% of UK patients > 60 years of age
🅒 predominantly composed of cholesterol in 75% of gallstones in the UK
🅓 usually pigment stones in hepatic cirrhosis
🅔 usually the result of reduced hepatic bile acid secretion

57
Gallstones are a recognised complication of
🅐 obesity
🅑 oral contraceptive therapy
🅒 chronic haemolytic anaemia
🅓 terminal ileal disease
🅔 rapid weight loss

58
The typical features of acute cholecystitis include
🅐 absence of obstruction of the cystic duct
🅑 sterile culture of bile 72 hours after onset
🅒 invariable association with gallstones
🅓 exacerbation of pain following morphine analgesics
🅔 radio-opaque gallstones on plain X-ray

59
The typical clinical features of acute cholecystitis include
🅐 jaundice, nausea and vomiting
🅑 colicky abdominal pain in spasms lasting about 5 minutes
🅒 right hypochondrial tenderness worse on inspiration
🅓 air in the biliary tree on plain X-ray
🅔 peripheral blood leucocytosis

60
The post-cholecystectomy syndrome is characteristically associated with
🅐 patients with previous acalculous cholecystitis
🅑 females with a history of abdominal pain > 5 years in duration
🅒 retained stones in the common bile duct
🅓 dysfunction of the sphincter of Oddi
🅔 early postoperative complications

61
The typical features of cholangiocarcinoma include
🅐 association with hepatic cirrhosis
🅑 abdominal pain and obstructive jaundice
🅒 serum alpha-fetoprotein in high titre
🅓 serum alkaline phosphatase > three times normal
🅔 surgically resectable in the majority of cases

62
Carcinoma of the gallbladder is
🅐 much commoner in males than females
🅑 usually squamous in cell type
🅒 associated with gallstones and calcification of the gallbladder
🅓 suggested by the presence of a palpable non-tender abdominal mass
🅔 surgically curable in most instances

11 DISEASES OF THE BLOOD

ANSWERS PAGE 234

1
In the normal formation of blood cells
Ⓐ fetal haematopoiesis does not take place in bone marrow
Ⓑ all lymphocytes originate in the bone marrow
Ⓒ haematopoiesis in adults extends to the femoral and humeral heads
Ⓓ the proerythroblast precedes the development of the normoblast
Ⓔ erythropoietin is produced by the Ito cells in the liver

2
Mature erythrocytes
Ⓐ contain blood group antigens in their cytoplasm
Ⓑ stain with methylene blue due to ribosomal production of haemoglobin
Ⓒ derive energy from glucose to fuel the Na^+/K^+ ionic pump
Ⓓ have a circulation half-life of about 120 days
Ⓔ contain carbonic anhydrase which facilitates carbon dioxide transport

3
Haemoglobin
Ⓐ F comprises two alpha and two delta chains
Ⓑ A_2 comprises two alpha and two gamma chains
Ⓒ has four porphyrin rings each containing ferrous iron
Ⓓ is an important buffer of carbonic acid
Ⓔ oxygen binding is increased by 2, 3-diphosphoglycerate within the red cells

4
Mature neutrophil granulocytes
Ⓐ typically comprise > 50% of the total peripheral blood white blood cells in adults
Ⓑ remain in the circulation for less than 12 hours
Ⓒ exhibit increased nuclear segmentation in infection
Ⓓ are derived from a different progenitor cell to that of monocytes
Ⓔ produce the vitamin B_{12} binding protein transcobalamin III

5
The following statements about white blood cells are correct
Ⓐ eosinophils are phagocytic and are involved in the killing of protozoa and helminths
Ⓑ basophils bind IgE antibody on their surface and are involved in hypersensitivity reactions
Ⓒ monocytes migrate into the tissues to become macrophages
Ⓓ B lymphocytes mediate cellular immunity
Ⓔ B lymphocytes comprise helper cells and suppressor cells

6
Typical causes of the following changes in the peripheral blood leucocyte count include
Ⓐ neutropenia in malaria
Ⓑ eosinopenia in Cushing's syndrome
Ⓒ basopenia in hyperthyroidism
Ⓓ lymphopenia in renal failure
Ⓔ basophilia in myeloproliferative disorders

7
Peripheral blood lymphocytosis would be an expected finding in
Ⓐ brucellosis
Ⓑ pneumococcal pneumonia
Ⓒ measles and rubella
Ⓓ Hodgkin's disease
Ⓔ chronic lymphatic leukaemia

8
Peripheral blood neutrophil leucocytosis would be an expected finding in
Ⓐ connective tissue disease
Ⓑ corticosteroid therapy
Ⓒ pregnancy
Ⓓ whooping cough
Ⓔ mesenteric infarction

9
Platelets
Ⓐ have a circulation lifespan of 10 hours in healthy subjects
Ⓑ are produced and regulated under the control of thrombopoietins
Ⓒ contain small nuclear remnants called Howell–Jolly bodies
Ⓓ decrease in number in response to aspirin therapy
Ⓔ release serotonin and von Willebrand factor (vWF)

10
The following statements about red blood cell morphology are true
Ⓐ hypochromia is pathognomonic of iron deficiency
Ⓑ polychromasia indicates active production of new red blood cells
Ⓒ poikilocytosis is invariably associated with anisocytosis
Ⓓ punctate basophilia is a typical feature of beta-thalassaemia
Ⓔ target cells are associated with hyposplenism and liver disease

11
Iron
Ⓐ content of blood is about 500 mg per litre
Ⓑ losses in the healthy male are about 3 mg per day
Ⓒ content of the adult body is about 5 g
Ⓓ is usually stored in hepatocytes as haemosiderin
Ⓔ in the healthy diet amounts to 10–15 mg per day

12
Peripheral blood findings in dietary iron deficiency include
Ⓐ microcytosis
Ⓑ ovalocytosis
Ⓒ mean corpuscular haemoglobin concentration < 50% of normal
Ⓓ Howell–Jolly bodies
Ⓔ thrombocytosis

13
In the treatment of iron deficiency anaemia with iron
Ⓐ folic acid should also be given if the anaemia is severe
Ⓑ treatment is stopped as soon as haemoglobin normalises
Ⓒ haemoglobin should rise by 1 g/L every 7–10 days
Ⓓ maximal reticulocyte count usually develops within 1–2 days
Ⓔ parenteral iron is usually more effective than oral iron

14
Hypochromic microcytic anaemia is a recognised finding in
Ⓐ haemolytic anaemia
Ⓑ primary sideroblastic anaemia
Ⓒ hypothyroidism
Ⓓ beta-thalassemia
Ⓔ rheumatoid arthritis

15

Normocytic normochromic anaemia is an expected feature of

Ⓐ alcoholic liver disease
Ⓑ chronic renal failure
Ⓒ rheumatoid arthritis
Ⓓ kwashiorkor
Ⓔ strict vegetarianism

16

Macrocytic anaemia is a typical finding in

Ⓐ folic acid deficiency
Ⓑ haemolytic anaemia
Ⓒ alcohol abuse
Ⓓ primary sideroblastic anaemia
Ⓔ myelodysplastic syndrome

17

Typical haematological findings in megaloblastic anaemia include

Ⓐ pancytopenia and oval macrocytosis
Ⓑ neutrophil leucocyte hypersegmentation
Ⓒ anisocytosis and poikilocytosis
Ⓓ reticulocytosis and polychromasia
Ⓔ excess urinary urobilinogen and bilirubinuria

18

Folate and vitamin B$_{12}$ deficiency both typically produce

Ⓐ subacute combined degeneration of the spinal cord
Ⓑ intermittent glossitis and diarrhoea
Ⓒ mild jaundice and splenomegaly
Ⓓ peripheral neuropathy
Ⓔ marked weight loss

19

Characteristic features of Addisonian pernicious anaemia include

Ⓐ onset before the age of 20 years
Ⓑ gastric parietal cell and intrinsic factor antibodies in the serum
Ⓒ increased serum bilirubin and lactate dehydrogenase concentrations
Ⓓ four-fold increase in the risk of developing gastric carcinoma
Ⓔ Schilling test usually reverts to normal with intrinsic factor

20

Causes of folic acid deficiency include

Ⓐ vegetarian diet
Ⓑ gluten enteropathy
Ⓒ pregnancy
Ⓓ haemolytic anaemia
Ⓔ antibiotic therapy

21

Typical features of the myelodysplastic syndromes include

Ⓐ presentation before the age of 30 years
Ⓑ macrocytic anaemia and pancytopenia
Ⓒ ring sideroblasts present on bone marrow cytology
Ⓓ chromosomal abnormalities in 50% of patients
Ⓔ risk of progression to an acute leukaemia

22

Recognised causes of pancytopenia include

Ⓐ systemic lupus erythematosus
Ⓑ indomethacin and sulphonamide therapy
Ⓒ hepatitis A infection
Ⓓ megaloblastic anaemia
Ⓔ myelodysplastic syndromes

23

Characteristic features of primary aplastic anaemia include

Ⓐ peak incidence about the age of 60 years
Ⓑ normocytic normochromic anaemia with thrombocytosis
Ⓒ bone marrow trephine is required to confirm the diagnosis
Ⓓ splenomegaly indicating extramedullary erythropoiesis
Ⓔ pancytopenia

24

Typical features suggesting intravascular haemolysis include

Ⓐ bilirubinuria and haemoglobinuria

Ⓑ methaemalbuminaemia and haemosiderinuria

Ⓒ increased serum haptoglobin concentration

Ⓓ increased plasma haemoglobin concentration

Ⓔ rigors and splenomegaly

25

Laboratory features suggesting haemolytic anaemia include

Ⓐ increased serum lactate dehydrogenase (LDH) concentration

Ⓑ conjugated hyperbilirubinaemia and bilirubinuria

Ⓒ peripheral blood neutrophil leucocytosis

Ⓓ peripheral blood polychromasia and macrocytosis

Ⓔ bone marrow erythroid hyperplasia

26

Non-immune haemolytic anaemia is a complication of

Ⓐ prosthetic heart valves

Ⓑ mycoplasmal pneumonia

Ⓒ megaloblastic anaemia

Ⓓ malarial infection

Ⓔ amoxycillin therapy

27

Typical features of hereditary spherocytosis include

Ⓐ splenomegaly

Ⓑ intravascular haemolysis

Ⓒ decreased red blood cell osmotic fragility

Ⓓ transient aplastic anaemia

Ⓔ deficiency of red cell spectrin

28

The typical clinical features of sickle-cell anaemia include

Ⓐ haemolytic and aplastic crises

Ⓑ neonatal spherocytic haemolytic anaemia

Ⓒ pulmonary, splenic and mesenteric infarcts

Ⓓ splenomegaly with hypersplenism

Ⓔ bone necrosis and salmonella osteomyelitis

29

In patients with sickle-cell disease, acute painful crises are likely to be precipitated by

Ⓐ high altitude

Ⓑ pregnancy

Ⓒ dehydration

Ⓓ systemic infection

Ⓔ hypothermia

30

The typical features of the beta-thalassaemias include

Ⓐ macrocytic anaemia

Ⓑ hepatosplenomegaly

Ⓒ pigment gallstones

Ⓓ neonatal haemolytic anaemia

Ⓔ chronic leg ulceration

31

The typical features of autoimmune haemolytic anaemia include

Ⓐ peripheral blood spherocytosis and splenomegaly

Ⓑ fever with haemoglobinuria and haemosiderinuria

Ⓒ increased serum haptoglobin concentration

Ⓓ positive Coomb's test

Ⓔ association with lymphoproliferative disease

32

The typical features of polycythaemia rubra vera include

Ⓐ peak prevalence in females aged > 60 years

Ⓑ splenomegaly, leucocytosis and thrombocytosis

Ⓒ headaches, pruritus and peptic ulcer dyspepsia

Ⓓ decreased leucocyte alkaline phosphatase score

Ⓔ increased blood viscosity associated with vascular disease

33

Recognised causes of leucoerythroblastic anaemia include

Ⓐ carcinomatosis

Ⓑ miliary tuberculosis

Ⓒ myelofibrosis

Ⓓ whooping cough

Ⓔ severe haemolysis

34

Characteristic features of acute leukaemia include

Ⓐ rapid onset of fever and anaemia

Ⓑ mouth ulceration and gingival hypertrophy

Ⓒ myalgia, arthralgia and skin rashes

Ⓓ microcytic anaemia and leucopenia

Ⓔ hypocellular bone marrow cytology

35

Acute lymphoblastic leukaemia (ALL)

Ⓐ has a peak prevalence in patients aged 20–30 years

Ⓑ typically produces cytoplasmic Auer rods in blast cells

Ⓒ has a median survival of 30 months with chemotherapy

Ⓓ is the most common of all acute leukaemias

Ⓔ is a typical complication of multiple myeloma

36

Clinical features of chronic myeloid leukaemia (CML) include

Ⓐ painful splenomegaly

Ⓑ sternal tenderness, gout and arthralgia

Ⓒ generalised lymphadenopathy

Ⓓ tendency to bleeding and bruising

Ⓔ median survival of 15 years with chemotherapy

37

The typical laboratory findings in chronic myeloid leukaemia include

Ⓐ leucoerythroblastic anaemia and thrombocytosis

Ⓑ peripheral blood neutrophilia, eosinophilia and basophilia

Ⓒ chromosomal translocation q-22/q+9

Ⓓ increased neutrophil leucocyte alkaline phosphatase (LAP) score

Ⓔ transformation to acute lymphoblastic leukaemia (ALL)

38

Typical features of chronic lymphocytic leukaemia include

Ⓐ onset in younger patients than in chronic myeloid leukaemia

Ⓑ development of autoimmune haemolytic anaemia

Ⓒ presentation with massive hepatosplenomegaly

Ⓓ lymphadenopathy associated with recurrent infections

Ⓔ median survival of 15 years following chemotherapy

39

The typical laboratory features in chronic lymphocytic leukaemia include

Ⓐ hyperuricaemia and thrombocytosis

Ⓑ hypogammaglobulinaemia

Ⓒ peripheral blood lymphocytosis in the absence of lymphoblasts

Ⓓ positive Coomb's test

Ⓔ transformation to acute leukaemia is more common than in chronic myeloid leukaemia

40

Allogeneic bone marrow transplantation is particularly useful in the treatment of

Ⓐ multiple myeloma

Ⓑ severe aplastic anaemia

Ⓒ alpha-thalassaemia

Ⓓ severe combined immunodeficiency disorder

Ⓔ chronic lymphatic leukaemia

41

Complications of allogeneic bone marrow transplantation include

Ⓐ acute graft-versus-host disease

Ⓑ severe infection

Ⓒ infertility

Ⓓ pneumonitis

Ⓔ malignant disease during long-term follow up

42

The presence of lymphadenopathy and splenomegaly would be expected findings in

Ⓐ multiple myeloma

Ⓑ chronic lymphocytic leukaemia

Ⓒ chronic myeloid leukaemia

Ⓓ infectious mononucleosis

Ⓔ myelofibrosis

43

The typical features of myelofibrosis include

Ⓐ absence of splenomegaly or lymphadenopathy

Ⓑ leucoerythroblastic blood film with tear-drop poikilocytes

Ⓒ increased leucocyte neutrophil alkaline phosphatase score

Ⓓ folic acid deficiency and hyperuricaemia

Ⓔ absent bone marrow megakaryocytes and thrombocytopenia

44

Recognised clinical features of multiple myeloma include

Ⓐ peak incidence between the ages of 30 and 50 years

Ⓑ secondary amyloidosis

Ⓒ median survival of about 10 years with chemotherapy

Ⓓ recurrent infections and pancytopenia

Ⓔ increased serum calcium, urate and blood urea

45

In differentiating multiple myeloma from a benign monoclonal gammopathy, the following findings would favour the diagnosis of multiple myeloma

Ⓐ monoclonal gammopathy with normal serum immunoglobulin levels

Ⓑ bone marrow plasmacytosis of > 20%

Ⓒ bilateral carpal tunnel syndrome

Ⓓ Bence Jones proteinuria

Ⓔ multiple osteolytic lesions on X-ray

46

A poor prognosis in multiple myeloma is suggested by the presence of

Ⓐ blood urea > 10 mmol/L after rehydration

Ⓑ decreased serum beta$_2$-microglobulin concentration

Ⓒ blood haemoglobin < 70 g/L

Ⓓ Bence Jones proteinuria

Ⓔ thrombocytopenia

47

Typical histopathological features of Hodgkin's disease include

Ⓐ Reed–Sternberg binucleate giant cells and lymphocytes

Ⓑ increased tissue eosinophils, neutrophils and plasma cells

Ⓒ increased fibrous stroma in the nodular sclerosing type

Ⓓ frequent involvement of the central nervous system

Ⓔ splenic involvement is rare in the absence of splenomegaly

48

The clinical features of Hodgkin's disease include

Ⓐ painless cervical lymphadenopathy
Ⓑ anaemia due to bone marrow involvement
Ⓒ impaired T cell function in the absence of lymphopenia
Ⓓ pruritus and alcohol-induced abdominal pain
Ⓔ overall median survival of 10 years

49

Typical characteristics of non-Hodgkin's lymphoma include

Ⓐ low-grade lymphomas rapidly produce symptoms due to high cell proliferation rates
Ⓑ bone marrow and splenic involvement are present from the onset
Ⓒ isolated involvement of gastric mucosa associated with *Helicobacter pylori* infection
Ⓓ the majority are T cell rather than B cell in origin
Ⓔ better prognosis in high-grade rather than low-grade lymphomas

50

Typical features of Waldenström's macroglobulinaemia include

Ⓐ the hyperviscosity syndrome
Ⓑ IgA paraproteinaemia
Ⓒ cold sensitivity and a progressive polyneuropathy
Ⓓ bone marrow infiltration with lymphoid cells and many mast cells
Ⓔ median survival of 5 years

51

Causes of non-thrombocytopenic purpura include

Ⓐ paraproteinaemia
Ⓑ Henoch–Schönlein purpura
Ⓒ ascorbic acid deficiency
Ⓓ folic acid deficiency
Ⓔ haemolytic-uraemic syndrome

52

Haemorrhagic disorders due to defective blood vessels include

Ⓐ von Willebrand disease
Ⓑ Ehlers–Danlos disease
Ⓒ septicaemia
Ⓓ Christmas disease
Ⓔ uraemia

53

Recognised causes of thrombocytosis include

Ⓐ myeloproliferative disorders
Ⓑ iron deficiency anaemia
Ⓒ hypersplenism
Ⓓ carcinomatosis
Ⓔ connective tissue disorders

54

Recognised causes of thrombocytopenia include

Ⓐ megaloblastic anaemia
Ⓑ acquired immunodeficiency syndrome
Ⓒ disseminated intravascular coagulation
Ⓓ von Willebrand disease
Ⓔ aspirin therapy

55

Typical features of idiopathic thrombocytopenic purpura include

Ⓐ IgG-mediated thrombocytopenia
Ⓑ peak prevalence in patients aged > 60 years old
Ⓒ prolongation of the bleeding time
Ⓓ marked splenomegaly
Ⓔ prompt response to corticosteroid therapy

56

The prothrombin time is typically prolonged in

Ⓐ disorders of the intrinsic pathway
Ⓑ factor X deficiency
Ⓒ factor VII deficiency
Ⓓ factor V deficiency
Ⓔ factor XII deficiency

57

The activated partial thromboplastin time (APTT) is typically prolonged in

Ⓐ disorders of the extrinsic pathway
Ⓑ factor VII deficiency
Ⓒ factor VII or X deficiency
Ⓓ factor XIII deficiency
Ⓔ factor IX, XI or XII deficiency

58

Disseminated intravascular coagulation is a complication of

Ⓐ amniotic fluid embolism
Ⓑ incompatible blood transfusion
Ⓒ hypovolaemic and anaphylactic shock
Ⓓ septicaemic shock
Ⓔ carcinomatosis

59

Features of disseminated intravascular coagulation include

Ⓐ thrombocytopenia
Ⓑ schistocytes in the peripheral blood
Ⓒ decreased serum fibrin degradation products (FDPs)
Ⓓ normal prothrombin time and normal thrombin time
Ⓔ prolongation of the activated partial thromboplastin time

60

The bleeding time is characteristically prolonged in

Ⓐ ascorbic acid deficiency
Ⓑ thrombocytopenia
Ⓒ haemophilia
Ⓓ warfarin therapy
Ⓔ von Willebrand disease

61

Haemorrhagic disorders due to decreased clotting factors include

Ⓐ hereditary haemorrhagic telangiectasia
Ⓑ Christmas disease
Ⓒ senile purpura
Ⓓ Henoch-Schönlein purpura
Ⓔ haemophilia

62

The following statements about severe haemophilia A are true

Ⓐ the disorder is inherited in an X-linked recessive mode
Ⓑ recurrent haemarthroses and haematuria are typical
Ⓒ activated partial thromboplastin time and prothrombin time are both prolonged
Ⓓ factor VIII has a biological half-life of about 12 days
Ⓔ desmopressin therapy increases factor VIII concentrations

63

The following statements about von Willebrand disease are true

Ⓐ the disorder is inherited in an X-linked recessive mode
Ⓑ it is characterised by a prolonged bleeding time
Ⓒ the von Willebrand factor (vWF) is synthesised by both platelets and endothelial cells
Ⓓ vWF is bound to factor VIII and forms bridges between platelets and endothelial cells
Ⓔ deficiency of vWF is best treated by desmopressin

64

The following statements about clotting factors are true

Ⓐ factor V is synthesised solely by the liver
Ⓑ factors II, VII, IX and X are activated by carboxylation of their glutamate residues
Ⓒ protein C and protein S interact to produce inhibition of factor Va
Ⓓ heparin enhances the inhibitory action of antithrombin on factor Xa and thrombin
Ⓔ warfarin acts by direct inhibition of vitamin K

65
Thrombophilia with a predisposition to recurrent venous thromboses is associated with
Ⓐ the antiphospholipid antibody syndrome
Ⓑ antithrombin deficiency
Ⓒ factor V Leiden
Ⓓ polycythaemia rubra vera
Ⓔ protein C deficiency

66
In the primary antiphospholipid antibody syndrome
Ⓐ antibodies impair enzymatic reactions in the coagulation cascade
Ⓑ an increased prevalence in venous but not arterial thromboses is characteristic
Ⓒ confirmation of the disorder is provided by the Russell viper venom test
Ⓓ tests for cardiolipin antibodies and/or lupus anticoagulant are usually negative
Ⓔ a peripheral blood thrombocytosis is a typical finding

67
Indications for warfarin anticoagulation include
Ⓐ venous thromboembolism
Ⓑ arterial embolism
Ⓒ myocardial infarction
Ⓓ atrial fibrillation
Ⓔ mechanical prosthetic heart valves

68
The following categories of patients require heparin for antithrombotic prophylaxis
Ⓐ patients about to undergo hip or knee surgery
Ⓑ patients with a previous history of DVT (deep venous thrombosis) who are about to undergo pelvic surgery
Ⓒ patients who are about to undergo pelvic or abdominal surgery for malignancy
Ⓓ patients with a previous history of DVT who are about to undergo dental extraction
Ⓔ patients admitted to hospital with a major cerebrovascular accident

69
The hazards of blood transfusion include
Ⓐ urticaria
Ⓑ congestive cardiac failure (CCF)
Ⓒ development of Rhesus antibodies in a Rhesus-negative patient
Ⓓ fever
Ⓔ acute intravascular haemolysis

70
Clinical features suggesting an acute haemolytic transfusion reaction include
Ⓐ onset within minutes of starting the transfusion
Ⓑ rigors and fever
Ⓒ chest and lumbar pain
Ⓓ sudden loss of consciousness
Ⓔ development of hypotension and shock

DISEASES OF THE CONNECTIVE TISSUES, JOINTS AND BONES

12

ANSWERS PAGE 242

1

Articular cartilage is

Ⓐ composed of chondrocytes
Ⓑ extremely vascular
Ⓒ rich in the proteoglycan aggrecan
Ⓓ devoid of a nerve supply
Ⓔ dependent on rapid collagen turnover for its capacity for repair

2

The synovial membrane

Ⓐ is composed principally of macrophages and fibroblast-like cells
Ⓑ secretes synovial fluid from the stellate cells of the intercellular matrix
Ⓒ receives its rich blood supply from the adjacent cartilage
Ⓓ is devoid of a nerve supply
Ⓔ has an intercellular matrix containing hyaluronan, chondroitin sulphate and tenascin

3

The following statements about bone are correct

Ⓐ there are two types of bone—cortical and trabecular
Ⓑ cortical bone predominates in the epiphyses
Ⓒ bone matrix is mainly composed of type I collagen
Ⓓ cortical bone is composed of Haversian systems
Ⓔ the lamellae of trabecular bone run parallel to the surface of the bone

4

The following diseases are associated with antinuclear and/or rheumatoid factor antibodies

Ⓐ infective endocarditis
Ⓑ autoimmune thyroiditis
Ⓒ Sjögren's syndrome
Ⓓ fibrosing alveolitis
Ⓔ ankylosing spondylitis

5

The autoantibodies listed below are associated with the following diseases

Ⓐ antinuclear antibodies—rheumatoid arthritis
Ⓑ anti-topoisomerase—progressive systemic sclerosis (PSS)
Ⓒ anti-SSA (anti-Ro)—Sjögren's syndrome
Ⓓ anti-centromere antibodies—dermatomyositis
Ⓔ antinuclear cytoplasmic antibodies—CREST syndrome

6

Antinuclear antibodies (ANA)

Ⓐ occur in 95% of patients with systemic lupus erythematosus (SLE)
Ⓑ of anti-ds-DNA type are specific to systemic lupus erythematosus
Ⓒ fluctuate in titre in parallel with clinical activity of disease
Ⓓ are rarely found in healthy subjects
Ⓔ typically occur in patients with polyarteritis nodosa

7

The biochemical features listed below characterise the following metabolic bone disorders

Ⓐ increased serum calcium, serum phosphate and serum alkaline phosphatase—osteoporosis

Ⓑ normal serum calcium and serum phosphate but increased serum alkaline phosphatase—Paget's disease

Ⓒ normal serum calcium and serum alkaline phosphatase, and decreased serum phosphate—osteomalacia

Ⓓ decreased serum calcium, serum phosphate and serum alkaline phosphatase—metastatic bone disease

Ⓔ decreased serum calcium and serum phosphate but increased serum alkaline phosphatase—osteomalacia

8

In the measurement of bone densitometry

Ⓐ conventional X-rays of the skeleton will detect early changes in bone mineral density

Ⓑ dual energy X-ray absorptiometry (DXA scanning) is the method of choice; it is associated with a radiation dose similar to that of a chest X-ray

Ⓒ bone mineral densitometry (BMD) is measured in grams of hydroxyapatite per square centimetre

Ⓓ the Z-score expresses the number of standard deviations by which a patient's measurement differs from age and sex matched controls subjects

Ⓔ the T-score expresses the number of standard deviations by which a patient's measurement differs from healthy young control subjects

9

Presentation with acute monoarthritis suggests the possibility of

Ⓐ crystal arthritis

Ⓑ trauma

Ⓒ bacterial infection

Ⓓ rheumatoid arthritis

Ⓔ enteropathic arthritis

10

The following statements about infective arthritis are true

Ⓐ the onset is typically insidious

Ⓑ preexisting arthritis is a recognised predisposing factor

Ⓒ small peripheral joints are involved more often than larger joints

Ⓓ *Haemophilus influenzae* is the commonest causative organism in adults

Ⓔ joint aspiration should be avoided given the risk of septicaemia

11

The typical features of gonococcal arthritis include

Ⓐ more commonly found in young males

Ⓑ pustular or vesicular rashes

Ⓒ tenosynovitis and asymmetrical polyarthritis

Ⓓ positive synovial fluid culture in most instances

Ⓔ chronic joint disease in the majority of cases

12

Tuberculous arthritis is

Ⓐ a common accompaniment of pulmonary tuberculosis in the UK

Ⓑ characterised by early, florid destructive joint changes on X-ray

Ⓒ typically associated with a strongly positive tuberculin skin test

Ⓓ usually best confirmed by joint aspiration

Ⓔ best managed by intra-articular antituberculous drugs

13
Polyarthralgia is a common presenting complaint in
- Ⓐ rubella
- Ⓑ depression
- Ⓒ hypothyroidism
- Ⓓ metabolic bone disease
- Ⓔ diabetes insipidus

14
The following disorders produce symptoms and signs in the joints
- Ⓐ Lyme disease
- Ⓑ acromegaly
- Ⓒ chondrocalcinosis
- Ⓓ chronic sarcoidosis
- Ⓔ amyloidosis

15
Common extra-articular manifestations of rheumatological disorders include
- Ⓐ episcleritis and keratoconjunctivitis sicca in rheumatoid arthritis
- Ⓑ erythema nodosum in enteropathic synovitis
- Ⓒ enthesitis in ankylosing spondylitis
- Ⓓ alopecia in systemic lupus erythematosus
- Ⓔ retinitis pigmentosa in psoriatic arthritis

16
The following features suggest a mechanical rather than inflammatory cause of back pain
- Ⓐ radiation of pain down the back of one leg to the ankle
- Ⓑ an elevated C-reactive protein (CRP)
- Ⓒ localised tenderness over the greater sciatic notch
- Ⓓ gradual mode of onset in an elderly patient
- Ⓔ back pain and stiffness exacerbated by resting

17
In a patient with low back pain
- Ⓐ X-ray changes of spina bifida occulta would explain the symptom
- Ⓑ loss of lumbar lordosis suggests neoplastic vertebral infiltration
- Ⓒ exacerbation of pain with exercise suggests sacroiliitis
- Ⓓ previous myelography suggests the possibility of arachnoiditis
- Ⓔ spontaneous resolution within 1 month is the commonest outcome

18
The typical findings in fibromyalgia include
- Ⓐ elevation of the ESR
- Ⓑ symptoms of fatigue and an irritable bowel
- Ⓒ coexistent anxiety and depression
- Ⓓ rapid, spontaneous resolution
- Ⓔ musculoskeletal pain without local tenderness

19
The following statements about musculoskeletal pains are true
- Ⓐ in inflammatory arthritis, pain is typically worse by day
- Ⓑ ligamentous strain produces pain which is usually only felt on movement
- Ⓒ the pain of impacted fractures is invariably worse on movement
- Ⓓ muscle pain is typically unaffected by isometric contraction
- Ⓔ in osteoarthrosis, pain is usually worse on resting

20
In a patient with neck pain
Ⓐ aggravation by sneezing suggests cervical disc prolapse

Ⓑ radiation to the occiput suggests disease affecting in the upper cervical vertebrae

Ⓒ associated bilateral arm paraesthesiae suggest angina pectoris as the most likely diagnosis

Ⓓ and otherwise normal joints, rheumatoid arthritis is excluded as a possible diagnosis

Ⓔ associated drop attacks suggest vertebral artery compression due to cervical spondylosis

21
Shoulder pain is a recognised feature of
Ⓐ myocardial ischaemia

Ⓑ supraspinatus tendonitis

Ⓒ bronchial carcinoma

Ⓓ pneumococcal pneumonia

Ⓔ cervical spondylosis

22
In a patient with shoulder pain
Ⓐ supraspinatus tendonitis is associated with a 'painful arc'

Ⓑ bicipital tendinitis is associated with a painful arc

Ⓒ shoulder pain developing beyond 90° abduction suggests infraspinatus tendinitis

Ⓓ shoulder pain in all directions of movement suggests capsulitis

Ⓔ subscapularis tendinitis is suggested by pain worsening on resisted abduction

23
In diffuse idiopathic skeletal hyperostosis (DISH)
Ⓐ there is ossification along the anterolateral aspect of at least four contiguous vertebrae

Ⓑ the condition has a peak prevalence in adolescents

Ⓒ excessive vitamin D intake is thought to be responsible for the condition

Ⓓ there is an association with type 2 diabetes mellitus

Ⓔ pain in the axial skeleton is characteristic

24
Osteoarthritis is
Ⓐ evident radiologically in at least 80% of patients > 65 years old

Ⓑ more likely to be generalised and severe in males

Ⓒ characterised by degeneration of cartilage and synovial inflammation

Ⓓ associated with increased collagen synthesis in the affected cartilage

Ⓔ best managed with anti-inflammatory doses of NSAIDs

25
The clinical features of primary (nodal) osteoarthrosis include
Ⓐ joint pain aggravated by rest and relieved by activity

Ⓑ proximal interphalangeal and metacarpal-phalangeal joint involvement

Ⓒ involvement of the hip, knee and spinal apophyseal joints

Ⓓ a strong family history of Heberden's nodes

Ⓔ microfractures of subchondral bone

26
Causes of secondary osteoarthritis include
Ⓐ acromegaly

Ⓑ septic arthritis

Ⓒ haemochromatosis

Ⓓ Perthes' disease

Ⓔ Ehlers–Danlos syndrome

27
Factors predisposing to hyperuricaemia and gout include
Ⓐ hypothyroidism
Ⓑ severe exfoliative psoriasis
Ⓒ chronic renal failure
Ⓓ polycythaemia rubra vera
Ⓔ therapy with loop diuretic agents

28
The clinical features of gout include
Ⓐ precipitation of an acute attack by allopurinol
Ⓑ cellulitis, tenosynovitis and bursitis
Ⓒ the abrupt onset of severe joint pain and tenderness
Ⓓ serum urate levels fall during an acute attack
Ⓔ loin pain and haematuria

29
In the treatment of gout
Ⓐ NSAID therapy increases urinary urate excretion
Ⓑ salicylates control symptoms and accelerate resolution of the acute attack
Ⓒ allopurinol inhibits xanthine oxidase and hence urate production
Ⓓ tophi should resolve with control of hyperuricaemia
Ⓔ allopurinol or probenecid should be given within 24 hours of onset of the acute attack

30
In pyrophosphate arthropathy
Ⓐ calcium pyrophosphate dihydrate crystals are deposited in the synovial cells
Ⓑ haemochromatosis is a recognised predisposing factor
Ⓒ the clinical appearances are similar to acute gout
Ⓓ the findings on synovial aspiration are indistinguishable from acute gout
Ⓔ intra-articular corticosteroid injections are contraindicated

31
Disorders associated with periarticular calcium deposition include
Ⓐ progressive systemic sclerosis
Ⓑ chronic haemodialysis
Ⓒ dermatomyositis
Ⓓ rotator cuff syndrome
Ⓔ Milwaukee shoulder/knee syndrome

32
The typical features of rheumatoid arthritis (RA) include
Ⓐ onset usually before the age of 30 years
Ⓑ a female to male ratio of 3:1
Ⓒ association with HLA-DR4
Ⓓ progression to bone and cartilage destruction
Ⓔ sparing of joints of the pelvic and shoulder girdle

33
Criteria for the diagnosis of rheumatoid arthritis include
Ⓐ morning stiffness lasting more than 1 hour
Ⓑ arthritis in both hip joints
Ⓒ the presence of rheumatoid nodules
Ⓓ symmetrical polyarthritis
Ⓔ positive rheumatoid factor test

34
Characteristic pathological changes in rheumatoid arthritis include
Ⓐ diffuse necrotising vasculitis
Ⓑ increased synovial fluid complement concentration
Ⓒ subcutaneous nodules with numerous giant cells
Ⓓ generalised lymphadenopathy
Ⓔ progression to amyloidosis

35
Typical features of active rheumatoid arthritis include
Ⓐ fever and weight loss
Ⓑ macrocytic anaemia
Ⓒ anterior uveitis
Ⓓ thrombocytopenia
Ⓔ generalised lymphadenopathy

36

The typical pattern of synovial disease in rheumatoid arthritis includes

Ⓐ early involvement of the sacroiliac joints

Ⓑ symmetrical peripheral joint involvement

Ⓒ spindling of the fingers and broadening of the forefeet

Ⓓ distal interphalangeal joint involvement of fingers and toes

Ⓔ atlantoaxial joint involvement

37

Extra-articular manifestations of rheumatoid arthritis include

Ⓐ cutaneous ulceration

Ⓑ pericardial and pleural effusions

Ⓒ amyloidosis

Ⓓ peripheral neuropathy

Ⓔ hypersplenism

38

The following statements about rheumatoid arthritis are true

Ⓐ joint pain and stiffness is typically aggravated by rest

Ⓑ the rheumatoid factor test is positive in about 70% of patients

Ⓒ joint involvement is additive rather than flitting

Ⓓ associated scleromalacia typically produces painful red eyes

Ⓔ Raynaud's and sicca syndrome suggest an alternative diagnosis

39

The clinical features of Felty's syndrome include

Ⓐ peak prevalence in the age group 20–30 years

Ⓑ previous long-standing rheumatoid arthritis

Ⓒ negative rheumatoid factor test

Ⓓ lymphadenopathy and splenomegaly

Ⓔ recurrent infections and leg ulcers

40

In the treatment of rheumatoid arthritis

Ⓐ bed rest should be avoided because of bony ankylosis

Ⓑ splinting of the affected joints reduces pain and swelling

Ⓒ associated anaemia responds promptly to oral iron therapy

Ⓓ systemic corticosteroids are contraindicated

Ⓔ non-steroidal anti-inflammatory drugs retard disease progression

41

Disease-modifying antirheumatic drugs (DMARD) in rheumatoid arthritis include

Ⓐ sulphasalazine

Ⓑ naproxen

Ⓒ D-penicillamine

Ⓓ sodium aurothiomalate

Ⓔ azathioprine

42

A poorer prognosis in rheumatoid arthritis is associated with

Ⓐ insidious onset of rheumatoid arthritis

Ⓑ high titres of rheumatoid factor early in the course of the disease

Ⓒ early development of subcutaneous nodules and erosive arthritis

Ⓓ extra-articular manifestations of the disease

Ⓔ onset with palindromic rheumatism

43

Recognised features of primary Sjögren's syndrome include

Ⓐ an increased incidence of lymphoma

Ⓑ dryness of the eyes, mouth and vagina

Ⓒ reduced lacrimal secretion rate

Ⓓ more males affected than females

Ⓔ a positive IgM rheumatoid factor in over 80% of patients

44

Typical features of seronegative spondyloarthritis include

Ⓐ asymmetrical oligoarthritis

Ⓑ involvement of cartilaginous joints

Ⓒ enthesitis of tendinous insertions

Ⓓ scleritis and episcleritis

Ⓔ mitral valve disease

45

Features associated with ankylosing spondylitis include

Ⓐ peak onset in the 2nd and 3rd decades

Ⓑ subcutaneous nodules

Ⓒ HLA-B27 in at least 90% of affected patients

Ⓓ faecal carriage of specific *Klebsiella* species

Ⓔ family history of psoriatic arthritis and Reiter's syndrome

46

Features suggesting ankylosing spondylitis include

Ⓐ early morning low back pain radiating to the buttocks

Ⓑ persistence of lumbar lordosis on spinal flexion

Ⓒ chest pain aggravated by breathing

Ⓓ 'squaring' of the lumbar vertebrae on X-ray

Ⓔ erosions of the symphysis pubis on X-ray

47

In the treatment of ankylosing spondylitis

Ⓐ systemic corticosteroid therapy is contraindicated

Ⓑ prolonged bed rest accelerates functional recovery

Ⓒ spinal radiotherapy modifies the course of the disease

Ⓓ spinal deformity is minimised with physiotherapy

Ⓔ hip joint involvement augurs a poorer prognosis

48

The typical features of Reiter's disease include

Ⓐ anterior uveitis develops more often than conjunctivitis

Ⓑ non-specific urethritis and prostatitis

Ⓒ symmetrical small joint polyarthritis

Ⓓ onset 1–3 weeks following bacterial dysentery

Ⓔ keratoderma blenorrhagica and nail dystrophy

49

In Reiter's disease

Ⓐ a peripheral blood monocytosis is commonly found

Ⓑ sacroiliitis and spondylitis develop in most patients

Ⓒ *Salmonella* or *Shigella* species can be cultured from joint aspirates

Ⓓ calcaneal spurs are not apparent radiologically

Ⓔ arthritis resolves within 3–6 months of onset

50

Psoriatic arthritis is

Ⓐ usually preceded by the development of psoriasis

Ⓑ likely to develop in 25% of patients with psoriasis

Ⓒ commoner in patients with psoriatic nail changes

Ⓓ associated with a poorer prognosis than rheumatoid arthritis

Ⓔ likely to respond to hydroxychloroquine

51

Recognised patterns of psoriatic arthritis include

Ⓐ asymmetrical oligoarthritis of the fingers and toes

Ⓑ distal interphalangeal joint involvement with nail dystrophy

Ⓒ sacroiliitis and spondylitis

Ⓓ rheumatoid-like symmetrical small joint arthritis

Ⓔ arthritis mutilans with telescoping of the digits

52

Diseases associated with seronegative spondyloarthritis include

Ⓐ Sjögren's syndrome
Ⓑ Whipple's disease
Ⓒ coeliac disease
Ⓓ ulcerative colitis
Ⓔ Behçet's disease

53

Recognised causes of juvenile arthritis include

Ⓐ sickle-cell disease
Ⓑ salmonellosis
Ⓒ acute leukaemia
Ⓓ Henoch–Schönlein purpura
Ⓔ meningococcal infection

54

The following statements about juvenile idiopathic arthritis are true

Ⓐ Still's disease usually presents with an unexplained arthritis
Ⓑ seropositive polyarthritis resembles adult rheumatoid arthritis
Ⓒ oligoarticular disease in girls is associated with chronic iritis
Ⓓ oligoarticular disease in boys resembles ankylosing spondylitis
Ⓔ a polyarticular pattern is seen most commonly

55

Typical features of systemic lupus erythematosus include

Ⓐ a higher prevalence in Caucasian than in African women
Ⓑ onset usually in the 4th and 5th decades
Ⓒ impaired function of suppressor T lymphocytes
Ⓓ increased prevalence of HLA-B8 and HLA-DR3
Ⓔ exacerbations occurring during pregancy and the puerperium

56

Characteristic clinical features of systemic lupus erythematosus (SLE) include

Ⓐ Raynaud's phenomenon
Ⓑ alopecia
Ⓒ an erythematous photosensitive facial rash
Ⓓ absence of renal complications
Ⓔ neuropsychiatric symptoms

57

Typical haematological findings in systemic lupus erythematosus include

Ⓐ leucocytosis and thrombocytosis
Ⓑ impaired coagulation
Ⓒ circulating anti-DNA and rheumatoid factor antibodies in high titre
Ⓓ elevated CH_{50}, C_3 and C_4 complement levels in peripheral blood
Ⓔ elevated C-reactive protein levels

58

Drug-induced systemic lupus erythematosus is associated with

Ⓐ NSAID exposure
Ⓑ hydralazine therapy
Ⓒ oral contraception
Ⓓ phenytoin therapy
Ⓔ phenothiazine therapy

59

In the management of systemic lupus erythematosus, the following are of proven value

Ⓐ NSAIDs for renal involvement
Ⓑ corticosteroid therapy for cerebral involvement
Ⓒ plasmapheresis for immune complex disease
Ⓓ hydroxychloroquine for skin and joint involvement
Ⓔ long-term corticosteroid therapy during periods of remission to prevent relapse

60

Typical features of mixed connective tissue disease include

Ⓐ proximal muscle weakness and tenderness

Ⓑ diffuse interstitial pulmonary fibrosis

Ⓒ antiribonucleoprotein antibodies in high titre

Ⓓ renal and neurological involvement

Ⓔ decreased serum creatine kinase concentration

61

The clinical features of progressive systemic sclerosis include

Ⓐ presentation with Raynaud's phenomenon

Ⓑ reflux oesophagitis and dysphagia

Ⓒ fibrosing alveolitis

Ⓓ ulceration, atrophy and subcutaneous calcification of the fingertips

Ⓔ anti-DNA antibodies and decreased serum complement levels

62

In polymyositis

Ⓐ there is an association with HLA-B8, HLA-DR3

Ⓑ antinuclear antibodies are characteristically absent

Ⓒ electromyography is helpful in differentiation from peripheral neuropathy

Ⓓ underlying malignancy is usually present if weight loss is marked

Ⓔ an erythematous rash on the knuckles, elbows, knees and face is typical

63

Features of giant cell arteritis include

Ⓐ a predominance in females > 60 years of age

Ⓑ pain in the jaw during eating

Ⓒ confluent involvement of affected arteries

Ⓓ difficulty in rising from the seated position

Ⓔ weight loss with normochromic anaemia and high ESR

64

In polymyalgia rheumatica

Ⓐ antinuclear and rheumatoid factor antibodies are present in high titre

Ⓑ temporal artery biopsy usually confirms the diagnosis

Ⓒ response to oral corticosteroids typically occurs within 7 days

Ⓓ corticosteroid therapy should be withdrawn after 6 months

Ⓔ sudden uniocular blindness suggests steroid-induced cataract

65

The features of classical polyarteritis nodosa include

Ⓐ more common in males

Ⓑ an association with circulating immune complexes containing hepatitis B virus

Ⓒ involvement of small arteries and arterioles

Ⓓ multiple peripheral nerve palsies

Ⓔ severe hypertension

66

Typical laboratory findings in systemic vasculitis include

Ⓐ peripheral blood lymphocytosis

Ⓑ high titres of anti-DNA antibodies

Ⓒ high titres of antineutrophil cytoplasmic antibodies

Ⓓ anaemia with an elevated MCV

Ⓔ haematuria on dipstick testing

67

The typical features of relapsing polychondritis include

Ⓐ both conductive and sensorineural deafness

Ⓑ episcleritis and scleritis

Ⓒ presentation with hoarseness and stridor

Ⓓ development of renal failure

Ⓔ valvular heart disease

68
Features of Kawasaki disease include
Ⓐ persistent fever
Ⓑ aneurysms of the coronary arteries
Ⓒ bilateral conjunctivitis
Ⓓ erythematous rash involving the palms and soles
Ⓔ cervical lymphadenopathy associated with erythema of the lips and tongue

69
Osteoporosis is
Ⓐ usually associated with normal serum calcium, phosphate and alkaline phosphatase
Ⓑ more likely to occur if menopause is early
Ⓒ commonly asymptomatic
Ⓓ a typical complication of untreated Addison's disease
Ⓔ more common in patients with chronic high alcohol intake

70
Common causes of osteoporosis include
Ⓐ gluten enteropathy
Ⓑ rheumatoid arthritis
Ⓒ pregnancy
Ⓓ anorexia nervosa
Ⓔ hypogonadism

71
Therapies useful in preventing recurrent vertebral fractures in osteoporosis include
Ⓐ regular exercise
Ⓑ oral phosphate supplementation
Ⓒ etidronate
Ⓓ vitamin D and calcium supplementation
Ⓔ corticosteroid

72
In osteomalacia
Ⓐ the finding of a proximal myopathy suggests an alternative diagnosis
Ⓑ bone involvement is characteristically painless
Ⓒ Chvostek's sign indicates that the underlying diagnosis may be hyperparathyroidism
Ⓓ due to renal disease, 25-hydroxycholecalciferol therapy is recommended
Ⓔ pseudofractures on X-ray are pathognomonic

73
Typical features of Paget's disease of bone include
Ⓐ onset before the age of 40 years
Ⓑ increased serum alkaline phosphatase and urinary hydroxyproline excretion
Ⓒ presentation with severe bone pain, especially in elderly patients
Ⓓ delayed healing of fractures
Ⓔ risk of development of osteogenic sarcoma

74
In a male patient with widespread metastatic bone disease
Ⓐ osteolytic deposits are likely to be due to prostatic carcinoma
Ⓑ the plasma calcium is typically elevated
Ⓒ bone pain is invariably present
Ⓓ the alkaline phosphatase is only elevated if pathological fracture occurs
Ⓔ cyproterone acetate retards progress of the disease

DISEASES OF THE SKIN

ANSWERS PAGE 251

13

1
The following statements about the skin are true
Ⓐ the surface area of an adult is approximately 2m²
Ⓑ the subcutis is composed predominantly of fat
Ⓒ keratinocytes comprise one-third of epidermal cell numbers
Ⓓ Langerhans cells synthesise vitamin D in the epidermis
Ⓔ sweat is produced solely by eccrine sweat glands

2
In the terminology of skin lesions
Ⓐ papules are solid skin elevations > 20 mm in diameter
Ⓑ nodules are solid skin masses > 5 mm in diameter
Ⓒ vesicles are fluid-containing skin elevations > 5 mm in diameter
Ⓓ petechiae are pinhead-sized macules of blood within the skin ˙
Ⓔ macules are small raised areas of skin of altered colour

3
The following are recognised causes of pigmented cutaneous lesions
Ⓐ a benign melanocytic naevus
Ⓑ malignant melanoma
Ⓒ seborrhoeic wart
Ⓓ dermatofibroma
Ⓔ pigmented basal cell carcinoma

4
Effects of topical corticosteroid therapy include
Ⓐ dermal atrophy most marked in the face and body folds
Ⓑ striae, particularly in the body folds
Ⓒ absence of hypothalamo–pituitary–adrenal axis suppression
Ⓓ decreased hair growth, particularly of the beard
Ⓔ spread of skin infection

5
Characteristic features of eczema include
Ⓐ epidermal oedema and intra-epidermal vesicles
Ⓑ delayed hypersensitivity reaction in seborrhoeic eczema
Ⓒ increased serum IgA concentration in discoid (nummular) eczema
Ⓓ eyelid and scrotal oedema in allergic contact eczema
Ⓔ persistence of childhood atopic eczema into adulthood

6
Typical sensitising agents in contact eczema include
Ⓐ aluminium
Ⓑ colophony
Ⓒ lanolin
Ⓓ rubber
Ⓔ ethanol

7

In the evaluation of a sudden widespread scaly rash

Ⓐ a fluctuating course since infancy suggests atopic eczema

Ⓑ involvement of extensor surfaces suggests psoriasis

Ⓒ a fir-tree distribution suggests pityriasis versicolor

Ⓓ absence of itch suggests pityriasis versicolor

Ⓔ absence of itch suggests lichen planus

8

The following are recognised causes of blistering at birth

Ⓐ herpes simplex infection

Ⓑ *Staphylococcus aureus* infection

Ⓒ bullous ichthyosiform erythroderma

Ⓓ epidermolysis bullosa

Ⓔ incontinentia pigmenti

9

The following blistering eruptions are typically associated with mucosal involvement

Ⓐ dermatitis herpetiformis

Ⓑ bullous pemphigoid

Ⓒ pemphigus

Ⓓ toxic epidermal necrolysis

Ⓔ porphyria cutanea tarda

10

The conditions listed below are typically associated with the following specific skin disorders

Ⓐ pernicious anaemia—pemphigus vulgaris

Ⓑ Crohn's disease—dermatitis herpetiformis

Ⓒ periumbilical rash—pemphigoid gestationis

Ⓓ intraepidermal blistering—pemphigus vulgaris

Ⓔ response to a gluten-free diet—bullous pemphigoid

11

The following are recognised causes of leg ulcers

Ⓐ leprosy

Ⓑ sickle-cell disease

Ⓒ diabetes mellitus

Ⓓ pyoderma gangrenosum

Ⓔ syphilis

12

The following cause alopecia with scarring

Ⓐ tinea capitis

Ⓑ alopecia areata

Ⓒ discoid lupus erythematosus

Ⓓ telogen effluvium

Ⓔ androgenetic alopecia

13

With regard to psoriasis

Ⓐ a child with one affected parent has a 50% chance of developing the disease

Ⓑ the cellular infiltrate is typically lymphocytic

Ⓒ guttate psoriasis may be preceded by beta-haemolytic streptococcal infection

Ⓓ nail pitting is associated with distal interphalangeal arthropathy

Ⓔ about 5% of patients develop arthropathy

14

Typical features of psoriasis include

Ⓐ well-defined erythematous plaques with adherent silvery scales

Ⓑ epidermal thickening and nucleated horny layer cells (parakeratosis)

Ⓒ induction of plaques by local trauma

Ⓓ an association with HLA-Cw6

Ⓔ exacerbation by propranolol and lithium carbonate therapy

15

The characteristic clinical features of psoriasis include

Ⓐ sparing of the skin over the head, face and neck

Ⓑ guttate psoriasis usually affects the elderly

Ⓒ nail changes with pitting and onycholysis

Ⓓ oligoarthritis particularly associated with nail changes occurring in 5% of cases

Ⓔ red non-scaly skin areas in the natal cleft and submammary folds

16

Appropriate therapeutic schedules in psoriasis include

Ⓐ dithranol cream for facial, genital and flexural plaques

Ⓑ steroid-antifungal combinations for flexural plaques

Ⓒ tar-steroid combinations during withdrawal of steroid creams

Ⓓ short-wave UVA exposure from sunbeds

Ⓔ combined psoralen and UVA (PUVA) photochemotherapy and isotretinoin

17

The typical features of acne vulgaris include

Ⓐ involvement of pilosebaceous glands and their ducts

Ⓑ distribution over the face and upper torso

Ⓒ infection with the skin commensal *Proprionobacterium acnes*

Ⓓ increased sebum production containing excess free fatty acids

Ⓔ open and closed comedones, inflammatory papules, nodules and cysts

18

Drug therapies associated with acneiform eruptions include

Ⓐ chlorinated hydrocarbons

Ⓑ corticosteroid therapy

Ⓒ androgenic or oestrogenic steroid therapy

Ⓓ lithium carbonate therapy

Ⓔ anticonvulsants

19

Therapies of proven value in acne vulgaris include

Ⓐ oral tetracycline or erythromycin drug therapy

Ⓑ topical preparations of benzoyl peroxide and retinoic acid

Ⓒ oral contraceptive pill

Ⓓ cyproterone acetate anti androge

Ⓔ oral isotretinoin ↑ keratogenic

20

The following drugs are associated with hyperpigmentation

Ⓐ amiodarone

Ⓑ phenothiazines

Ⓒ phenytoin

Ⓓ mepacrine

Ⓔ L-dopa

21

The characteristic features of rosacea include

Ⓐ predominantly affects adolescents

Ⓑ increased secretion of sebum

Ⓒ facial erythema, telangiectasia, pustules and papules

Ⓓ rhinophyma, conjunctivitis and keratitis

Ⓔ non-responsive to oral tetracycline therapy

22

The typical features of lichen planus include

Ⓐ involvement of the skin, nails, hair and mucous membranes

Ⓑ dense subepidermal lymphocytic infiltration on histology

Ⓒ itchy, purplish, polygonal, shiny skin papules

Ⓓ hypopigmentation at sites of previous lesions

Ⓔ complete resolution following topical steroid therapy

23

Systemic causes of pruritus include

Ⓐ oral contraceptives and pregnancy

Ⓑ hypothyroidism and hyperthyroidism

Ⓒ lymphoproliferative and myeloproliferative diseases

Ⓓ iron deficiency anaemia

Ⓔ opiate and antidepressant drug therapy.

24

Skin diseases associated with marked pruritus include

Ⓐ cutaneous vasculitis

Ⓑ lichen planus

Ⓒ atopic eczema

Ⓓ seborrhoeic keratosis

Ⓔ dermatitis herpetiformis

25

Skin diseases associated with blistering eruptions include

Ⓐ erythema multiforme

Ⓑ dermatitis herpetiformis

Ⓒ pemphigoid

Ⓓ pemphigus vulgaris

Ⓔ guttate psoriasis

26

Skin diseases associated with photosensitivity include

Ⓐ variegate and hepatic porphyrias

Ⓑ atopic eczema

Ⓒ drug reactions to phenothiazine, thiazide and tetracycline

Ⓓ pyoderma gangrenosum

Ⓔ pityriasis rosea

27

The typical features of erythema multiforme include

Ⓐ target-like skin lesions of the hands and feet

Ⓑ skin eruption lasting 6–12 weeks

Ⓒ absence of vesiculation or blistering

Ⓓ involvement of the eyes, genitalia and mouth

Ⓔ association with underlying systemic malignancy

28

Recognised causes of erythema multiforme include

Ⓐ herpes simplex infection

Ⓑ mycoplasmal pneumonia

Ⓒ sulphonamide therapy

Ⓓ systemic lupus erythematosus

Ⓔ pregnancy

29

The typical features of erythema nodosum include

Ⓐ red hot tender nodules over the shins

Ⓑ lesions disappear over 1–2 weeks

Ⓒ fever, malaise and polyarthralgia

Ⓓ oral and genital mucosal ulceration

Ⓔ predominantly affects the elderly

30

Recognised causes of erythema nodosum include

Ⓐ sarcoidosis

Ⓑ beta-haemolytic streptococcal infection

Ⓒ inflammatory bowel disease

Ⓓ tuberculosis

Ⓔ contraceptive drug therapy

31

Cutaneous manifestations of systemic malignancy include

Ⓐ generalised pruritus

Ⓑ acanthosis nigricans

Ⓒ late-onset dermatomyositis

Ⓓ generalised hyperpigmentation

Ⓔ seborrhoeic eczema

32

Typical features of melanocytic naevi include

Ⓐ usually present from birth

Ⓑ development after the age of 40 years

Ⓒ junctional naevi are smooth, papillomatous, hairy nodules

Ⓓ intradermal naevi are circular, brown macules < 10 mm in diameter

Ⓔ 30% life-time risk of malignant transformation

33
Typical features of malignant melanoma include
Ⓐ changing appearance of a preceding melanocytic naevus
Ⓑ diameter of the lesion > 5 mm
Ⓒ irregular colour, border and elevation
Ⓓ personal or family history of melanoma
Ⓔ painless, expanding, subungual area of pigmentation

34
The following suggest that a pigmented lesion is a malignant melanoma
Ⓐ asymmetry
Ⓑ irregular border
Ⓒ irregular colour
Ⓓ diameter > 0.5 cm
Ⓔ irregular elevation

35
In the UK, malignant melanoma is
Ⓐ increasing in incidence
Ⓑ more common before puberty than after puberty
Ⓒ more common in males than females
Ⓓ invariably pigmented
Ⓔ associated with a 2-year survival in metastatic disease of 50%

36
The typical features of seborrhoeic keratosis include
Ⓐ appearance before the age of 30 years
Ⓑ discrete irregular lesions in light-exposed skin areas
Ⓒ yellow-brown, pedunculated lesions on the trunk or face
Ⓓ lesions exhibit greasy scaling and tiny keratin plugs
Ⓔ eventual transition to squamous cell carcinoma

37
The typical features of basal cell carcinoma include
Ⓐ predominantly affects the elderly
Ⓑ metastatic spread to the lungs if untreated
Ⓒ occurrence in areas exposed to light or X-irradiation
Ⓓ papule with surface telangiectasia or ulcerated nodule
Ⓔ unresponsive to radiotherapy

38
The typical features of squamous cell carcinoma include
Ⓐ occurrence in areas exposed to light or X-irradiation
Ⓑ arise from malignant transformation of the Langerhans cells
Ⓒ preceded by leukoplakia on the lips, mouth or genitalia
Ⓓ metastatic spread to the liver and lungs
Ⓔ unresponsive to radiotherapy

39
In disorders of the nail
Ⓐ koilonychia suggests B_{12} or folate deficiency
Ⓑ onycholysis is associated with psoriasis
Ⓒ leuconychia is a feature of severe liver disease
Ⓓ splinter haemorrhages usually indicate the presence of infective endocarditis
Ⓔ Beau's lines disappear faster from fingernails than from toenails

14 DISEASES OF THE NERVOUS SYSTEM

ANSWERS PAGE 255

1
In the investigation of neurological disease
Ⓐ the dominant rhythm on the EEG in health is the alpha rhythm
Ⓑ the alpha rhythm persists when the eyes are closed
Ⓒ the EEG is usually abnormal between seizures
Ⓓ the normal conduction velocity in motor nerves is 5–6 m/s
Ⓔ metabolic myopathies are characterised by normal EMG findings

2
In the investigation of nervous system disease
Ⓐ MRI is preferred for visualisation of the posterior fossa
Ⓑ MRI provides more detailed analysis of grey but not white matter
Ⓒ CT is preferred in the examination of the orbit
Ⓓ MRI avoids exposure to ionising radiation
Ⓔ inter-observer variability is low in carotid Doppler ultrasound

3
The following statements about the cerebrospinal fluid of a healthy person are correct
Ⓐ opening pressure is 50–180 mm/H_2O
Ⓑ glucose is usually < 25% of blood level
Ⓒ protein content is usually < 0.5 g/L
Ⓓ white cell count is usually < 4 mm³
Ⓔ oligoclonal IgG bands are absent

4
Dysphonia would be an expected finding in a patient with
Ⓐ myasthenia gravis
Ⓑ supranuclear bulbar palsy
Ⓒ Parkinson's disease
Ⓓ cerebellar disease
Ⓔ lesions of Broca's area

5
Dysarthria would be an expected finding in a patient with
Ⓐ bilateral recurrent laryngeal nerve palsies
Ⓑ supranuclear bulbar palsy
Ⓒ cerebellar disease
Ⓓ myasthenia gravis
Ⓔ lesion of Wernicke's area

6
Upper motor neuron involvement is characterised by
Ⓐ extensor plantar responses
Ⓑ absent abdominal reflexes
Ⓒ muscle fasciculation
Ⓓ increased muscle tone and tendon reflexes
Ⓔ plantar flexion of the great toe in response to rapid dorsiflexion of the toes

7
Lower motor neuron involvement is characterised by
Ⓐ flaccid muscle tone
Ⓑ the rapid onset of muscle wasting
Ⓒ absent or decreased tendon reflexes
Ⓓ clonus
Ⓔ weakness affecting adductors more than abductors of shoulder

8

Recognised features of extrapyramidal tract disease include

Ⓐ intention tremor

Ⓑ 'clasp-knife' rigidity

Ⓒ choreoathetosis

Ⓓ delayed relaxation of the tendon reflexes

Ⓔ delayed initiation of movements

9

The lateral spinothalamic tract of the spinal cord

Ⓐ transmits pain sensation from the same side of the body

Ⓑ crosses to the opposite side in the medial lemniscus

Ⓒ transmits contralateral light touch sensation

Ⓓ stratifies fibres from the lowest spinal segments innermost

Ⓔ crosses from the thalamus to the contralateral parietal lobe

10

Loss of tendon reflexes is characteristic of

Ⓐ proximal myopathy

Ⓑ peripheral neuropathy

Ⓒ syringomyelia

Ⓓ myasthenia gravis

Ⓔ tabes dorsalis

11

The segmental innervation of the following tendon reflexes is

Ⓐ biceps jerk—C5–C6

Ⓑ triceps jerk—C6–C7

Ⓒ supinator jerk—C5–C6

Ⓓ knee jerk—L3–L4

Ⓔ ankle jerk—L5–S1

12

The following statements about bladder innervation are correct

Ⓐ sacral cord lesions usually produce urinary retention

Ⓑ thoracic cord lesions produce urinary urge incontinence

Ⓒ pelvic nerve parasympathetic stimulation causes bladder emptying

Ⓓ pudendal nerve lesions produce automatic bladder emptying

Ⓔ the L1–L2 segment sympathetic outflow mediates bladder relaxation

13

Typical findings in cerebellar disease include

Ⓐ dysmetria

Ⓑ dysarthria

Ⓒ intention tremor

Ⓓ increased muscle tone

Ⓔ pendular nystagmus

14

Right homonymous hemianopia usually results from damage to the

Ⓐ left optic tract

Ⓑ left optic radiation

Ⓒ optic chiasma

Ⓓ right lateral geniculate body

Ⓔ left optic nerve

15

Features suggesting a third cranial nerve palsy include

Ⓐ paralysis of abduction

Ⓑ absence of facial sweating

Ⓒ complete ptosis

Ⓓ pupillary dilatation

Ⓔ absence of the accommodation reflex

16
Paralysis of the fourth cranial nerve produces
- Ⓐ weakness of the inferior oblique muscle
- Ⓑ pupillary dilatation
- Ⓒ impaired downward gaze in adduction
- Ⓓ elevation and abduction of the eye
- Ⓔ nystagmus more marked in the abducted eye

17
Paralysis of the sixth cranial nerve
- Ⓐ produces impaired adduction of the eye
- Ⓑ produces enophthalmos
- Ⓒ is a characteristic feature of Wernicke's encephalopathy
- Ⓓ results from disease of the upper pons
- Ⓔ is a recognised feature of posterior fossa tumour

18
Drooping of the upper eyelid results from a lesion of the
- Ⓐ levator palpebrae superioris
- Ⓑ third cranial nerve
- Ⓒ cervical sympathetic outflow
- Ⓓ seventh cranial nerve
- Ⓔ parabducens nucleus

19
Absence of pupillary constriction in either eye on shining a light into the right pupil suggests
- Ⓐ bilateral Argyll Robertson pupils
- Ⓑ bilateral Holmes–Adie pupils
- Ⓒ right optic nerve lesion
- Ⓓ right oculomotor nerve lesion
- Ⓔ bilateral Horner's syndrome

20
Recognised causes of impaired facial sensation include
- Ⓐ cavernous sinus disease
- Ⓑ trigeminal neuralgia
- Ⓒ acoustic neuroma
- Ⓓ lesion of the posterior limb of the internal capsule
- Ⓔ lesion of the upper cervical cord segments

21
Features of an intracranial lower motor neuron lesion of the facial nerve include
- Ⓐ inability to wrinkle the forehead
- Ⓑ increased lacrimation on the affected side
- Ⓒ upward deviation of the eye on attempted eyelid closure
- Ⓓ deafness due to loss of the nerve to the stapedius muscle
- Ⓔ loss of taste over the anterior two-thirds of the tongue

22
Characteristic features of pseudobulbar palsy include
- Ⓐ dysarthria
- Ⓑ dysphagia
- Ⓒ emotional lability
- Ⓓ wasting and fasciculation of the tongue
- Ⓔ absence of the jaw jerk

23
The following statements about the Glasgow coma scale are correct
- Ⓐ the best response to an arousal stimulus should be measured
- Ⓑ appropriate motor responses to verbal commands = score 6
- Ⓒ spontaneous eye opening = score 4
- Ⓓ verbal responses with normal speech and orientation = score 5
- Ⓔ the minimum total score = 3

24
The diagnosis of brain death is supported by
- Ⓐ pin-point pupils
- Ⓑ absent corneal reflexes
- Ⓒ absent vestibulo-ocular responses to caloric testing
- Ⓓ absence of spontaneous respiration
- Ⓔ preservation of the cough and gag reflexes

25
Typical features of prefrontal lobe lesions include
Ⓐ positive grasp reflex
Ⓑ astereognosis
Ⓒ sensory dysphasia
Ⓓ olfactory hallucinations
Ⓔ social disinhibition

26
Typical features of posterior parietal lobe lesions include
Ⓐ lower homonymous quadrantanopia
Ⓑ constructional apraxia
Ⓒ perceptual rivalry
Ⓓ motor dysphasia
Ⓔ agnosia and acalculia

27
Typical causes of papilloedema include
Ⓐ migraine
Ⓑ central retinal vein thrombosis
Ⓒ cranial arteritis
Ⓓ chronic ventilatory failure
Ⓔ chronic glaucoma

28
In the evaluation of a patient with headache
Ⓐ thunderclap headache is invariably associated with subarachnoid haemorrhage
Ⓑ patients with viral meningitis invariably display meningism
Ⓒ the presence of concurrent focal limb weakness excludes migraine
Ⓓ improvement with simple analgesia suggests tension headache
Ⓔ headache on waking suggests raised intracranial pressure

29
Migrainous neuralgia (cluster headache) is
Ⓐ more common in females than in males
Ⓑ the commonest form of migraine
Ⓒ associated with Horner's syndrome in some patients
Ⓓ likely to be cured by prophylactic propranolol treatment
Ⓔ likely to respond well to sumatriptan therapy

30
In the evaluation of a patient with true vertigo
Ⓐ short lived symptoms favour a labyrinthine cause
Ⓑ the presence of nystagmus excludes viral labyrinthitis
Ⓒ associated paroxysmal tinnitus suggests Ménière's disease
Ⓓ positional vertigo fatigues rapidly when due to central cause
Ⓔ temporal lobe epilepsy should be considered

31
Features suggesting vasovagal faint rather than epilepsy in a patient with a blackout include
Ⓐ an olfactory aura
Ⓑ confusion following the event
Ⓒ headache following the event
Ⓓ memory loss surrounding the event
Ⓔ urinary incontinence

32
In the analysis of gait
Ⓐ circumduction of a leg suggests pyramidal weakness
Ⓑ a high-stepping gait suggests foot drop
Ⓒ inability to walk heel-to-toe suggests cerebellar disease
Ⓓ difficulty negotiating doorways suggests parkinsonism
Ⓔ a waddling gait suggests proximal muscle weakness

33

Jerking nystagmus that changes in direction with the direction of gaze is

Ⓐ compatible with cerebellar hemisphere disease

Ⓑ indicative of a brain-stem disorder

Ⓒ compatible with a vestibular nerve lesion

Ⓓ typically accompanied by vertigo and tinnitus

Ⓔ likely to continue following closure of the eyes

34

The characteristic features of trigeminal neuralgia include

Ⓐ pain lasting several hours at a time

Ⓑ pain precipitated by touching the face and/or chewing

Ⓒ absence of the corneal reflex

Ⓓ predominance in young females

Ⓔ response to anticonvulsants

35

The typical features of Ménière's disease include

Ⓐ sudden onset of vertigo, nausea and vomiting

Ⓑ progressive sensorineural deafness and tinnitus

Ⓒ rotatory jerking nystagmus and ataxic gait

Ⓓ positional nystagmus usually persists between attacks

Ⓔ restoration of hearing following effective treatment

36

Typical causes of vertigo include

Ⓐ cardiac arrythmia

Ⓑ acoustic neuroma

Ⓒ vestibular neuronitis

Ⓓ gentamicin drug therapy

Ⓔ otitis media

37

Wasting and fasciculation of the tongue is a feature of

Ⓐ pseudobulbar palsy

Ⓑ myasthenia gravis

Ⓒ motor neuron disease

Ⓓ nasopharyngeal carcinoma

Ⓔ Paget's disease of the skull

38

Typical features of generalised epilepsy include

Ⓐ loss of consciousness accompanied by symmetrical EEG discharge

Ⓑ invariable presence of an aura

Ⓒ lesion demonstrable on CT brain scanning

Ⓓ induction by photic stimulation

Ⓔ induction by hyperventilation

39

The clinical features of tonic clonic seizures include

Ⓐ prodromal phase lasting hours or days

Ⓑ onset with an audible cry due to the aura

Ⓒ sustained spasm of all muscles lasting 30 seconds

Ⓓ interrupted jerking movements lasting 1–5 minutes

Ⓔ flaccid post-ictal state with bilateral extensor plantars

40

The typical features of absence (petit mal) seizures include

Ⓐ loss of consciousness lasting up to 10 seconds

Ⓑ onset around age 25–30 years

Ⓒ synchronous three per second spike and wave activity on EEG

Ⓓ later development of tonic clonic seizures in 50% of patients

Ⓔ sleepiness lasting several hours post-ictally

41

Characteristic features of temporal lobe epilepsy include

Ⓐ complex partial seizure with loss of awareness

Ⓑ hallucinations of smell, taste, hearing or vision

Ⓒ *déjà vu* phenomena associated with intense emotion

Ⓓ progression to tonic clonic seizure

Ⓔ hemiparesis lasting several hours post-ictally

42

The following statements about epilepsy are correct

Ⓐ treatment should be started following a single witnessed seizure

Ⓑ 25% of patients will have a further seizure within 1 year of a first seizure

Ⓒ trigger factors for epilepsy include sleep deprivation, physical and mental exhaustion

Ⓓ the lifetime risk of a single seizure is 20%

Ⓔ sharp waves on EEG are highly specific for epilepsy

43

A patient with seizures in the UK

Ⓐ cannot drive a private car for a year following a single seizure

Ⓑ can hold a heavy goods vehicle license if all seizures occurred before the age of 5 years

Ⓒ can drive a private car during the withdrawal of anticonvulsant therapy

Ⓓ can drive a heavy goods vehicle only if seizure-free for 5 years

Ⓔ can drive a private car if seizures have only occurred during sleep in the previous 3 years

44

The following statements about anticonvulsants are correct

Ⓐ plasma level monitoring is particularly useful in sodium valproate therapy

Ⓑ primidone is likely to cause sideroblastic anaemia

Ⓒ clonazepam is the first line treatment of absence seizures

Ⓓ sodium valproate is the first line treatment in primary generalised tonic clonic seizures

Ⓔ carbamazepine is a recognised cause of hyponatraemia

45

The management of grand mal epilepsy should include

Ⓐ hospital admission following episodes

Ⓑ return to driving after 1 year free of all seizures

Ⓒ irrevocable loss of a heavy goods vehicle driving licence

Ⓓ combined primidone and phenobarbitone therapy

Ⓔ phenytoin, carbamazepine or sodium valproate therapy

46

Features suggesting epilepsy as the cause of blackouts include

Ⓐ impairment of vision heralding the attack

Ⓑ tongue-biting during the attack

Ⓒ eye-witness account of clonic jerking movements during the attack

Ⓓ attacks aborted by lying supine

Ⓔ attacks confined to the sleeping hours

47

Clinical features of raised intracranial pressure include

Ⓐ tachycardia and hypotension

Ⓑ dizziness and lightheadedness

Ⓒ headache aggravated by bending and straining

Ⓓ behavioral and personality changes

Ⓔ sixth or third cranial nerve palsies

48

The following statements about primary brain tumours are correct

Ⓐ meningiomas are the most common type in the middle-aged

Ⓑ gliomas are the most common type in childhood

Ⓒ most childhood brain tumours arise within the posterior fossa

Ⓓ presentation with adult-onset partial seizures is typical

Ⓔ acoustic neuromas usually present in the 6th and 7th decades

49

Papilloedema due to raised intracranial pressure typically produces

Ⓐ severe visual impairment at presentation

Ⓑ an arcuate scotoma progressing to 'tunnel' vision

Ⓒ pain and tenderness in the affected eye

Ⓓ retinal haemorrhages around the optic disc if rapid in onset

Ⓔ contralateral optic atrophy in tumours of the anterior cranial fossa

50

Typical features of migraine include

Ⓐ family history of migraine

Ⓑ onset before the age of puberty

Ⓒ headache is always unilateral and throbbing

Ⓓ premonitory symptoms include teichopsia

Ⓔ hemiparaesthesiae or hemiparesis at onset

51

There is a major risk of cerebral embolism associated with

Ⓐ calf vein thrombosis

Ⓑ atrial fibrillation

Ⓒ atrial myxoma

Ⓓ infective endocarditis

Ⓔ acute rheumatic fever

52

Typical causes of transient cerebral ischaemic attacks include

Ⓐ carotid artery stenosis

Ⓑ atrial fibrillation

Ⓒ hypotension

Ⓓ intracerebellar haemorrhage

Ⓔ intracerebral tumour

53

Clinical features suggesting lacunar stroke include

Ⓐ homonymous hemianopia

Ⓑ motor or sensory dysphasia

Ⓒ facial weakness and arm monoparesis

Ⓓ isolated hemiparesis or hemianaesthesia

Ⓔ history of hypertension or diabetes mellitus

54

Clinical features suggesting intracerebral haemorrhage include

Ⓐ abrupt onset of severe headache followed by coma

Ⓑ third cranial nerve palsy

Ⓒ retinal haemorrhages and/or papilloedema

Ⓓ onset of stroke on waking from sleep

Ⓔ tinnitus, deafness and vertigo

55

The following statements about stroke are correct

Ⓐ 65% of completed strokes are due to cerebral infarction

Ⓑ most strokes are complete in < 6 hours

Ⓒ 20% of cerebral infarcts are secondary to cardiogenic embolism

Ⓓ following an ischaemic stroke, aspirin reduces the risk of death or further stroke by 25%

Ⓔ 20% of patients with carotid territory symptoms have a major (> 70%) stenosis

56

Typical manifestations of brain stem infarction include

Ⓐ pin-point pupils
Ⓑ vertigo and diplopia
Ⓒ sensory dysphasia
Ⓓ severe headache
Ⓔ bidirectional jerking nystagmus

57

Functional recovery following stroke is more likely to be poor if

Ⓐ coma is prolonged for more than 3 days
Ⓑ the stroke is haemorrhagic rather than embolic in origin
Ⓒ associated hypertension is severe
Ⓓ there is a conjugate gaze palsy
Ⓔ hemiplegia is left-sided rather than right-sided

58

Typical features of chronic subdural haematoma in adults include

Ⓐ recall of a recent head injury
Ⓑ urinary incontinence and ataxia
Ⓒ epilepsy without previous headaches
Ⓓ hemiplegia and hemianopia of sudden onset
Ⓔ fluctuating confusional state

59

Intracerebral abscess is a typical complication of

Ⓐ infective endocarditis
Ⓑ bronchiectasis
Ⓒ frontal sinusitis
Ⓓ otitis media
Ⓔ head injury

60

The typical features of chronic intracerebral abscess include

Ⓐ high fever, weight loss and peripheral blood leucocytosis
Ⓑ epilepsy persisting after successful treatment of the abscess
Ⓒ bradycardia and papilloedema
Ⓓ headache, vomiting and confusion
Ⓔ positive blood and CSF cultures

61

The typical features of adult tuberculous meningitis include

Ⓐ headache and vomiting
Ⓑ fever associated with neck stiffness
Ⓒ cranial nerve palsies associated with coma
Ⓓ miliary tuberculosis is often present
Ⓔ CSF cell count > 400 neutrophil leucocytes per ml

62

In the treatment of adult pyogenic meningitis

Ⓐ penicillin therapy should be given intrathecally initially
Ⓑ chloramphenicol therapy should be considered for penicillin-allergic patients
Ⓒ antibiotic therapy should not be given before CSF analysis has been undertaken
Ⓓ parenteral fluid therapy should be instituted immediately
Ⓔ the onset of a purpuric rash suggests drug allergy is likely

63

Recognised causes of viral meningitis include

Ⓐ herpes simplex
Ⓑ poliomyelitis
Ⓒ arenavirus
Ⓓ echo and Coxsackie viruses
Ⓔ measles and mumps viruses

64

Typical features of adult viral encephalitis include

Ⓐ acute onset of headache and fever
Ⓑ partial epilepsy and coma rapidly ensue
Ⓒ decreased CSF glucose concentration
Ⓓ temporal lobe EEG abnormalities are pathognomonic of herpes simplex infection
Ⓔ meningism

65
Typical features of herpes zoster include
A a rash that heals without scarring
B permanent dermatomal sensory impairment
C infection is confined to the posterior root ganglia
D pain is the first symptom before a rash appears
E treatment with acyclovir prevents post-herpetic neuralgia

66
Syphilis should be considered in the differential diagnosis of
A late-onset epilepsy
B progressive dementia
C stroke in young patients
D truncal or limb ataxia
E septic meningitis

67
Typical features of tabes dorsalis include
A paroxysmal abdominal and girdle pains
B loss of pain sensation of the nose, perineum and feet
C bilateral ptosis and Argyll Robertson pupils
D urinary incontinence with absent ankle and plantar reflexes
E high-stepping, stamping gait with muscle hypotonia

68
Epidemiological characteristics of multiple sclerosis include
A predominant occurrence in males
B association with HLA-A3, B7 and Dw2/DR2
C a prevalence of 1 in 2000 of the UK population
D more prevalent in the tropics than in temperate climates
E lesions within the CNS are confined to the grey matter

69
The typical features of multiple sclerosis include
A invariable progression with relapses and remission
B onset often occurs before the age of puberty
C choreoathetosis and parkinsonism
D urinary urgency, frequency and incontinence
E epilepsy, dysphasia or hemiplegia

70
Useful investigations in diagnosing multiple sclerosis include
A visual and somatosensory evoked potentials
B magnetic resonance brain scanning
C CSF analysis for oligoclonal IgG bands
D electroencephalography
E electromyography

71
The typical features of parkinsonism include
A hypokinesia
B dementia
C intention tremor
D 'lead-pipe' rigidity
E impaired upward gaze

72
Findings inconsistent with idiopathic Parkinson's disease include
A unilateral onset of the disorder
B emotional lability
C oculogyric crises
D extensor plantar responses
E impaired pupillary accommodation reflexes

73

Parkinsonism is a typical feature complicating

Ⓐ encephalitis lethargica

Ⓑ phenothiazine and butyrophenone therapy

Ⓒ Wilson's disease

Ⓓ repetitive head injury in boxers

Ⓔ methyl-phenyl-tetrahydropyridine exposure

74

In the management of Parkinson's disease

Ⓐ anti-cholinergic therapy is the best first line therapy for hypokinesis

Ⓑ L-dopa should be introduced as soon as diagnosis is made

Ⓒ sialorrhoea invariably indicates overuse of L-dopa

Ⓓ dopamine receptor agonists, unlike anti-cholinergies, do not cause confusion

Ⓔ dyskinesia is a frequent dose limiting side effect of L-dopa

75

The characteristic features of Huntington's disease include

Ⓐ autosomal recessive inheritance

Ⓑ clinical onset before the age of puberty

Ⓒ progress of dementia arrested with tetrabenazine therapy

Ⓓ choreiform movements of the face and arms particularly

Ⓔ cardiomyopathic changes on echocardiography

76

The clinical features of motor neuron disease include

Ⓐ insidious onset in elderly males

Ⓑ progressive distal muscular atrophy

Ⓒ progressive bulbar palsy

Ⓓ upper motor neuron signs in the lower limbs

Ⓔ lower motor neuron signs in the upper limbs

77

The differential diagnosis in motor neuron disease (MND) includes

Ⓐ syringomyelia

Ⓑ diabetic amyotrophy

Ⓒ cervical myelopathy

Ⓓ paraneoplastic syndrome

Ⓔ meningovascular syphilis

78

Typical features of cervical radiculopathy include

Ⓐ pathognomic X-ray abnormalities of the cervical spine

Ⓑ radicular pain in the arm and shoulder

Ⓒ painful limitation of movements of the cervical spine

Ⓓ C8–T1 sensory and/or motor loss in the upper limb

Ⓔ neurosurgical intervention is often required

79

The following statements about spinal cord compression are correct

Ⓐ metastatic disease is a more common cause than primary tumour

Ⓑ the CSF protein concentration is likely to be normal

Ⓒ local spinal pain and tenderness usually precedes motor weakness

Ⓓ urinary urgency is commonly the presenting feature

Ⓔ myelography is the best and most appropriate investigation

80

Recognised causes of paraplegia include

Ⓐ intracranial parasagittal meningioma

Ⓑ vitamin B_{12} deficiency

Ⓒ tuberculosis of the thoracic spine

Ⓓ anterior spinal artery thrombosis

Ⓔ spinal neurofibromas and gliomas

81

The clinical features of the Brown–Séquard syndrome include

Ⓐ pain and temperature sensory loss in the contralateral leg

Ⓑ proprioceptive sensory loss in the ipsilateral leg

Ⓒ an extensor plantar response in the ipsilateral leg

Ⓓ hyperreflexia and weakness of the contralateral leg

Ⓔ hyperaesthetic dermatome on the opposite side of the lesion

82

In the treatment of established paraplegia

Ⓐ prophylactic antibiotics are indicated to prevent urinary sepsis

Ⓑ pressure sores are not likely to occur unless sensation is lost

Ⓒ urinary retention usually requires long-term catheterisation

Ⓓ flexor spasms and contractures are usually unavoidable

Ⓔ constipation requires dietary treatment and regular enemas

83

The typical features of syringomyelia include

Ⓐ slow insidious progression of the disease

Ⓑ dissociate sensory loss with normal touch and position sense

Ⓒ loss of one or more upper limb tendon reflexes is invariable

Ⓓ wasting of the small muscles of the hands

Ⓔ hyperreflexia of the lower limbs and extensor plantar responses

84

Recognised features of neurofibromatosis include

Ⓐ autosomal dominant inheritance

Ⓑ café-au-lait spots

Ⓒ association with multiple endocrine neoplasias

Ⓓ intraspinal and intracranial neuromas and meningiomas

Ⓔ nerve deafness

85

The following statements about dementia are correct

Ⓐ 20% of the population aged over 80 years suffer a dementing illness

Ⓑ inheritance of the apolipoprotein ε_4 allele is associated with multi-infarct dementia

Ⓒ cerebral acetylcholinesterase inhibitors arrest progression of the disease

Ⓓ Alzheimer's disease is characterised by the presence of neurofibrillary tangles

Ⓔ associated parkinsonism suggests possible Lewy body disease

86

The neurological manifestations of severe vitamin B_{12} deficiency include

Ⓐ mononeuritis multiplex

Ⓑ optic atrophy

Ⓒ confusion and dementia

Ⓓ spastic paraparesis

Ⓔ sensory ataxia

87

Typical features of the carpal tunnel syndrome include

Ⓐ remission during pregnancy

Ⓑ wasting of the dorsal interossei and lumbricals

Ⓒ pain producing night waking

Ⓓ association with acromegaly and hypothyroidism

Ⓔ complication of both rheumatoid arthritis and amyloidosis

88
Recognised causes of mononeuritis multiplex include
Ⓐ rheumatoid arthritis
Ⓑ sarcoidosis
Ⓒ polyarteritis nodosa
Ⓓ diabetes mellitus
Ⓔ systemic lupus erythematosus

89
The patterns of sensory loss listed below suggest the following peripheral nerve lesion
Ⓐ lateral palm and thumb, index and half of ring finger—ulnar nerve
Ⓑ medial palm and little finger, half ring finger—median nerve
Ⓒ dorsum of thumb—radial nerve
Ⓓ dorsum of foot—peroneal nerve
Ⓔ lateral border of thigh—obturator nerve

90
Recognised causes of a generalised polyneuropathy include
Ⓐ bronchial carcinoma
Ⓑ rheumatoid arthritis
Ⓒ vitamin B_{12} deficiency and folate deficiency
Ⓓ amiodarone therapy
Ⓔ diabetes mellitus

91
Clinical features typical of the following polyneuropathies include
Ⓐ predominantly motor loss—lead poisoning
Ⓑ predominantly sensory loss—post-inflammatory polyneuropathy
Ⓒ painful sensory impairment—alcohol abuse
Ⓓ sparing of the cranial nerves—sarcoidosis
Ⓔ prominent postural hypotension—diabetes mellitus

92
The following findings suggest a likely cause of a peripheral neuropathy
Ⓐ peripheral blood punctate basophilia
Ⓑ atrophic glossitis and weight loss
Ⓒ hyponatraemia with urinary osmolality of 300 mOsm/kg
Ⓓ recent discovery of Kayser–Fleischer corneal rings
Ⓔ family history of neurofibromatosis

93
The typical features of Guillain–Barré polyneuropathy include
Ⓐ onset within 4 weeks of an acute infective illness
Ⓑ severe back pain and peripheral paraesthesiae
Ⓒ ascending flaccid paralysis with areflexia
Ⓓ sparing of the respiratory and facial nerves
Ⓔ normal CSF protein concentration and cell count

94
Non-metastatic neurological complications of malignancy include
Ⓐ meralgia paraesthetica
Ⓑ carpal tunnel syndrome
Ⓒ cerebellar ataxia
Ⓓ progressive dementia
Ⓔ myasthenic syndrome

95
Characteristic features of myasthenia gravis include
Ⓐ motor dysphasia
Ⓑ circulating anti-acetylcholine receptor antibodies
Ⓒ onset of the disease between the ages of 15 and 50 years
Ⓓ muscle wasting
Ⓔ intermittent diplopia and ptosis

96

In the treatment of myasthenia gravis

A pupillary miosis, salivation and sweating typify excessive therapy

B pyridostigmine therapy is best given with propantheline once per day

C thymectomy is mandatory as soon as the diagnosis is confirmed

D corticosteroid therapy produces a transient myasthenic crisis

E the prognosis is significantly worse if associated with thymoma

97

The typical features of Duchenne muscular dystrophy include

A presentation in the 3rd year of life

B calf muscle hypertrophy

C difficulty in rising from the floor

D normal serum creatine phosphokinase concentration

E death is usually due to cardiac and respiratory failure

98

Typical causes of proximal myopathy include

A hypothyroidism

B type 1 diabetes mellitus

C Cushing's syndrome

D Addisonian pernicious anaemia

E chronic alcohol abuse

PRINCIPLES OF CRITICAL CARE MEDICINE

15

ANSWERS PAGE 265

1

The following results in a healthy adult breathing room air would be normal

Ⓐ FiO_2 = 0.2 ml/L
Ⓑ minute volume = 15 L/min
Ⓒ SaO_2 = 97%
Ⓓ PaO_2 = 14 kPa
Ⓔ VO_2 (oxygen consumption) = 250 ml/min

2

The following statements about oxygen transport in the blood are correct

Ⓐ the amount of oxygen carried by haemoglobin is equal to that dissolved in the plasma
Ⓑ an increase in $PaCO_2$ shifts the oxygen/haemoglobin dissociation curve to the right
Ⓒ the optimum haemoglobin concentration in a critically ill adult male is 15 g/dl
Ⓓ at a PaO_2 = 3.5 kPa, approximately 10% of the haemoglobin will be saturated
Ⓔ increasing the haemoglobin concentration of the blood will increase its oxygen content but not its partial pressure of oxygen

3

The following statements about oxygen consumption are correct

Ⓐ VO_2 (global oxygen consumption) can be calculated from the PaO_2 and the $PaCO_2$
Ⓑ mixed venous oxygen saturation (SvO_2) is the pulmonary arterial oxygen saturation
Ⓒ SvO_2 reflects the amount of oxygen not consumed by the tissues
Ⓓ oxygen saturation of venous blood from differing tissues is identical
Ⓔ VO_2 rises 10–15% for every 1°C rise in body temperature

4

In septic shock

Ⓐ a high mixed venous oxygen saturation (SvO_2) would be an expected finding
Ⓑ blood lactate concentration is characteristically decreased
Ⓒ an increase in cardiac filling pressure induces a supranormal increase in cardiac output
Ⓓ systemic vascular resistance typically decreases
Ⓔ supranormal global oxygen delivery is not associated with increased oxygen consumption

5

The following statements about shock syndromes are correct

Ⓐ in severe hypovolaemia, a source of blood/fluid loss is invariably apparent clinically
Ⓑ in cardiogenic shock, the peripheries are characteristically warm
Ⓒ massive pulmonary embolism typically presents with shock
Ⓓ anaphylactic shock is associated with profound allergen-induced systemic vasoconstriction
Ⓔ arteriovenous shunting is a significant contributory factor in septic shock

6

Typical clinical features of acute circulatory failure due to anaphylactic shock include

Ⓐ elevated jugular venous pressure
Ⓑ warm dry skin
Ⓒ stridor
Ⓓ confusion
Ⓔ polyuria

7

Acute circulatory failure with an elevated central venous pressure are typical findings in

Ⓐ acute pancreatitis

Ⓑ massive pulmonary embolism

Ⓒ ruptured ectopic pregnancy

Ⓓ acute right ventricular infarction

Ⓔ pericardial tamponade

8

In a shocked patient

Ⓐ 250 ml of normal saline should be given rapidly indicated if the CVP < 7 cm

Ⓑ a high haematocrit suggests anaphylactic shock

Ⓒ the CVP gives a reliable guide to filling pressures in the right and left heart

Ⓓ intravenous sodium bicarbonate should be considered if respiratory acidosis is severe

Ⓔ negative blood cultures exclude septic shock

9

Diagnostic criteria for the systemic inflammatory response syndrome (SIRS) include

Ⓐ temperature > 38°C or < 36°C

Ⓑ respiratory rate > 30/min

Ⓒ heart rate > 90/min

Ⓓ white cell count > 12 000 or < 40 000/mm^3

Ⓔ $PaCO_2$ < 32 mmHg

10

In a patient with suspected septic shock

Ⓐ the lower urinary tract is the commonest source of infection

Ⓑ a normal transthoracic electrocardiogram excludes endocarditis

Ⓒ intravenous access sites need only be changed if cutaneous evidence of infection is visible

Ⓓ prior treatment with histamine receptor antagonists makes pneumonia a more likely cause

Ⓔ corticosteroid therapy is of no proven benefit

11

The adult respiratory distress syndrome (ARDS) is characterised by

Ⓐ maintenance of a normal PaO_2 despite profound dyspnoea

Ⓑ increased pulmonary compliance

Ⓒ a normal chest X-ray

Ⓓ greatly elevated pulmonary artery wedge pressure

Ⓔ elevated right heart pressure

12

Adult respiratory distress syndrome is associated with

Ⓐ alveolar oedema with a protein content 20 g/L

Ⓑ systemic hypotension

Ⓒ severe dyspnoea with rhonchi rather than crepitations

Ⓓ widespread 'fluffy' or 'soft' opacification on chest X-ray

Ⓔ thrombocytopenia and disseminated intravascular coagulation

13

The following strategies are beneficial in the management of adult respiratory distress syndrome (ARDS)

Ⓐ nursing the patient prone

Ⓑ corticosteroid therapy

Ⓒ loading the patient with intravenous fluids

Ⓓ maintaining the FiO_2 at 1.0 for prolonged periods during mechanical ventilation

Ⓔ using positive end expiratory pressure during mechanical ventilation

14

The following statements about pulmonary artery wedge pressure (PAWP) monitoring are correct

Ⓐ PAWP provides an indirect measure of left atrial pressure

Ⓑ the normal range is 15–20 mmHg

Ⓒ the PAWP is reduced in acute left ventricular failure

Ⓓ complications of monitoring include pulmonary artery rupture

Ⓔ the optimum PAWP in acute circulatory failure is 12–15 mmHg

15
The following statements about monitoring of pulmonary function are correct

Ⓐ oxygen saturation (SaO_2) should be maintained in the range 75–85%

Ⓑ the oxygenation index (PaO_2/FiO_2) is a useful measure of gas exchange

Ⓒ end-tidal alveolar CO_2 concentrations measures the effectiveness of ventilation

Ⓓ measurement of oxygen saturation requires arterial blood sampling

Ⓔ a decreasing cardiac output is likely to induce an abrupt fall in SaO_2

16
The following statements about the normal circulation are correct

Ⓐ cardiac output (Q_t) is equal to the product of stroke volume and heart rate

Ⓑ venous return is the major factor determining the afterload

Ⓒ systemic vascular resistance approximates to the pulmonary vascular resistance

Ⓓ a reduction in afterload moves the Starling curve to the left

Ⓔ pulmonary vascular resistance (PVR) = [pulmonary artery pressure minus the left atrial pressure] divided by the cardiac output

17
The expected effects of the following vasoactive drugs include

Ⓐ sodium nitroprusside—reduction in systemic vascular resistance

Ⓑ prostacyclin—increased pulmonary vascular resistance

Ⓒ isoprenaline—sinus tachycardia

Ⓓ dopamine—sinus bradycardia

Ⓔ adrenaline—increased splanchnic blood flow

18
The following statements about the management of respiratory problems are correct

Ⓐ the work of normal breathing uses under 5% of total body oxygen consumption

Ⓑ in a critically-ill patient, the work of breathing > 25% of total body oxygen consumption

Ⓒ pulmonary oedema increases pulmonary compliance

Ⓓ functional residual capacity is typically decreased in severe pneumonia

Ⓔ beta-adrenoreceptor agonists can increase as well as decrease the work of breathing

19
The following statements about artificial respiratory support are correct

Ⓐ intermittent positive pressure ventilation (IPPV) permits spontaneous breathing

Ⓑ IPPV can only be pressure controlled

Ⓒ positive end expiratory pressure (PEEP) increases functional residual capacity

Ⓓ continuous positive airway pressure (CPAP) facilitates spontaneous breathing

Ⓔ CPAP increases the clearance of bronchial secretions

20
In the management of raised intracranial pressure (ICP)

Ⓐ normal ICP is from –2 to +5 mmHg

Ⓑ cerebral perfusion pressure = mean systemic arterial pressure minus intracranial pressure

Ⓒ modest hyperglycaemia facilitates a decrease in ICP

Ⓓ temporary hyperventilation reduces ICP

Ⓔ the patient should be nursed with 30° head-up tilt

21

The following statements about mechanical respiratory support are correct

Ⓐ cardiac output increases with positive end expiratory pressure (PEEP)

Ⓑ PEEP helps correct V/Q mismatch

Ⓒ continuous positive airways pressure (CPAP) requires intubation

Ⓓ barotrauma only occurs with PEEP

Ⓔ intermittent ventilation is useful in the transition to non-assisted ventilation

PRINCIPLES OF ONCOLOGICAL AND PALLIATIVE CARE

16

ANSWERS PAGE 268

1

The histological features useful in distinguishing benign from malignant lesions include

Ⓐ the degree of cellular pleomorphism
Ⓑ the presence of aberrations in nuclear morphology
Ⓒ the number of cell mitoses
Ⓓ presence of cellular invasion into surrounding tissues
Ⓔ the number of mitochondria in the cell cytoplasm

2

Useful serum tumour markers associated with the following diseases include

Ⓐ human chorionic gonadotrophin in testicular seminoma
Ⓑ alpha-fetoprotein in primary hepatocellular carcinoma
Ⓒ carcinoembryonic antigen in bronchial adenoma
Ⓓ placental alkaline phosphatase in cervical carcinoma
Ⓔ Ca-125 in breast carcinoma

3

The following statements about the predictive value of screening tests are true

Ⓐ the positive predictive value is dependent on the prevalence of the disease
Ⓑ the negative predictive value is dependent on the specificity of the test
Ⓒ the sensitivity is inversely related to specificity
Ⓓ specificity = % patients with a positive test in patients with the disease
Ⓔ sensitivity = % patients with a negative test in subjects without the disease

4

The paraneoplastic syndromes listed below are typical of the following tumours

Ⓐ inappropriate ADH activity— adenocarcinoma of lung
Ⓑ parathyroid hormone activity—squamous cell carcinoma of lung
Ⓒ polymyositis—gastric carcinoma
Ⓓ myasthenia-like syndrome—small cell anaplastic lung carcinoma
Ⓔ acanthosis nigricans—gastric carcinoma

5

The following statements about tumour staging and response to therapy are correct

Ⓐ the TNM system defines only tumour size and the number of metastases
Ⓑ T0 indicates undetectable tumour proven only by aspirate cytology
Ⓒ functional status at diagnosis partly predicts prognosis
Ⓓ a partial response to therapy = > 50% reduction in tumour size
Ⓔ no response to therapy = < 50% reduction in tumour size

6

In the Ann Arbor staging of lymphomas

Ⓐ intrathoracic and intra-abdominal lymphadenopathy = stage III
Ⓑ splenomegaly and intra-abdominal lymphadenopathy = stage IIIS
Ⓒ diffuse hepatic or bone marrow involvement = stage IV
Ⓓ gastric and splenic involvement = stage IIS
Ⓔ pulmonary hilar lymphadenopathy with fever = stage IB

7

In the TNM staging of bronchial carcinoma

Ⓐ TX indicates positive cytology

Ⓑ T2 indicates tumour size > 3 cm and/or extension to hilar nodes

Ⓒ malignant pleural effusion would be staged as T4

Ⓓ N1 indicates extension to the ipsilateral mediastinum

Ⓔ M0 indicates the absence of metastases

8

The following statements about radiotherapy are true

Ⓐ ionising radiation damages cell nuclear DNA

Ⓑ 1 gray of absorbed radiation = 10 joule per kilogram of tissue

Ⓒ brachytherapy is radiotherapy delivered by an external photon beam

Ⓓ megavoltage teletherapy is used for skin tumours

Ⓔ hypoxia enhances tissue sensitivity to irradiation

9

The following statements about chemotherapy are true

Ⓐ methotrexate is an antifolate blocking nucleotide synthesis

Ⓑ vincristine is an alkylating agent blocking DNA transcription

Ⓒ doxorubicin is a plant alkaloid which disrupts mitotic spindles

Ⓓ taxotere is a nitrosourea which blocks pyrimidine synthesis

Ⓔ melphalan is an alkylating agent which blocks DNA replication

10

The general principles governing the use of combination chemotherapy include

Ⓐ the toxic effects of each drug should be closely similar

Ⓑ each drug should have a similar mode of action

Ⓒ each drug should be of proven efficacy individually

Ⓓ drugs used in combination should not have adverse interactions

Ⓔ the minimum effective dose of each drug should be used

11

Malignant diseases that are potentially curable using combination chemotherapy include

Ⓐ melanoma

Ⓑ squamous cell bronchial carcinoma

Ⓒ choriocarcinoma

Ⓓ oesophageal carcinoma

Ⓔ soft tissue sarcoma

12

Malignant diseases refractory to current chemotherapeutic agents include

Ⓐ rhabdomyosarcoma

Ⓑ Wilms tumour

Ⓒ testicular teratoma

Ⓓ Ewing's sarcoma

Ⓔ Burkitt's lymphoma

13

The adverse effects listed below are associated with the following chemotherapy drugs

Ⓐ alopecia—cyclophosphamide

Ⓑ acute leukaemia—methotrexate

Ⓒ cardiomyopathy—doxorubicin

Ⓓ pulmonary fibrosis—cisplatin

Ⓔ neuropathy—vincristine

14
Endocrinological therapies useful in the treatment of the malignant disorders include

Ⓐ gonadotrophin releasing hormone for prostatic carcinoma
Ⓑ thyroxine for papillary thyroid carcinoma
Ⓒ progesterone for endometrial carcinoma
Ⓓ aminoglutethamide for testicular teratoma
Ⓔ tamoxifen for breast carcinoma

15
In the management of pain in patients with malignant diseases

Ⓐ analgesia is best used on an 'as required' basis
Ⓑ NSAID therapy is particularly valuable in bone pain
Ⓒ morphine is more highly soluble than diamorphine
Ⓓ dextropropoxyphene and dihydrocodeine are equipotent
Ⓔ opiate and phenothiazine combinations should be the used routinely

16
The following drugs have clinically useful anti-emetic properties

Ⓐ lorazepam
Ⓑ domperidone
Ⓒ ondansetron
Ⓓ dexamethasone
Ⓔ etoposide

17 PRINCIPLES OF GERIATRIC MEDICINE

ANSWERS PAGE 270

1

Expected physiological changes associated with normal ageing include

Ⓐ decreased calcium phosphate content per 100 g bone

Ⓑ increased tissue sensitivity to insulin

Ⓒ reduced numbers of pacing cells within the sinoatrial node

Ⓓ increased glomerular filtration rate (GFR)

Ⓔ decreased suppressor T cell function

2

Expected neurophysiological changes associated with normal ageing include

Ⓐ cortical neuronal loss

Ⓑ cochlear degeneration

Ⓒ loss of anterior horn cells

Ⓓ increased postural sway on standing

Ⓔ wasting of the dorsal columns

3

The causes of urinary incontinence in the elderly include

Ⓐ impaired mobility

Ⓑ diuretic therapy

Ⓒ severe constipation

Ⓓ parietal lobe disease

Ⓔ urinary tract infection

4

In a patient with urinary incontinence

Ⓐ stress incontinence is characterised by the inability to inhibit the micturition reflex

Ⓑ stress incontinence is likely to resolve with bladder retraining exercises

Ⓒ the finding of a procidentia is likely to explain urge incontinence

Ⓓ the finding of a palpable bladder is typical of stress incontinence

Ⓔ the finding of benign prostatic hypertrophy is unlikely to explain frequency and nocturia

5

Drugs useful in the management of patients with urinary incontinence include

Ⓐ loperamide

Ⓑ oxybutynin

Ⓒ bisacodyl

Ⓓ oestrogen

Ⓔ indoramin

6

Likely causes of recurrent falls in the elderly include

Ⓐ accidental slips and trips

Ⓑ postural hypotension

Ⓒ vasovagal syncope

Ⓓ Parkinson's disease

Ⓔ drop attacks

7

Susceptibility to hypothermia in healthy elderly individuals is associated with

Ⓐ an increased core-skin temperature gradient

Ⓑ reduced ability to detect small changes in room temperature

Ⓒ an impaired ability to shiver effectively in response to cooling

Ⓓ impaired cellular responses to thyroid hormones

Ⓔ impaired thermoregulation due to autonomic dysfunction

8
When compared to healthy young people, elderly patients with recurrent falls have

Ⓐ reduced variability of step length
Ⓑ reduced step frequency
Ⓒ increased step width
Ⓓ increased step length
Ⓔ greater anteroposterior sway in women than in men

9
Typical features of acute confusional states include

Ⓐ impaired consciousness particularly in the evening
Ⓑ impaired attention, concentration and speed of thought
Ⓒ impaired memory, registration, recall and retention
Ⓓ illusions, hallucinations and delusions
Ⓔ anxiety, irritability and depression

10
Acute confusion in the elderly is likely to be the result of

Ⓐ adverse drug reaction
Ⓑ hypothermia
Ⓒ bronchopneumonia
Ⓓ myocardial infarction
Ⓔ cerebral infarction

11
Typical features of dementia include

Ⓐ loss of intellectual function without impaired consciousness
Ⓑ impairment of judgement, abstract thought and problem-solving
Ⓒ impairment of long-term memory without loss of short-term memory
Ⓓ personality change with disinhibition and loss of social awareness
Ⓔ psychomotor retardation, anxiety and depression

12
Recurrent dizziness in the elderly is likely to be the result of

Ⓐ adverse drug reaction
Ⓑ postural hypotension
Ⓒ Ménière's disease
Ⓓ vertebrobasilar insufficiency
Ⓔ sick sinus syndrome

18 PRINCIPLES OF MEDICAL PSYCHIATRY

ANSWERS PAGE 272

1
Prevalence rates of psychiatric illness in the UK include
Ⓐ 5% of the general adult population
Ⓑ 75% of patients attending their general practitioner
Ⓒ 25% of patients attending a hospital outpatient clinic
Ⓓ 25% of patients admitted to general medical wards
Ⓔ schizophrenia in 5% of the population

2
Aetiological factors in psychiatric illness include
Ⓐ family history of psychiatric illness
Ⓑ parental loss or disharmony in childhood
Ⓒ stressful life events and difficulties
Ⓓ chronic physical ill-health
Ⓔ social isolation

3
Important factors in the assessment of mental state include
Ⓐ appearance and behaviour
Ⓑ mood state
Ⓒ speech and thought content
Ⓓ abnormal perceptions and beliefs
Ⓔ cognitive function

4
Intellectual impairment should be suspected in the presence of
Ⓐ disordered thought content
Ⓑ auditory hallucination
Ⓒ inappropriate optimism and elation
Ⓓ disorientation in time and place
Ⓔ impaired serial 7s test and arithmetic ability

5
The following psychiatric definitions are true
Ⓐ delusions—unreasonably persistent, firmly-held, false beliefs
Ⓑ illusions—abnormal perceptions of normal external stimuli
Ⓒ hallucinations—abnormal perceptions without external stimuli
Ⓓ depersonalisation—perception of altered reality
Ⓔ phobia—abnormal fear leading to avoidance behaviour

6
Cardinal elements in behavioural therapy include
Ⓐ systematic desensitisation
Ⓑ flooding
Ⓒ operant conditioning
Ⓓ exploration of repressed unpleasant experiences
Ⓔ modification of negative patterns of thinking

7
Cardinal elements in cognitive therapy include
Ⓐ restructuring psychological conflicts and behaviour
Ⓑ identification of negative patterns of automatic thoughts
Ⓒ awareness of connections between thoughts, mood and behaviour
Ⓓ reorientation of negative views of the past, present and future
Ⓔ personality assessment and transactional analysis

8

The following statements about psychiatric drug treatments are true

Ⓐ risperidone selectively blocks dopamine receptors more than serotonin receptors

Ⓑ tricyclic antidepressants block synaptic reuptake of noradrenaline and serotonin

Ⓒ the adverse effects of tricyclic antidepressants result from their anticholinergic effects

Ⓓ monoamine oxidase inhibitors are more potent antidepressants than tricyclics

Ⓔ lithium carbonate inhibits catechol-*O*-methyltransferase to prevent recurrent depression

9

The following statements about antipsychotic drugs are true

Ⓐ phenothiazines block central nervous dopamine D_2 receptors

Ⓑ dystonia and dyskinesia are attributable to cholinergic side-effects

Ⓒ long-term ocular complications include corneal and lenticular opacities

Ⓓ galactorrhoea suggests an alternative explanation rather than an adverse drug effect

Ⓔ patients prescribed clozapine therapy should have monitoring of the full blood count

10

The typical features of depression include

Ⓐ depressed mood for most of the day

Ⓑ insomnia or hypersomnia

Ⓒ loss of pleasure, self-esteem and hope

Ⓓ loss of energy, libido and interest

Ⓔ psychomotor retardation and suicidal thoughts

11

Clinical features of generalised anxiety disorders include

Ⓐ feelings of worthlessness and excessive guilt

Ⓑ depersonalisation and derealisation

Ⓒ feelings of apprehension and impending disaster

Ⓓ breathlessness, dizziness, sweating and palpitation

Ⓔ claustrophobia and agoraphobia

12

Diseases mimicking anxiety disorders include

Ⓐ alcohol withdrawal

Ⓑ hyperthyroidism

Ⓒ hypoglycaemia

Ⓓ temporal lobe epilepsy

Ⓔ phaeochromocytoma

13

Alcohol abuse should be suspected in patients presenting with

Ⓐ painless diarrhoea and/or vomiting

Ⓑ atrial fibrillation and/or hypertension

Ⓒ weight gain and/or gout

Ⓓ peripheral neuropathy and/or epilepsy

Ⓔ infertility and/or insomnia

14

The typical features of alcohol dependence include

Ⓐ expansion of the drinking repertoire

Ⓑ increasing tolerance to alcohol *initially?,*

Ⓒ subjective compulsion to drink *but*

Ⓓ use of alcohol to relieve withdrawal *dramatically*
symptoms *↓ later in*

Ⓔ recurrent withdrawal symptoms *disorder*

15
The typical features of alcohol withdrawal include
A early-morning waking with anxiety and tremor
B visual or auditory hallucinations
C amnesia and epileptic seizures
D depression and morbid jealousy
E ataxia, nystagmus and ophthalmoplegia

16
Recognised features of benzodiazepine withdrawal include
A heightened sensory perception
B hallucinations and delusions
C epilepsy and ataxia
D manic-depressive-like disorder
E poverty of ideas and speech

17
Typical features of dissociative disorder include
A conscious attempt to manipulate and/or malinger
B previous history of multiple recurrent somatic complaints
C co-existent disease of the nervous system
D gait disturbance or sensory or motor disorder in the limbs
E pseudo-seizures, blindness or aphonia

18
Typical features of the following somatisation disorders include
A repeated medical consultations for unexplained physical symptoms
B morbid preoccupation with the possibility of physical illness in hypochondriacal disorder
C irritable bowel syndrome in patients with somatoform autonomic dysfunction
D severe persistent pain in patients with somatoform pain disorder
E association with abnormal illness behaviour from childhood

19
Typical features of anorexia nervosa include
A only adolescent girls are affected
B amenorrhoea or loss of libido > 3 months
C weight loss > 25% or weight < 25% below normal
D normal perception of body weight and image
E retardation of physical sexual development

20
Typical features of bulimia nervosa include
A age of onset at puberty
B dramatic weight loss
C lack of control of binge-eating
D self-induced vomiting and purgation
E hospital admission required to control the disorder

21
Factors associated with recurrent attempted suicide include
A female sex
B socioeconomic status
C social deprivation
D loss of a parent in childhood
E sexual abuse in childhood

22
Factors associated with a higher suicide risk following attempted suicide include
A females aged < 45 years
B self-poisoning rather than more violent methods of self-harm
C absence of a suicide note or previous suicide attempts
D chronic physical or psychiatric illness
E living alone and/or recently separated from partner

23

Psychiatric illness rather than an organic brain disorder is suggested by

Ⓐ onset for the first time at the age of 55

Ⓑ a family history of major psychiatric illness

Ⓒ no previous history of psychiatric illness

Ⓓ recent occurrence of a major adverse life event

Ⓔ episodes of dysphasia and impaired short-term memory

24

Under the provisions of the Mental Health Act, 1983 (England and Wales)

Ⓐ the signatures of one doctor and a relative/social worker are required under section 4 in order to secure an emergency admission lasting for up to 72 hours

Ⓑ the signatures of two doctors and a relative/social worker are required under section 2 in order to secure admission for assessment and treatment lasting for up to 28 days

Ⓒ the signature of only the doctor in charge is required under section 5 in order to detain a patient in hospital for up to 72 hours

Ⓓ the signature of a nurse of REM status is required under section 5 in order to detain a patient in hospital for up to 6 hours

Ⓔ the signature of a policeman is required under section 136 in order to secure an emergency admission of a person for a 72-hour period of assessment, if they are found in a public place and thought to be mentally ill and in need of safety

25

Authorisation for hospital detention of a mentally ill patient under the provisions of the Mental Health (Scotland) Act 1984 requires the signature of

Ⓐ the doctor in charge under section 25 lasting for 72 hours

Ⓑ one nurse of RMN status under section 25 lasting for 2 hours

Ⓒ two doctors and a relative under section 18 for non-urgent admission for up to 6 months

Ⓓ one doctor and a relative under section 26 for treatment lasting up to 28 days

Ⓔ a policeman can detain a person thought to be mentally ill and in need of safety for a 72-hour period of assessment under section 118

19 PRINCIPLES OF DRUG THERAPY AND MANAGEMENT OF POISONING

ANSWERS PAGE 275

1
The following statements about drug metabolism are true

Ⓐ apparent volume of distribution = volume of total body water

Ⓑ first order elimination = exponential decline in plasma drug concentration

Ⓒ drug clearance = amount of the drug removed from plasma per hour

Ⓓ first-pass elimination = pre-systemic elimination of drugs after absorption

Ⓔ bioavailability = amount of the drug bound to specific receptors

2
The following statements about pharmacokinetics are true

Ⓐ 50% of steady-state concentration is achieved in one half-life

Ⓑ the plasma half-life = plasma elimination half-life

Ⓒ steady state is achieved after approximately five half-lives

Ⓓ urinary excretion is increased when the drug is in a non-ionised state

Ⓔ plasma drug concentrations are greater after i.v. than after oral administration

3
The following statements about drug absorption are true

Ⓐ the rate of oral drug absorption is reduced if nausea or pain are present

Ⓑ only 10% of drugs given by pressurised aerosols reach the lungs

Ⓒ buccal and transdermal routes avoid first-pass hepatic metabolism

Ⓓ rectal administration avoids pre-systemic hepatic elimination

Ⓔ drug absorption within the stomach is enhanced by food or alcohol

4
The following examples of pharmacokinetic variability are true

Ⓐ lipid-soluble drug bioavailability is enhanced by food

Ⓑ chronic liver disease reduces the bioavailability of propranolol

Ⓒ hypoalbuminaemia decreases drug concentrations in the free unbound form

Ⓓ impaired neonatal glucuronidation increases chloramphenicol toxicity

Ⓔ amoxicillin therapy increases plasma concentrations of oral contraceptives

5
Examples of pharmacokinetic interactions include

Ⓐ allopurinol inhibits the metabolism of azathioprine

Ⓑ amitriptyline delays gastric emptying and the rate of drug absorption

Ⓒ digoxin and verapamil compete for renal tubular secretion

Ⓓ effect of methotrexate is inhibited by NSAID therapy

Ⓔ antibiotics alter gut flora, disrupting enterohepatic drug cycling

6
The following drugs inhibit drug metabolism by reducing hepatic enzyme activities

Ⓐ carbamazepine

Ⓑ ciprofloxacin

Ⓒ metronidazole

Ⓓ allopurinol

Ⓔ erythromycin

7
The following drugs should be avoided in moderate or severe renal failure
- Ⓐ gentamicin
- Ⓑ oxytetracycline
- Ⓒ morphine
- Ⓓ mesalazine
- Ⓔ metformin

8
The following drugs exhibit high rates of hepatic clearance
- Ⓐ codeine phosphate
- Ⓑ diazepam
- Ⓒ simvastatin
- Ⓓ propranolol
- Ⓔ warfarin

9
The actions of the following drugs are enhanced in liver disease
- Ⓐ warfarin
- Ⓑ metformin
- Ⓒ chloramphenicol
- Ⓓ sulphonylureas
- Ⓔ naproxen

10
The following statements about drug prescribing in elderly patients are true
- Ⓐ the error rate in patients taking prescribed drugs is similar to that found in younger adults
- Ⓑ adverse drug reactions are more likely to occur than in younger adults
- Ⓒ an increased proportion of body fat increases the accumulation of lipid-soluble drugs
- Ⓓ drug excretion is typically increased due to impaired urinary concentrating ability
- Ⓔ drug metabolism of paracetamol reduces with advancing age

11
The following are statutory requirements for the prescription for controlled drugs
- Ⓐ prescriptions must be typewritten not written by hand
- Ⓑ prescriptions must specify the patient's name and address
- Ⓒ prescriptions must specify the prescriber's name and address
- Ⓓ prescriptions must state the dosage in both words and numbers
- Ⓔ prescriptions must be signed and dated by the prescriber

12
The following statements about non-accidental self-poisoning are true
- Ⓐ at least 30% of episodes involve more than one drug (excluding alcohol)
- Ⓑ 50% of episodes are associated with alcohol intoxication
- Ⓒ most patients are intent on suicide and do not plan to survive
- Ⓓ the majority of patients are middle-aged or elderly
- Ⓔ the majority of patients repeat self-poisoning within 12 months

13
Clinical features suggestive of self-poisoning include
- Ⓐ coma in patients under the age of 35 years
- Ⓑ strabismus and nystagmus in young patients
- Ⓒ evidence of self-injury (e.g. scars on the forearms)
- Ⓓ evidence of needle tracks
- Ⓔ circumoral acneiform rash

14

Immediate measures in the management of self-poisoning include

Ⓐ identification of the ingested poison
Ⓑ maintenance of the airway and respiratory function
Ⓒ maintenance of blood pressure and circulatory function
Ⓓ induction of vomiting by salt water
Ⓔ use of specific antagonists in comatose patients

15

The following statements about gut decontamination in poisoned patients are true

Ⓐ gastric lavage is indicated in most patients with self-poisoning
Ⓑ the position of the lavage tube should be checked under X-ray control
Ⓒ in comatose patients, endotracheal intubation must precede lavage
Ⓓ patients should be given syrup of ipecacuanha if gastric lavage is refused
Ⓔ conscious patients should be given activated charcoal by mouth

16

The use of oral activated charcoal is indicated following poisoning with

Ⓐ paracetamol
Ⓑ acetyl salicylic acid
Ⓒ ferrous sulphate
Ⓓ ethylene glycol
Ⓔ lithium carbonate

17

The treatments listed below are clinically useful in poisoning with the following

Ⓐ forced alkaline diuresis—salicylates
Ⓑ dimercaprol—heavy metal poisons
Ⓒ flumazenil—opioid analgesics
Ⓓ N-acetylcysteine—paracetamol
Ⓔ desferrioxamine—iron salts

18

Typical features 6–8 hours after paracetamol poisoning include

Ⓐ nausea and vomiting
Ⓑ coma and internuclear ophthalmoplegia
Ⓒ prolongation of the prothrombin time
Ⓓ metabolic acidosis and hypoglycaemia
Ⓔ prevention of liver damage with N-acetylcysteine therapy

19

Typical features 8 hours after salicylate poisoning in an adult include

Ⓐ coma and dilated pupils in adults
Ⓑ deafness, tinnitus and blurred vision
Ⓒ hypokalaemia and respiratory alkalosis
Ⓓ hyperventilation, sweating and restlessness
Ⓔ an empty stomach before gastric lavage

20

Typical features following benzodiazepine poisoning include

Ⓐ ataxia, dysarthria, nystagmus and drowsiness
Ⓑ severe systemic hypotension and respiratory depression
Ⓒ nausea, vomiting and diarrhoea
Ⓓ convulsions, muscle spasms and papilloedema
Ⓔ resolution of symptoms and signs within < 12 hours of poisoning

21

Typical features following amphetamine poisoning include

Ⓐ restlessness and excitement
Ⓑ bradycardia and hypotension
Ⓒ skin blisters on dependent areas
Ⓓ paranoid delusions and hallucinations
Ⓔ non-cardiogenic pulmonary oedema

22

Typical features following tricyclic antidepressant poisoning include

Ⓐ coma, hyperreflexia and extensor plantar responses

Ⓑ warm, dry skin and dry mouth

Ⓒ pin-point pupils

Ⓓ hallucinations and urinary retention

Ⓔ convulsions and cardiac tachyarrhythmias

23

Poisoning with drugs containing dextropropoxyphene produces

Ⓐ hyperventilation and agitation

Ⓑ coma with pin-point pupils and hypotonia

Ⓒ hypotension and hypothermia

Ⓓ high plasma paracetamol concentration

Ⓔ absence of a response to naloxone therapy

24

Typical features of morphine poisoning include

Ⓐ nausea, vomiting and pallor

Ⓑ coma with widely-dilated pupils

Ⓒ hypoventilation and respiratory arrest

Ⓓ hypotension and hypothermia

Ⓔ non-cardiac pulmonary oedema

25

Typical features of elemental iron poisoning include

Ⓐ nausea, vomiting and abdominal pain

Ⓑ tachypnoea and tachycardia

Ⓒ acute gastrointestinal haemorrhage

Ⓓ encephalopathy and circulatory failure

Ⓔ upper gastrointestinal obstruction presenting 6 weeks post-ingestion

26

Typical features of lithium carbonate poisoning include

Ⓐ nausea, vomiting and diarrhoea

Ⓑ ataxia, vertigo and muscle rigidity

Ⓒ prompt response to oral activated charcoal therapy

Ⓓ hypernatraemia and hypokalaemia

Ⓔ prolongation of the QRS and QT intervals and AV block on ECG

27

Typical features of carbon monoxide poisoning include

Ⓐ nausea, vomiting and constipation

Ⓑ marked central cyanosis

Ⓒ hypotension and myocardial ischaemia

Ⓓ cognitive impairment and personality changes following recovery

Ⓔ parkinsonian features following recovery

28

Findings consistent with ethanol poisoning include

Ⓐ dysarthria, ataxia and nystagmus

Ⓑ hypoglycaemia

Ⓒ hypothermia

Ⓓ hyponatraemia and metabolic acidosis

Ⓔ aspiration pneumonia

29

Methanol poisoning characteristically produces

Ⓐ the features of ethanol intoxication

Ⓑ abdominal pain, vomiting and convulsions

Ⓒ fixed dilated pupils and papilloedema

Ⓓ severe metabolic acidosis due to lactic acid

Ⓔ severe toxicity only in volumes > 100 ml

30

In ethylene glycol poisoning

Ⓐ toxicity is primarily due to ethylene glycol rather than its metabolites

Ⓑ papilloedema and ophthalmoplegia are typical features

Ⓒ lactic acidosis and renal failure frequently develop

Ⓓ hypokalaemia and hypercalcaemia are typical

Ⓔ treatment with alcohol may be valuable

PART 2
ANSWERS

1 THE MOLECULAR AND CELLULAR BASIS OF DISEASE

1
- **A** T In addition there are 2 X chromosomes in females and 1 X and 1 Y in males
- **B** T In contrast to somatic cell nuclei which are diploid
- **C** F Haploid male cell (sperm) may contain an X or a Y chromosome
- **D** F Occurs during meiosis
- **E** F One X chromosome is inactive and appears as the Barr body in the nucleus

2
- **A** T The most common form of numerical chromosome aberration
- **B** T
- **C** T Liveborn frequency is 0.6%
- **D** F Gene expression can be affected by the parental origin of the abnormal chromosome
- **E** T No genetic material is lost

3
- **A** T The anticodon is the complementary sequence to a triplet codon
- **B** T There are 20 amino acids in total
- **C** T In the large 60S ribosomal subunit
- **D** F There are only three stop codons
- **E** T The start codon is AUG

4
- **A** F 10^{-9} to 10^{-12}
- **B** F May be repaired before replication
- **C** T Resulting from a failure to correct deaminated cytosine
- **D** T As may pyrimidine dimerisation
- **E** T

5
- **A** T Defines the eukaryotic state
- **B** T In addition to protein synthesis
- **C** F Golgi apparatus has a role in protein metabolism
- **D** T Which may change as cells age
- **E** T Reflecting their critical role in aerobic metabolism

6
- **A** T The small ribosomal subunit is responsible for mRNA binding
- **B** T Protein degradation also occurs within lysosomes
- **C** T Although conformation cannot currently be accurately predicted
- **D** T
- **E** T

7
- **A** F During the S (synthetic) phase
- **B** F They are joined at the centromere
- **C** T Once in mitosis
- **D** T There may be several chiasmata per chromosomal pair
- **E** T And may relate to a cell's finite capacity to divide

8
- **A** F Small lipid soluble molecules can move in such a manner
- **B** F Transport against gradients is possible
- **C** F They may open only in response to a specific signal
- **D** T Partly dependent on polymerisation of filamentous actin
- **E** F Facilitates sodium influx

9

Ⓐ F Signalling cascades converge on common pathways limiting cellular responses

Ⓑ T Important in the development of tolerance to some drugs

Ⓒ T Also control movement of larger molecules (e.g. cholesterol)

Ⓓ T And convert ATP

Ⓔ T Rendering a molecule enzymatically active as a kinase

10

Ⓐ T Via phosphorylation

Ⓑ F If this checkpoint is missed, DNA repair may not occur

Ⓒ T An actively regulated process

Ⓓ T But in some cells (e.g. thymocytes) can occur during any phase

Ⓔ F Apoptotic cells are engulfed by local macrophages

11

Ⓐ T Epstein–Barr virus

Ⓑ T Human papillomavirus

Ⓒ F

Ⓓ T Herpesvirus 8

Ⓔ F

12

Ⓐ F They are genes which facilitate neoplastic growth

Ⓑ T Proto-oncogenes (e.g. *erbB* in breast carcinoma)

Ⓒ T Loss of a 'tumour suppressor' gene

Ⓓ F Decline in apoptosis may allow malignant transformation (e.g. *APC* in colon cancer)

Ⓔ T But often require two, especially if the oncogene works via loss of tumour suppression

13

Ⓐ T Perhaps due to synthesis of a growth factor

Ⓑ T Apoptosis may also become less frequent

Ⓒ T Promoting polyploidy

Ⓓ T

Ⓔ T Facilitating malignant tissue growth

14

Ⓐ F 6 hours

Ⓑ T They are highly responsive to chemotactic mediators such as IL-8

Ⓒ F They have a critical role in the orchestration of the inflammatory response

Ⓓ F Parasitic infection

Ⓔ T Via e.g. fibroblast growth factor

15

Ⓐ T Acute inflammatory tissue injury

Ⓑ F

Ⓒ T Chronic allergic infiltrate with lymphocytes and eosinophils

Ⓓ T

Ⓔ T Chronic inflammatory response with lymphocytes and macrophages

16

Ⓐ F Within 2 hours

Ⓑ T Starting at 6 hours

Ⓒ F Vasodilatation occurs secondary to cytokine formation

Ⓓ T E.g. LFA-1

Ⓔ T Some also attract neutrophils via complement activation

17

Ⓐ T Particularly bacteria

Ⓑ T Also capable of phagocytosis

Ⓒ T Also activated by interferons

Ⓓ T Opsonisation facilitates phagocytosis

Ⓔ T Also induces T cell proliferation

18
- **Ⓐ F** Large granular lymphocytes
- **Ⓑ T** And cells which act as mediators of delayed hypersensitivity
- **Ⓒ T** E.g. via production of interleukin-4
- **Ⓓ T** Possess the CD4 marker
- **Ⓔ F** Amplifies T cell proliferation

19
- **Ⓐ F** B lymphocytes
- **Ⓑ T** And in the respiratory tract and other mucosae
- **Ⓒ T** Responsible for fetal passive immunity
- **Ⓓ F** Only 20%, IgG = 70%+
- **Ⓔ T** Involved in B lymphocyte maturation and regulation

20
- **Ⓐ T**
- **Ⓑ F** A function of IgM predominantly
- **Ⓒ T** IgG also fixes complement
- **Ⓓ F** No direct defensive role
- **Ⓔ F** This is a function of IgD

21
- **Ⓐ T** Attracted by T cell eosinophilic chemotactic factor
- **Ⓑ T** Most severe when antigen injected
- **Ⓒ T** Many vasoactive products are released
- **Ⓓ T** Preferably i.m.; used in lower doseage i.v.
- **Ⓔ F** Can be induced by cold or local skin trauma

22
- **Ⓐ T** Specific T_{DTH} lymphocytes are involved
- **Ⓑ F** Intracellular location (e.g. tuberculosis, leprosy, syphilis)
- **Ⓒ T** Granulomatous reactions such as sarcoidosis
- **Ⓓ T** Jewellery and garment clips
- **Ⓔ F** Cells are predominantly epidermal

23
- **Ⓐ T** Due to recruitment of inflammatory mediators
- **Ⓑ T** Also on the antigen/antibody ratio and the nature of antigen
- **Ⓒ F** 6–24 hours after exposure
- **Ⓓ F** 10 days after exposure
- **Ⓔ F** IgG antibodies

24
- **Ⓐ T** Also asthma
- **Ⓑ T** Also myasthenia gravis
- **Ⓒ T** An immune complex mediated disease
- **Ⓓ F** Rheumatoid arthritis is a complex inflammatory response
- **Ⓔ T** Mediated via T cells

25
- **Ⓐ T** As in older age
- **Ⓑ T** E.g. sperm in vas deferens occlusion
- **Ⓒ T** E.g. Group A haemolytic streptococci
- **Ⓓ T** E.g. methyldopa
- **Ⓔ T** Expression of MHC class II surface antigens important

26
- **Ⓐ F** Normal
- **Ⓑ F** There are no mature lymphocytes
- **Ⓒ T** But susceptibility to infection remains
- **Ⓓ T** Linked to HLA DR3
- **Ⓔ F** Not B cell-dependent

27
- **Ⓐ T** Viral infections are frequently fatal in infants
- **Ⓑ T** B cell function is normal
- **Ⓒ T** Absent circulating T cells
- **Ⓓ T** Causing neonatal hypocalcaemic convulsions
- **Ⓔ T** Fetal thymic graft can help

28
A F RNA retrovirus
B T With decreased numbers and abnormal function
C T Also show reduced responses to some antigens
D T With subsequent impaired killing and cytokine secretion
E T Antiplatelet antibodies are detectable

29
A F H_1 receptors only
B T Useful in asthma
C F No direct immunosuppressive action
D T Also suppress macrophage function
E T A non-cytotoxic effect

30
A T 2–6 months
B F Inactivated toxin is used
C T Like tetanus
D F Active immunisation
E F Contraindicated due to danger of dissemination

31
A F Cell mediated immunity is the more important
B F HLA antigen groups have the major role
C T Lymphocytes carry all class I and II MHC antigens
D T 1 in 4 in siblings
E T Graft versus host disease

32
A T Glomerular basement membrane antibodies
B T Parietal cell antibodies
C T Acetylcholine receptor antibodies
D T TSH receptor antibodies
E T Anti-mitochondrial antibodies

33
A F Mutations result in diseases, but polymorphisms do not
B F By definition, no disease results
C T
D T Or if an identical amino acid is produced
E T E.g. ABO blood group polymorphisms

34
A T
B F Parent is almost always affected
C F An equal chance
D F Unaffected children are free of the mutant gene
E F Some affected individuals are clinically normal—'non-penetrance'

35
A F 75% will carry the gene, 25% will be normal homozygotes
B F Children of either sex could be affected
C T
D T 25% chance that a single child will be affected
E F 25% chance of a grandchild being affected

36
A T
B T
C T
D T
E T

37
A T Absence of male to male transmission is a key feature of all X-linked inheritance
B T
C T If the X chromosome is inherited from the father
D F 50% of his sisters will be carriers and 50% normal
E T All the female children of an affected grandfather would carry the gene

38
- **Ⓐ F** Autosomal recessive mode of inheritance
- **Ⓑ T**
- **Ⓒ T**
- **Ⓓ F** Autosomal recessive mode of inheritance
- **Ⓔ T** As are familial hypercholesterolaemia, adult polycystic disease and Huntington's disease

39
- **Ⓐ F** X-linked dominant mode of inheritance
- **Ⓑ T** Haemophilia is also an X-linked recessive trait
- **Ⓒ F** Autosomal dominant mode of inheritance
- **Ⓓ F** Autosomal recessive mode of inheritance
- **Ⓔ T**

40
- **Ⓐ T** Like other aminoacidopathies such as phenylketonuria
- **Ⓑ F** Only congenital erythropoietic porphyria is not inherited as an autosomal dominant
- **Ⓒ T** Early onset hereditary ataxia associated with cardiac abnormalities
- **Ⓓ T** Abnormal copper metabolism leads to neurological and hepatic damage
- **Ⓔ T** Congenital defect of bilirubin uptake and conjugation

41
- **Ⓐ F** Multifactorial disorder
- **Ⓑ T** Autosomal recessive
- **Ⓒ F** Multifactorial disorder
- **Ⓓ T** Autosomal recessive
- **Ⓔ T** Autosomal dominant

42
- **Ⓐ T** In two strands
- **Ⓑ T** Rendering vaccine development more difficult
- **Ⓒ T**
- **Ⓓ T** Co-receptor variation determines disease progression
- **Ⓔ F** Susceptibility to viral effects varies

43
- **Ⓐ F** Typically over 10 years in humans
- **Ⓑ F** Predominantly protein
- **Ⓒ T** As in sporadic Creutzfeldt–Jakob disease (CJD)
- **Ⓓ T**
- **Ⓔ T** And then acts as a template for production of more insoluble protein

44
- **Ⓐ F** Peripheral blood lymphocytes are the most convenient source for chromosome study
- **Ⓑ F** 47,XX,+21
- **Ⓒ T**
- **Ⓓ T**
- **Ⓔ F** 47,XY,+18

45
- **Ⓐ F** Enzymes cleave DNA
- **Ⓑ T**
- **Ⓒ T** Minute quantities can now be detected with PCR techniques
- **Ⓓ T**
- **Ⓔ T**

46
- **Ⓐ T** This is the most common human aneuploidy
- **Ⓑ F** Only about 5% are translocations
- **Ⓒ T**
- **Ⓓ F** Most siblings will be chromosomally normal
- **Ⓔ F** Polyploidy = chromosome number is a multiple of 23 (e.g. triploidy = 69 chromosomes)

47
- **Ⓐ F** Cardiac abnormalities are rare
- **Ⓑ F** Intelligence is usually normal, but mild mental retardation may be seen
- **Ⓒ F** Affected individuals are typically tall
- **Ⓓ F** FSH and LH are typically elevated in hypergonadotrophic hypogonadism
- **Ⓔ T** A secondary phenomenon seen in many types of gonadal failure

48
- **Ⓐ F** Multifactorial disorder more frequent in males
- **Ⓑ T** Risk is greater for children of affected individuals of the less commonly affected sex
- **Ⓒ T** Presence of additional affected family members increase risk
- **Ⓓ F** In contrast with the chromosomal disorder Down's syndrome
- **Ⓔ T** Risks are higher for relatives of an individual with a more severe malformation

49
- **Ⓐ F** TSH is measured
- **Ⓑ T** Permitting genetic counselling
- **Ⓒ T**
- **Ⓓ F** Used in sickle-cell anaemia
- **Ⓔ T** Some affected subjects exhibit retinal abnormalities

50
- **Ⓐ T** 95% of patients with AS carry this antigen
- **Ⓑ F** Association with blood group O
- **Ⓒ T**
- **Ⓓ T**
- **Ⓔ T** HLA B27 is also associated with ankylosing spondylitis

2 DISEASES DUE TO INFECTION

1
- **A** F Airborne spread
- **B** T In some air-conditioning systems
- **C** T as in *Campylobacter* infection
- **D** T Particularly in the elderly or immunosuppressed
- **E** F but syphilis may be transmitted in maternal blood

2
- **A** T Amoebic dysentery
- **B** T
- **C** F Useful in e.g. brucellosis, tuberculosis
- **D** F Useful in brucella and other infections
- **E** T And also in tuberculosis

3
- **A** T From the urine of rats or dogs
- **B** F *Mycobacterium bovis*
- **C** T From lice, fleas, ticks, mites
- **D** T From ticks
- **E** F Faecal-oral spread

4
- **A** T
- **B** T
- **C** T Like hepatitis A
- **D** F Hepatitis B is transmitted parenterally and sexually
- **E** T

5
- **A** F Three times during the first 6 months of life
- **B** T
- **C** F At 12–24 months
- **D** T
- **E** T

6
- **A** F
- **B** T Also contraindicated in other immunosuppressed states
- **C** T
- **D** F
- **E** T Diminishes the effectiveness of live vaccines

7
- **A** T Inactivated vaccine also available
- **B** F
- **C** F
- **D** T Do not give to immunosuppressed patients
- **E** F

8
- **A** T Active immunisation also available
- **B** T In susceptible injured patients
- **C** T Post-exposure protection
- **D** F
- **E** T

9
- **A** T
- **B** T
- **C** T
- **D** T
- **E** T

10
- **A** T Chancres also occur in syphilis
- **B** T
- **C** T
- **D** T
- **E** F Rickettsial infection produces an eschar (necrotic sore) at the site of bite

11

Ⓐ T

Ⓑ T And Epstein–Barr virus infection

Ⓒ F An occasional cause

Ⓓ F Rare cause

Ⓔ T Due to a variety of organisms

12

Ⓐ T Common causes include *Escherichia coli*

Ⓑ F Most resolve spontaneously

Ⓒ F Avoid, may cause toxic dilatation of the bowel

Ⓓ T

Ⓔ F Reserve for susceptible individuals

13

Ⓐ T E.g. malaria

Ⓑ T E.g. abattoir workers and Q fever

Ⓒ T E.g. inland water skiiers and leptospira

Ⓓ T E.g. penicillin hypersensitivity

Ⓔ T E.g. farmers and brucellosis

14

Ⓐ T Also includes asymptomatic patients

Ⓑ F Classed as group A infection

Ⓒ F Group C includes conditions meeting CDC/WHO case definition

Ⓓ T

Ⓔ F Group A are asymptomatic

15

Ⓐ T Affects the tongue and mouth

Ⓑ T especially *Pneumocystis carinii*

Ⓒ T

Ⓓ T Sometimes with atypical mycobacteria

Ⓔ T

16

Ⓐ T

Ⓑ F Male homosexuality is the commonest risk factor in the UK

Ⓒ F Greater effect on T lymphocytes

Ⓓ F CD4 helper T cells are principally involved

Ⓔ F Prognosis is worse with Kaposi's sarcoma

17

Ⓐ F Majority occur during parturition

Ⓑ F Under 50% chance

Ⓒ T 10–20% additional risk for breastfed babies

Ⓓ F Zidovudine can reduce transmission rate

Ⓔ F Heterosexual transmission is the major mode world-wide (75%)

18

Ⓐ F Typically milder and more slowly progressive

Ⓑ T

Ⓒ F Confined to West Africa and India

Ⓓ T

Ⓔ T Fewer than the number of subtypes described with HIV 1 virus

19

Ⓐ T ELISA testing therefore widely used as a screening test

Ⓑ F 6–12 weeks or longer

Ⓒ F May have transplacentally acquired maternal antibody

Ⓓ T Sometimes used as a confirmatory test

Ⓔ T Because of delay in seroconversion in some patients

20

Ⓐ F Some are protease inhibitors

Ⓑ F

Ⓒ T But not replication

Ⓓ F As with zidovudine

Ⓔ F Survival rates improve with combination regimens

21

Ⓐ F Around 0.3% risk of transmission

Ⓑ F Around 80% reduction in risk of seroconversion

Ⓒ T And if the inoculum is larger

Ⓓ F 1–2 hours

Ⓔ T

22
Ⓐ T Also causes pulmonary disease
Ⓑ F Poor inflammatory response masks classical features
Ⓒ T And serum/CSF culture
Ⓓ T
Ⓔ F CSF monocytosis is typical

23
Ⓐ T
Ⓑ F Profuse diarrhoea, but usually with abdominal pain
Ⓒ T In about one third of patients
Ⓓ T
Ⓔ F Poorly responsive to anti-parasitic drug therapy

24
Ⓐ F Tuberculosis is very common
Ⓑ F Dry cough and dyspnoea
Ⓒ F Crackles would be unusual
Ⓓ T In 95% of cases
Ⓔ F Normal chest X-ray is found in 10% of cases

25
Ⓐ T
Ⓑ T The catarrhal phase
Ⓒ F They precede the rash
Ⓓ T
Ⓔ F Contact should be avoided for 7 days after the onset of the rash

26
Ⓐ T A togavirus
Ⓑ F Constitutional symptoms and polyarthritis are both worse in adults
Ⓒ T
Ⓓ T
Ⓔ T Greatest risk is in the first 4 weeks

27
Ⓐ T Termination should be offered if infection proven
Ⓑ F
Ⓒ F
Ⓓ T
Ⓔ F

28
Ⓐ T
Ⓑ F Infectivity is generally low
Ⓒ T
Ⓓ F Pain suggests pancreatitis or oophoritis
Ⓔ F It is usually unilateral and postpubertal

29
Ⓐ T especially HS type 2
Ⓑ T HS type 1
Ⓒ T HS type 1
Ⓓ F Varicella zoster virus
Ⓔ T HS type 1—'herpetic whitlow'

30
Ⓐ T
Ⓑ T And malaise and anorexia
Ⓒ F
Ⓓ T
Ⓔ T Especially if there is dysphagia or breathing difficulty

31
Ⓐ T
Ⓑ T
Ⓒ T
Ⓓ T
Ⓔ F Adults are more severely affected

32
Ⓐ F Usually in adults or the immunosuppressed
Ⓑ T
Ⓒ F May occur in mumps
Ⓓ T
Ⓔ T

33
Ⓐ T Especially that of dogs and foxes
Ⓑ F Average 4–8 weeks
Ⓒ T It is usually fatal
Ⓓ T
Ⓔ T

34
- **A** F Sub-Saharan West Africa
- **B** F typically via infected urine or body fluids
- **C** F Tribavarin may be useful
- **D** T In severe cases
- **E** F 3–6 days

35
- **A** F Yellow fever is a flarivirus enzootic in monkeys and transmitted by mosquitoes
- **B** F 3–6 days
- **C** F There is leucopenia
- **D** T
- **E** F Supportive therapy only

36
- **A** F Infects many other animals
- **B** F High level of antigenic shift associated with pandemic infection
- **C** T
- **D** F 1–3 days
- **E** T Occurs in children given aspirin therapy

37
- **A** F Major cause of lower respiratory tract infection in children
- **B** F Immunofluorescence of throat swabs may be useful
- **C** F Offers no protection
- **D** T Also pneumonia
- **E** F Cough is usually a dominant feature

38
- **A** T There are 30 strains
- **B** T Vesicular rash in children
- **C** T In Bornholm disease
- **D** F Together with echoviruses, cause 90% of cases
- **E** T Particularly in cerebrospinal fluid

39
- **A** T
- **B** T Fever may remit on day 4–5 ('saddleback')
- **C** T But non-specific
- **D** T Rash starts peripherally
- **E** F No vaccine is available

40
- **A** T *Chlamydia psittaci*
- **B** F *Rickettsia prowazekii*
- **C** T *Chlamydia trachomatis*
- **D** T *Chlamydia trachomatis*
- **E** F *Coxiella burnetii*

41
- **A** F Often, no symptoms occur before vision fails
- **B** T With entropion and trichiasis
- **C** T
- **D** T Oral tetracycline is also effective
- **E** F It is due to corneal scarring

42
- **A** T 4–14 days
- **B** T Non specific
- **C** T As in other 'atypical' pneumonia
- **D** F
- **E** F Tetracycline is effective

43
- **A** T Due to cold agglutinins
- **B** T
- **C** T The commonest clinical problem
- **D** T Rare complication of pneumonia
- **E** T

44
- **A** T Lice and fleas
- **B** T With widespread clinical manifestations
- **C** T
- **D** F Under 40%
- **E** T

45
- **A** T Especially butchers and abattoir workers
- **B** T
- **C** F Acute Q fever is a flu-like illness
- **D** T
- **E** F Responds to tetracyclines, rifampicin or chloramphenicol

46
Ⓐ T *Ixodes* species of tick
Ⓑ T An annular red lesion
Ⓒ T Or meningitis or radiculopathy
Ⓓ T Not in acute stages
Ⓔ T And cephalosporins

47
Ⓐ T Louse- or tick-borne
Ⓑ F Typically under 3 weeks
Ⓒ T
Ⓓ T
Ⓔ T

48
Ⓐ F 4–21 days
Ⓑ T
Ⓒ T With abrupt onset
Ⓓ F *L. canicola* infection usually presents as aseptic meningitis
Ⓔ T Mortality is 15–20%

49
Ⓐ T
Ⓑ T
Ⓒ T Warts
Ⓓ T Anogenital lesions
Ⓔ T Wart-like lesions

50
Ⓐ F Due to infection with *Treponema pallidum*
Ⓑ F Infectivity persists if untreated
Ⓒ T
Ⓓ T But may be up to 90 days
Ⓔ F Takes at least two years to develop

51
Ⓐ T Perhaps with lymphadenopathy
Ⓑ T Differentiate from viral warts
Ⓒ T 'Snail-track' ulcers
Ⓓ F Meningeal involvement is rare
Ⓔ F Cardiac involvement is a feature of late disease

52
Ⓐ F The tests are typically positive
Ⓑ T
Ⓒ T Due to dorsal column spinal disease
Ⓓ T Typically with calcification
Ⓔ F

53
Ⓐ F 2–10 days
Ⓑ T Dysuria, discharge or no symptoms
Ⓒ T
Ⓓ T With septicaemia
Ⓔ T Or cefotaxime or spectinomycin

54
Ⓐ T In about 50% of cases
Ⓑ T Less common than *C. trachomatis*
Ⓒ T Suggesting Reiter's disease
Ⓓ F
Ⓔ F Tetracycline or erythromycin

55
Ⓐ F These are seen in granuloma inguinale
Ⓑ T
Ⓒ T Tender lymph nodes
Ⓓ T
Ⓔ T

56
Ⓐ T More often herpes simplex
Ⓑ T *Haemophilus ducreyi* infection
Ⓒ T
Ⓓ T With oral ulcers, iritis and arthropathy
Ⓔ F

57
Ⓐ F Type 2 more often than type 1
Ⓑ T Healing is more rapid in recurrent attacks
Ⓒ T
Ⓓ T
Ⓔ F Shortens first attacks and may prevent recurrence

58
Ⓐ T Most commonly in children
Ⓑ T The face is spared
Ⓒ F *Streptococcus pyogenes* (group A)
Ⓓ F Suggests an alternative diagnosis
Ⓔ F Suggests diphtheria

59
Ⓐ T *Streptococcus pyogenes*
Ⓑ F Systemic upset is common
Ⓒ T The rash has a palpably raised edge
Ⓓ F More common in the elderly
Ⓔ T

60
Ⓐ T In 90% of cases
Ⓑ T
Ⓒ T Often secondary to viral infection
Ⓓ T Often complicating vaginal infection
Ⓔ T

61
Ⓐ F It does not follow ingestion of infected foodstuffs
Ⓑ T There is severe systemic upset
Ⓒ T Perhaps with renal failure
Ⓓ F
Ⓔ T Similar to scarlet fever

62
Ⓐ T
Ⓑ T Due to vasodilatation
Ⓒ F Due to peripheral vasodilation and capillary damage
Ⓓ F Leucopenia may suggest a poor prognosis
Ⓔ F Urgent antibiotic therapy after taking the appropriate cultures

63
Ⓐ F May occur in either
Ⓑ T Suggests anterior nasal infection and myocarditis
Ⓒ T Streptococcal exudate is easily removed
Ⓓ T Occasionally with peripheral polyneuritis
Ⓔ F There is rarely a marked fever at onset

64
Ⓐ F Tissue fixed toxin cannot be neutralised
Ⓑ F Requires adrenaline, fluid and antihistamine
Ⓒ F Causes fever, urticaria and joint pains
Ⓓ F Isolation is vital
Ⓔ F Recovery is complete in survivors

65
Ⓐ T
Ⓑ T A highly infectious stage
Ⓒ T Lasting one or more weeks
Ⓓ F Swabs from the posterior nasopharyngeal wall are better
Ⓔ F

66
Ⓐ T
Ⓑ T With rapid progression
Ⓒ T Septicaemia usually precedes meningitis
Ⓓ F
Ⓔ F Chemoprophylactic treatment of close contacts is preferred

67
Ⓐ F May be as long as several weeks
Ⓑ T Causing trismus
Ⓒ F They are painful
Ⓓ T
Ⓔ F Not often achieved

68
Ⓐ F Antitoxin is given intravenously
Ⓑ F Antitoxin should be given as soon as possible
Ⓒ T
Ⓓ F It is necessary to control spasms
Ⓔ T Metronidazole if allergic to penicillin

69
Ⓐ F 12–72 hours after ingestion
Ⓑ T
Ⓒ T
Ⓓ T Diplopia may be the earliest symptom
Ⓔ F Bound toxin cannot be neutralised

70
- **A** T Farmers, butchers and dealers in wool, hides and bone meal
- **B** F 1–3 days
- **C** T Painless but itchy
- **D** T
- **E** F The organism is widely sensitive

71
- **A** F 3 weeks
- **B** T And joint pains and anorexia
- **C** T But rarely
- **D** T Due to localised granulomatous disease
- **E** F Neutropenia and lymphocytosis

72
- **A** T 3–6 days or less
- **B** F Transmitted in rodents by fleas
- **C** F Bubonic plague is commoner
- **D** T The bubo is the affected lymph node mass
- **E** T

73
- **A** T Usually asymptomatic carriers
- **B** F 10–14 days
- **C** T And relative bradycardia
- **D** T
- **E** T

74
- **A** T May remain infectious for years
- **B** T Septicaemia is characteristic during the first week
- **C** T
- **D** T Especially in patients with sickle-cell disease
- **E** T

75
- **A** T Abrupt onset
- **B** T
- **C** F The rash may be more pronounced
- **D** F
- **E** F Intestinal complications are less frequent

76
- **A** F Bacteraemia in the first week
- **B** F More likely in second or third week
- **C** F Leucopenia is typical
- **D** F There are frequent false negatives
- **E** F It may suggest a septicaemic focus

77
- **A** T Salmonella has similar incubation
- **B** T A toxin-mediated food poisoning
- **C** T Or chemical poisoning
- **D** T Typically *E. coli* type 0157
- **E** T

78
- **A** F *Shigella sonnei*
- **B** T
- **C** F Faecal contamination of food and milk is most important
- **D** F Bloodstained purulent stools with abdominal pain
- **E** F Antibiotics are often unnecessary—trimethoprim or ciprofloxacin

79
- **A** T
- **B** F Hours rather than days
- **C** T Typically without abdominal pain
- **D** T Fluid replacement must be prompt
- **E** F Typically a metabolic acidosis

80
- **A** T Via ribosomal binding
- **B** T And hence nucleic acid synthesis
- **C** F Affect cell wall synthesis
- **D** T As with penicillins
- **E** T Via ribosomal binding

81
- **A** T Deposited in fetal teeth and bone
- **B** T Precipitate haemolysis
- **C** T Risk of 'grey baby' syndrome
- **D** T Rash likely to occur
- **E** F Often useful

82

A T By interfering with their cell wall synthesis

B T Resistance by β-lactamase-producing organisms is common

C T Used in combination with amoxycillin as co-amoxiclav

D F Hypersensitivity may be shared

E F Never give penicillin intrathecally

83

A F Tetracyclines are bacteriostatic

B T Causes tooth discoloration in the fetus and child

C T Except for doxycycline and minocycline which can be used in renal failure

D T Calcium chelates tetracycline

E T And coxiellae and brucella

84

A T Especially in the elderly

B T Loop diuretics increase the ototoxic risk

C T Serum levels and duration of therapy correlate with risk of toxicity

D F No anti-anaerobic activity

E F If they are given, plasma concentrations must be carefully monitored

85

A T

B F Hence less likely to disrupt bowel flora

C T

D T In appropriate dosage

E F

86

A T Especially useful in *H. influenzae* meningitis

B T Although ciprofloxacin is the drug of choice

C T Gentamicin, ceftazidime or ciprofloxacin are preferred

D F Azlocillin plus gentamicin

E F Tetracycline plus rifampicin for 4 weeks

87

A T

B F Tetracycline plus rifampicin is better

C T Active against most of the enterobacteria

D F Only moderate activity

E F

88

A T 'Grey baby' syndrome due to poor hepatic conjugation

B T

C T Typically in patients with AIDS

D T

E F Also inactive against *Ureaplasma urealyticum*, a cause of urethritis

89

A T

B T Or ciprofloxacin for meningococcal or *H. influenzae* infections

C T

D F Avoid except in combination with other drugs

E T To prevent endocarditis

90

A T

B T Used in prophylaxis of influenza A

C T Also active in Lassa fever

D T Used in AIDS

E T Like aciclovir, useful orally or parenterally

91

A T

B F The organism cannot be grown in artificial media

C F There is no risk of infection in tuberculoid leprosy

D T

E F Characteristic of the tuberculoid form

92
- **A** T Sweat glands are also affected
- **B** T Infective risk is non-existent
- **C** T Perhaps with anaesthetic cutaneous macules
- **D** F This is type 2 lepra reaction seen in lepromatous leprosy
- **E** F This would suggest lepromatous disease

93
- **A** F Infectivity is high
- **B** F Is multi-bacillary disease
- **C** T No cell-mediated immune response
- **D** F Suggests tuberculoid disease
- **E** F Macules occur, but sensation is retained

94
- **A** T Sporozoites enter the liver within 30 minutes
- **B** T
- **C** T Duration of the pre-patent period varies
- **D** F Only P. vivax and P. ovale persist in this form
- **E** F Fertilisation occurs in the mosquito

95
- **A** F They may be transmitted by blood transfusion
- **B** F Only P. vivax and P. ovale have this
- **C** F Release of red blood cell schizonts produces symptoms
- **D** F They only parasitise these cells at certain stages
- **E** F P. falciparum may parasitise capillary endothelium in some sites

96
- **A** F Onset is insidious, fever without pattern and often low
- **B** F Haemolysis is predominant
- **C** T Especially in brain, kidney, liver, lungs and gut
- **D** T Severe infection is rare
- **E** T

97
- **A** T
- **B** T
- **C** T P. malariae may persist but clinical recrudescence is rare
- **D** T Especially in P. vivax and P. ovale
- **E** T

98
- **A** T May develop many months after exposure
- **B** F Subacute course with intermittent loose stools
- **C** F Lesions are often most marked in the caecum
- **D** T Flask-shaped ulcers
- **E** F One third of individuals in endemic areas are symptomless carriers

99
- **A** T Due to mucosal ulceration
- **B** T Rarely due to transdiaphragmatic rupture
- **C** T Very rare
- **D** T May mimic carcinoma
- **E** T Especially in homosexuals

100
- **A** F Free amoebae or cysts are rarely found
- **B** F Exudate in the stool should be examined for trophozoites
- **C** T Ultrasound-guided aspiration is useful
- **D** T Or tinidazole
- **E** T

101
- **A** F 1–3 weeks
- **B** F Usually by ingestion of contaminated water
- **C** T
- **D** T Mimics other malabsorptive conditions such as coeliac disease
- **E** T Tinidazole is even more effective

102
- **Ⓐ T** Immunocompromised patients are most at risk
- **Ⓑ T** Most infections are asymptomatic
- **Ⓒ T** Termination is suggested in seronegative mothers with first trimester infection
- **Ⓓ T** Can also cause thrombocytopenia
- **Ⓔ T**

103
- **Ⓐ T**
- **Ⓑ T** Occasionally longer in *T. gambiense* infections
- **Ⓒ T** At the site of the bite
- **Ⓓ T**
- **Ⓔ T** Unless cerebral infection has developed

104
- **Ⓐ T** Also spread by infected blood transfusions
- **Ⓑ T** Infection is also associated with regional lymphadenopathy
- **Ⓒ T**
- **Ⓓ T** Megaoesophagus and megacolon
- **Ⓔ T** Established tissue damage cannot be reversed

105
- **Ⓐ T** Also spread from infected blood transfusions
- **Ⓑ F** 1 month to 10 years
- **Ⓒ F** Splenomegaly is characteristic
- **Ⓓ F** Diagnosis by examination of stained smears of bone marrow, spleen or liver
- **Ⓔ T** Pentamidine is an alternative

106
- **Ⓐ T** Secondary to initial cutaneous ulceration
- **Ⓑ F** Typically painless and not involving nodes
- **Ⓒ F** This occurs in visceral leshmaniasis
- **Ⓓ F**
- **Ⓔ F** Typically positive except in diffuse cutaneous leishmaniasis

107
- **Ⓐ T** *Schistosoma haematobium, S. japonicum* and *S. mansoni*
- **Ⓑ F** Eggs are passed in urine and/or stool
- **Ⓒ T** With local papular dermatitis
- **Ⓓ F** Portal hypertension is not seen in *S. haematobium*
- **Ⓔ T** Or oxamniquine or metrifonate

108
- **Ⓐ F** Pulmonary disease also occurs
- **Ⓑ T** Due to early egg deposition in the bladder mucosa
- **Ⓒ F** Adult worms can live for 20 years
- **Ⓓ T**
- **Ⓔ F** *S. japonicum* is prevalent in this area

109
- **Ⓐ T** And in regions of South America
- **Ⓑ T** Due to deposition of eggs in colonic mucosa
- **Ⓒ F** Portal hypertension is seen, but liver failure is rare
- **Ⓓ T**
- **Ⓔ F** The small bowel is unaffected

110
- **Ⓐ T** A major public health problem in the Yellow River basin
- **Ⓑ F** Infection is by cutaneous penetration
- **Ⓒ T** Both the small and large bowel may be affected
- **Ⓓ T** Central nervous system involvement in about 5% of infections
- **Ⓔ F** *S. japonicum* produces more eggs— infective consequences are worse

111
- **Ⓐ F** *T. saginata* is the beef tapeworm
- **Ⓑ F** Usually asymptomatic
- **Ⓒ F** But worms may seen in faeces
- **Ⓓ F**
- **Ⓔ T** Prevention is by thorough cooking of beef

112
Ⓐ T May be many years before clinical manifestations appear
Ⓑ T Usually an asymptomatic event
Ⓒ T Right lobe of the liver is the commonest site
Ⓓ F Care must also be taken during excision
Ⓔ F But further enlargement may be prevented

113
Ⓐ F Seen in the colon
Ⓑ T Worms may be visible
Ⓒ T
Ⓓ F The small bowel is unaffected
Ⓔ T Cross infection and autoinfection are common

114
Ⓐ F Food contaminated by mature ova
Ⓑ T Pneumonitis with peripheral eosinophilia
Ⓒ T Due to large masses of worms
Ⓓ F Abdominal discomfort
Ⓔ T Or piperazine or mebendazole therapy

115
Ⓐ T Producing itchy cutaneous rash
Ⓑ T With pain, diarrhoea, steatorrhea and weight loss
Ⓒ T
Ⓓ T Intensely itchy
Ⓔ T Seen in HIV

116
Ⓐ T
Ⓑ F Clinical manifestations are due to dead or dying larvae
Ⓒ T Visceral larva migrans and ocular granulomas
Ⓓ T Tissue and blood eosinophilia
Ⓔ T Or albendazole

117
Ⓐ F Results from ingestion of partially cooked infected pork or ham
Ⓑ T With local symptoms and systemic upset
Ⓒ T During larval invasion
Ⓓ T
Ⓔ T Severe infections can be fatal

118
Ⓐ F The vector is a fly, *Chrysops* species
Ⓑ F 3 months minimum
Ⓒ T Following the movement of adult worms
Ⓓ T Occasionally
Ⓔ T

119
Ⓐ T A painful bite
Ⓑ F Worms can live for over 15 years
Ⓒ T The nodules contain adult worms
Ⓓ T
Ⓔ T

120
Ⓐ T
Ⓑ F Most are non-infectious within 24 hours of antibiotic therapy
Ⓒ T
Ⓓ F Infectious for 1 week after swellings appear
Ⓔ T

121
Ⓐ F Urease levels in the gastric mucosa are increased due to the presence of HP (CLO test)
Ⓑ F HP eradication has no clinically significant effect on oesophagitis
Ⓒ T Hence concomitant acid-lowering drug therapy in eradication regimes
Ⓓ T Eradication rates are increased from 65% to 90% by therapy with these two antibiotics
Ⓔ T Recurrence rates are > 90% without HP eradication

122

Ⓐ F Zoonoses endemic in pigs, domestic animals and birds

Ⓑ T

Ⓒ T Especially with *Y. pseudotuberculosis*

Ⓓ T Especially with *Y. enterocolitica*

Ⓔ F Tetracycline or gentamicin are more useful

3 DISEASES OF THE CARDIOVASCULAR SYSTEM

1
- **A T** Typical chest pain occurring at rest does not exclude myocardial ischaemia
- **B F** May also radiate to the shoulders, arms or back
- **C F** Rapid resolution is atypical—pain usually lasts for minutes
- **D F** Oesophageal pain may mimic angina—precipitation by swallowing may be useful
- **E T** Can disappear as exercise continues—'second wind' effect ('walk through' angina)

2
- **A F** Suggests episodic bradycardia—Adams–Stokes attacks
- **B F** Nausea and lightheadedness typically precede vasovagal attacks
- **C F** Exertional syncope is a feature of severe aortic stenosis
- **D F** Elderly patients do not usually lose consciousness during a fall
- **E T** Circulatory collapse or arrhythmia in massive embolism

3
- **A T** Due to severe reduction in cardiac output
- **B T** 'Cardiac cachexia'—however, weight gain due to oedema is more common
- **C T** Due to hepatic and gastrointestinal congestion
- **D T** Diuresis is induced by adopting the supine position
- **E T** A manifestation of pulmonary congestion

4
- **A F** Supplied by the right coronary artery in 90%
- **B T** These receptors also mediate inotropic responses
- **C F** Varies between 15 and 30 mmHg in health
- **D F** Restricts electrical connections between the atria and ventricles to the AV node
- **E F** The product of heart rate and ventricular stroke volume

5
- **A F** Measured from the start of the P wave to the start of the R wave
- **B T**
- **C T** Heart rate = 1500 / R-R interval (mm) or 300/R-R interval (cm)
- **D T** Reflecting the electrical dominance of the left ventricle
- **E F** Represents atrial depolarisation

6
- **A F** 'Double peak' pulse is found in mixed aortic stenosis and regurgitation
- **B F** Found in severe airways obstruction or pericardial tamponade
- **C T** Also typical of aortic regurgitation, pregnancy and therapy with nitrates et al
- **D F** Pulsus alternans is beat-to-beat variation in pulse volume with a regular rate
- **E F** Suggests severe aortic stenosis

7

Ⓐ F The right internal jugular vein is the best manometer

Ⓑ F Measured from the manubriosternal junction (angle of Louis)

Ⓒ F Venous tone increases with anxiety

Ⓓ F The rise may be more obvious in patients with cardiac failure

Ⓔ T On inspiration, heart rate rises, JVP falls and systemic arterial blood pressure falls

8

Ⓐ F Indicate atrial systole against a closed tricuspid valve and are seen in atrioventricular dissociation

Ⓑ T Also seen in pulmonary hypertension

Ⓒ T Better termed *cv* waves are synchronous with right ventricular systole

Ⓓ T Kussmaul's sign is associated with pulsus paradoxus

Ⓔ F There can be no *a* waves in atrial fibrillation

9

Ⓐ T Measured in L/min (70/min × 700ml = 5L/min)

Ⓑ F Also by sympathetic—both have dominant vasodilating effect

Ⓒ T But endothelial-derived relaxing factor (EDRF) mediated vasodilatation occurs in normal vessels

Ⓓ F Must be >70%

Ⓔ T Others include adenosine, prostaglandins and nitric oxide

10

Ⓐ F Occurs in mid-diastole due to rapid ventricular filling

Ⓑ T Due to variations in stroke volume

Ⓒ F Typically loud in mitral stenosis

Ⓓ T Due to delayed closure of the aortic valve compared with the pulmonary valve

Ⓔ F Coincides with atrial contraction and hence cannot occur in atrial fibrillation

11

Ⓐ F Records falsely higher BP measurements

Ⓑ T

Ⓒ F Disappearance of the sound marks phase V diastolic pressure

Ⓓ F Hence the need to record and use phase V as the diastolic pressure

Ⓔ F Random BP measurements correlate well with cardiovascular risk

12

Ⓐ F Proceeds from endocardium to epicardium

Ⓑ F Produces a negative deflection

Ⓒ T Absent in left bundle branch block (BBB)

Ⓓ T Hence the predominant S wave as depolarisation moves away from AVR

Ⓔ T An aid to the diagnosis of left ventricular hypertrophy

13

Ⓐ F The heart rate is unreliable in making this distinction

Ⓑ F Suggests an SVT

Ⓒ T Suggests atrioventricular dissociation

Ⓓ F Occurs with both especially if left ventricular function is abnormal

Ⓔ F ECG complexes in ventricular tachycardia are typically broader than 0.14 s

14

Ⓐ F The CTR should not be > 0.5

Ⓑ F False negative tests occur in 15–20%

Ⓒ T

Ⓓ T Pressure gradients can be extrapolated from measuring intracardiac flow velocities

Ⓔ T Ejection fraction is usually measured using this technique

15

A F Typically, the R-R interval variability decreases

B T The commonest cause of supraventricular tachyarrhythmias

C T Important to remember when assessing 24 hour ECG recordings

D F This suggests complete heart block; sinus arrest is characterised by missing P waves

E T Characteristic and predisposes to systemic emboli from intracardiac clot

16

A F Adenosine therapy can terminate an attack but has no role in prophylaxis

B T

C T Thought to be due to atrial natriuretic peptide release

D F

E F Bundle branch block can occur during rapid ventricular rates—'rate-dependent aberrance'

17

A T Re-entrant circuit includes AV node and the accessory bundle

B T

C T Consider WPW in young patients with episodes of atrial fibrillation

D F PR interval is shortened and a delta wave is seen in the QRS complex

E F Differential effects on the normal and anomalous pathways can increase cardiac rate

18

A F A regular tachycardia

B F Carotid sinus massage slows conduction in the AV node and may slow ventricular rate

C F An ectopic atrial focus with abnormal P waves

D T

E F QRS complexes are usually narrow

19

A T

B F Underlying structural heart disease is common and promotes the recurrence of AF

C T Warfarin therapy reduces the annual risk to about 1.5%

D T Episodes of sinus bradycardia or sinus arrest may coexist making drug therapy difficult

E T Indicating concomitant AV nodal disease, a common finding in elderly patients

20

A F A greater risk reduction is achieved with warfarin therapy

B T

C T The onset of AF may precipitate heart failure

D F Cardioversion should only be avoided if the patient is not taking anticoagulant therapy

E T A common cause and left ventricular function is usually normal

21

A T The pulse is irregular with weak or missed beats

B F Often occur in and are noticed by individuals with structurally normal hearts

C F Usually become more frequent during exertion

D T

E F No beneficial effect on subsequent mortality

22

A T Often ischaemic heart disease

B T A class III agent

C F A prolonged QT interval predisposes to recurrent VT

D F No effect on cardiac rate

E F The treatment of choice in acute heart failure with VT

23

Ⓐ F Arterial pulses are absent

Ⓑ T Also consider hypomagnesaemia

Ⓒ F Do not delay—it is easier to treat early than late

Ⓓ F

Ⓔ F Cardioversion is vital—prior lignocaine may diminish responsiveness to DC shock

24

Ⓐ T Strange but true

Ⓑ F Ventricular fibrillation is the commonest underlying arrhythmia

Ⓒ T A cause of 'electro-mechanical' dissociation

Ⓓ F Adrenaline should be given intravenously

Ⓔ T

25

Ⓐ T Also advise stopping smoking and avoidance of excessive consumption of tea or coffee

Ⓑ F Ambulatory or stress ECG monitoring or electrophysiological testing may be needed

Ⓒ T More often used, however, in bradycardias

Ⓓ F Single drug therapy is preferable to avoid adverse effects

Ⓔ F Control of ischaemia or heart failure can avert the need for antiarrhythmic therapy

26

Ⓐ F Prolongs the refractory period of conducting tissue; shortens it in cardiac muscle

Ⓑ F Often converts atrial flutter to atrial fibrillation

Ⓒ T

Ⓓ F Potentiated by hypokalaemia

Ⓔ T Increases myocardial excitability

27

Ⓐ T And lignocaine therapy

Ⓑ T Calcium channel blocking effect on smooth muscle

Ⓒ T

Ⓓ F An adverse effect of amiodarone therapy

Ⓔ T

28

Ⓐ T E.g. lignocaine-like drugs

Ⓑ T

Ⓒ T E.g. amiodarone

Ⓓ T E.g. verapamil, nifedipine

Ⓔ T E.g. sotalol and amiodarone

29

Ⓐ F TOE is better but still not 100% sensitive

Ⓑ T Clearly visualised by position of probe behind left atrium

Ⓒ F 1 m/sec

Ⓓ F Fixed and free floating thrombus can be identified

Ⓔ T The modified Bernoulli equation

30

Ⓐ T In common with other class III drugs

Ⓑ T

Ⓒ F Effective in both

Ⓓ F

Ⓔ F Can be safely used in heart failure

31

Ⓐ T Conversely, a short PR interval produces a loud first heart sound

Ⓑ F Fixed PR = Mobitz type II; variable PR (Wenckebach's phenomenon) = Mobitz type 1

Ⓒ F PR intervals gradually increase

Ⓓ T Due to AV dissociation

Ⓔ F Can be narrow if the escape rhythm arises from within the bundle of His

32

Ⓐ F Pacing has no effect on symptoms or prognosis

Ⓑ F Mobitz type II with symptoms is usually paced

Ⓒ T Mortality is reduced only if AV block is the underlying problem

Ⓓ T

Ⓔ F May respond to atropine and is often transient unlike in anterior infarcts

33

Ⓐ F May result from right ventricular hypertrophy

Ⓑ F No axis shift unless associated with left bundle hemiblock

Ⓒ F Causes enhanced physiological splitting; fixed splitting suggests an ASD

Ⓓ T Causes reversed splitting

Ⓔ F **L**eft **A**nterior hemiblock produces **L**eft **A**xis deviation

34

Ⓐ T As does a tearing quality

Ⓑ T As does variation with respiration

Ⓒ T The syndrome is a form of costochondritis

Ⓓ F And oesophageal pain may also be precipitated by exercise

Ⓔ F May occur in severe pain from any cause

35

Ⓐ T Cyclical variation in QRS amplitude

Ⓑ T This is pulsus paradoxus

Ⓒ F May rise—Kussmaul's sign

Ⓓ F As little as 75–100 ml

Ⓔ F May look normal but the cardiac shadow may appear globular

36

Ⓐ T Higher filling pressures are necessary to maintain cardiac output

Ⓑ F Pulmonary artery wedge pressure measurements are much better

Ⓒ T Heart rate and contractility are increased by high dose dopamine

Ⓓ T

Ⓔ F Occasionally used when either hypovolaemia or RV infarction is suspected

37

Ⓐ F High flow oxygen in concentrations > 35% should be administered

Ⓑ T Also has a vasodilating effect

Ⓒ T

Ⓓ F Can safely be used with systolic pressures > 90 mmHg

Ⓔ F Both preload and afterload are reduced

38

Ⓐ T And hypokalaemia

Ⓑ T Feature of cardiac cachexia

Ⓒ T Due to right ventricular failure and hepatic congestion

Ⓓ F But it may exacerbate heart failure if present

Ⓔ T Occurs in 50% of heart failure patients

39

Ⓐ F Angiotensin I to angiotensin 2

Ⓑ T Converted to enalaprilat in the liver

Ⓒ F Cough is a more common side-effect of ACE inhibitors—probably due to bradykinin accumulation

Ⓓ F Omitting diuretics pretreatment minimises risk

Ⓔ T A combination which also impairs the efficacy of ACE inhibitors and should be avoided

40

Ⓐ T   Via direct renal effects and aldosterone release
Ⓑ F   Angiotensin II is more important
Ⓒ F   Usually suggests free water excess
Ⓓ F   Marked increase in sympathetic neural activity
Ⓔ T   Occurs in response to atrial distension

41

Ⓐ T   And reduces mortality
Ⓑ F   Other factors favouring thromboembolism outweigh this effect
Ⓒ F   Prognosis is unchanged
Ⓓ F   There is evidence that they reduce mortality in some patients
Ⓔ F   Has a modest positive inotropic effect in sinus rhythm

42

Ⓐ F   Both minor, non-specific manifestations
Ⓑ F   Both minor
Ⓒ T   Suggest central nervous system involvement and carditis
Ⓓ F   Erythema marginatum is the classical rash
Ⓔ T   Both are major manifestations

43

Ⓐ T   First symptoms appear at valve areas of around 2cm²
Ⓑ F   Only in 50% of patients
Ⓒ F   Produces a double right heart border and an enlarged left atrial appendage
Ⓓ F   Embolic risk over 10 years is 10% compared with 35% if atrial fibrillation is present
Ⓔ T   Mitral regurgitation is a contraindication

44

Ⓐ F   Early diastolic murmurs suggest aortic or pulmonary regurgitation
Ⓑ F   Present only if there is severe calcification and immobility of the valve
Ⓒ T   Due to right ventricular hypertrophy
Ⓓ F   Tapping but undisplaced apex beat; displacement suggests mitral regurgitation
Ⓔ F   Occurs just after the second heart sound

45

Ⓐ T
Ⓑ T   Due to pulmonary hypertension
Ⓒ F   Reduced by afterload reduction (e.g. ACE inhibitor therapy)
Ⓓ T
Ⓔ T

46

Ⓐ F   Typically causes aortic regurgitation
Ⓑ T   Due to papillary muscle or chordal damage
Ⓒ T
Ⓓ T   Classical triad of changing murmur, fever and emboli
Ⓔ T   Rare cause of an acute myocarditis

47

Ⓐ F   Early systolic click implies the stenosis is valvular
Ⓑ F   Suggests coexistent aortic regurgitation
Ⓒ T   Implies left ventricular hypertrophy
Ⓓ T
Ⓔ F   Quiet S2 if the valve is heavily calcified and immobile

48

Ⓐ T   Also Reiter's disease and psoriatic arthritis
Ⓑ T   Due to cystic medial necrosis
Ⓒ T   Typically affects the ascending aorta
Ⓓ F   Produces the 'machinery murmur'
Ⓔ T   Rare granulomatous arteritis of the aorta

49

ⓐ F Austin Flint murmur due to turbulence around the anterior mitral cusp

ⓑ F Flow murmur due to an increased stroke volume

ⓒ F A left parasternal heave suggests right ventricular hypertrophy

ⓓ T Hence the increase in pulse pressure

ⓔ F Suggests severe acute regurgitation with rapid equalisation of aortic/LV pressures

50

ⓐ F Best heard in inspiration

ⓑ F Both may cause ascites

ⓒ F A prominent *a* wave and slow *y* descent

ⓓ F Stenosis may produce a presystolic hepatic pulsation

ⓔ T The pulmonary valve may also be affected

51

ⓐ F Acyanotic unless associated with a VSD and right to left shunt

ⓑ T

ⓒ F Pulmonary component of S2 is usually soft

ⓓ T Due to right ventricular hypertrophy and stenosis

ⓔ T Post-stenotic dilatation of the pulmonary artery

52

ⓐ T *Streptococcus viridans* alone accounts for 30–40% of cases

ⓑ T

ⓒ F About 30% have no identifiable predisposing cardiac lesion

ⓓ T

ⓔ F Vegetations may be too small to be detected

53

ⓐ F Sensitivity of blood cultures does not correlate well with peaks of fever

ⓑ F Onset of therapy is best judged by illness severity

ⓒ F Total duration of antibiotic therapy is typically 4 weeks

ⓓ T Also suggests abscess or drug resistance

ⓔ T The mortality rate without surgery is high in such patients

54

ⓐ F Risk is decreased by oestrogen therapy

ⓑ T Effect is measurable within 6 months of stopping

ⓒ T Not more than 21 units per week

ⓓ T

ⓔ F Both confer increased risk

55

ⓐ F Usually normal

ⓑ F Fall in blood pressure suggests significant ischaemia

ⓒ F False negatives may occur

ⓓ F Useful in patients with convincing history but normal ETT

ⓔ F Important to exclude anaemia and valvular stenosis

56

ⓐ F But it improves the prognosis

ⓑ F Extensive first pass hepatic metabolism

ⓒ T Common adverse effect

ⓓ F A nitrate free period should be achieved

ⓔ F Nitrates, calcium antagonists and β-blockers are all equally efficacious

57

Ⓐ F No effect on mortality

Ⓑ F Used to dilate graft stenoses

Ⓒ F About 55% are asymptomatic

Ⓓ T Also useful in triple vessel coronary artery disease

Ⓔ F Spontaneous improvement is common due to the growth of a collateral circulation

58

Ⓐ F Frequently occurs de novo

Ⓑ T Should therefore be actively managed

Ⓒ T

Ⓓ F Exercise testing must be deferred until symptoms have settled

Ⓔ F Usually resolves with therapy but angioplasty and surgery may become necessary

59

Ⓐ T Due to activation of the autonomic nervous system

Ⓑ T

Ⓒ T Suggests a large infarct

Ⓓ T

Ⓔ T 15% of infarcts are believed to be clinically 'silent'

60

Ⓐ T Both could occur in response to pain and anxiety

Ⓑ F Suggests mitral stenosis

Ⓒ F Suggests an inferior myocardial infarction

Ⓓ T Suggests left ventricular impairment

Ⓔ F Suggests hepatic enzyme induction (e.g. alcoholic liver disease)

61

Ⓐ T Vascular events are reduced by 25%

Ⓑ F

Ⓒ F

Ⓓ T Limit infarct expansion

Ⓔ T Reduce mortality by 25%

62

Ⓐ F The risk–benefit ratio of thrombolytic therapy patients > 80 years is unknown

Ⓑ F More beneficial if ST elevation is present

Ⓒ T

Ⓓ F Should be administered on basis of ECG and clinical impression

Ⓔ T Much more antigenic than genetically-engineered thrombolytic agents

63

Ⓐ T 30% reduction in short-term mortality

Ⓑ T The earlier thrombolysis is given the better the results

Ⓒ T Intramuscular injections predispose to haematoma

Ⓓ F Similarly, nitrate therapy has no effect on the early mortality rate

Ⓔ F mobilisation should begin on day 2 in the absence of cardiac failure

64

Ⓐ F Only if symptoms are associated

Ⓑ F Suppressing ectopic beats has no effect on subsequent ventricular fibrillation (VF) rate or survival

Ⓒ F May respond to thrombolysis, atropine or resolve spontaneously

Ⓓ F Cardioversion should immediately follow a praecordial thump

Ⓔ T More likely to be successful than drug treatment

65

Ⓐ T Of which half occur within the first 20 minutes, often before help arrives

Ⓑ T Rehabilitation programmes can be helpful

Ⓒ T

Ⓓ T Limiting infarct size improves prognosis

Ⓔ F Late VF has a poorer prognosis

66
- **A** F Early studies established a link between mortality and a single BP reading
- **B** F Elevated systolic BP is associated with increased cardiovascular mortality
- **C** T
- **D** T
- **E** F Only 5% have secondary hypertension

67
- **A** F In contrast to coarctation of the aorta
- **B** T Conn's syndrome
- **C** T
- **D** T And pregnancy
- **E** F In contrast to hypothyroidism

68
- **A** F Suggests connective tissue disease
- **B** F Suggests coarctation of the aorta
- **C** F A non-specific finding in hypertension
- **D** F Suggests renal artery stenosis
- **E** F Suggest polycystic kidney disease

69
- **A** F Arteriolar thickening, irregularity and tortuosity are detectable
- **B** T
- **C** T Hypertension predisposes to atheroma formation
- **D** T
- **E** F Hypertension predisposes to intracerebral and subarachnoid haemorrhage

70
- **A** F Hypokalaemic alkalosis suggests this diagnosis
- **B** F Exclusion requires renal arteriography or radionuclide renography
- **C** F Urinary metanephrines are measured in suspected phaeochromocytoma
- **D** T To detect renal disease or coexistent diabetes
- **E** T Other causes are rare

71
- **A** F Occurs in many hypertensives
- **B** F Indicates left ventricular hypertrophy
- **C** T
- **D** T Papilloedema may occur
- **E** T Mortality is 80% untreated

72
- **A** F Rapid reduction is more dangerous than beneficial
- **B** F If used, the dose must be carefully titrated to response
- **C** F Sublingual nifedipine may be effective
- **D** T Such as frusemide, nifedipine or sodium nitroprusside
- **E** F They impair renal function given bilateral disease

73
- **A** T
- **B** F Smoking is the most important remediable risk factor
- **C** F
- **D** F Good evidence of efficacy in the elderly
- **E** T Excessive consumption of alcohol is a significant factor in 10–15% of hypertensives

74
- **A** T
- **B** T Common particularly in asymptomatic patients
- **C** T But rare
- **D** T Conn's syndrome is suggested by a hypokalaemic alkalosis
- **E** T May also develop during follow-up

75
- **A** F Up to 1 month
- **B** F They cross the blood-brain barrier
- **C** T Monitoring is therefore important
- **D** F Hyperuricaemia and gout may be precipitated
- **E** T

76

Ⓐ F At the left sternal edge
Ⓑ T Late systolic murmur may also occur in hypertrophic obstructive cardiomyopathy
Ⓒ F An early diastolic decrescendo murmur
Ⓓ T With a loud first sound and, if the valve is pliant, an opening snap
Ⓔ T Continuous 'to and fro' murmur

77

Ⓐ T And 20% of females
Ⓑ F Plaque rupture with secondary thrombosis and spasm
Ⓒ T Remainder to non-cardiac causes
Ⓓ T But often after myocardial damage has been sustained
Ⓔ T Predominantly a disease of the very elderly

78

Ⓐ T Reducing preload and afterload
Ⓑ F May cause vasoconstriction by blocking β_2-receptors
Ⓒ F Reflex tachycardia may occur
Ⓓ F May be a problem with nitrates
Ⓔ F No definite evidence that any class of drugs superior

79

Ⓐ F Buccal nitrates are also effective
Ⓑ F Subcutaneous low molecular weight heparin also effective
Ⓒ T
Ⓓ T Coronary artery bypass grafting would be preferred
Ⓔ F Reflex tachycardia may occur

80

Ⓐ T
Ⓑ F ECG changes are non-specific
Ⓒ T Especially doxorubicin and daunorubicin
Ⓓ T
Ⓔ T And influenza, HIV and others

81

Ⓐ T Heart failure and a small heart
Ⓑ T Systolic function is well preserved
Ⓒ T Amyloid can also cause a dilated cardiomyopathy
Ⓓ T Hypereosinophilic syndrome (Loeffler's endocarditis)
Ⓔ F Heart is usually of normal size

82

Ⓐ T But previous ischaemic heart disease may be silent
Ⓑ F Suggests a previous anterior myocardial infarct as the cause
Ⓒ T
Ⓓ F Regional dyskinesis suggests underlying coronary artery disease
Ⓔ T Non-specific

83

Ⓐ T 50% of cases are autosomal dominant
Ⓑ T Mimicking aortic stenosis
Ⓒ T
Ⓓ T Left ventricular outflow obstruction and secondary mitral regurgitation
Ⓔ F Suggests calcific aortic stenosis

84

Ⓐ F Sharp pain worsened by posture and movement
Ⓑ F Localisation and character vary greatly
Ⓒ T In contrast to ischaemia
Ⓓ F May occur in pericarditis complicating acute myocardial infarction
Ⓔ F Widespread ECG changes

85

Ⓐ T And other malignant diseases
Ⓑ T And other connective tissue diseases
Ⓒ F Coxsackie B virus
Ⓓ T Rare in the UK
Ⓔ F Causes fetal cardiac disease in pregnant women

86

Ⓐ F Left heart failure is unusual
Ⓑ T But pericardial calcification may be seen
Ⓒ F Often no relevant previous history of disease
Ⓓ T These are classical features
Ⓔ T With 'systolic collapse' of the jugular venous pressure

87

Ⓐ F With a left to right shunt
Ⓑ T Usually due to a shunt through a ventricular septal defect
Ⓒ F No shunt
Ⓓ T Right to left shunt through a ventricular septal defect
Ⓔ F Left to right shunt

88

Ⓐ F This only happens if the shunt reverses
Ⓑ F Typically presents with a murmur in an otherwise healthy infant
Ⓒ F Continuous 'machinery' murmur is typical (systolic and diastolic)
Ⓓ T A rare sign
Ⓔ T

89

Ⓐ T Frequently coexists
Ⓑ F Cardiac failure is more likely to develop in infancy
Ⓒ T A useful but unusual finding
Ⓓ T Rib notching is due to enlarged collateral vessels
Ⓔ F Left (not right) ventricular hypertrophy develops

90

Ⓐ T Due to a patent fossa ovalis
Ⓑ F Occurs late, and rarely
Ⓒ F Splitting is fixed and wide
Ⓓ T In primum defect there may be left axis deviation
Ⓔ F Surgery is indicated when the pulmonary/systolic flow ratio is > 3:2

91

Ⓐ F It is pansystolic
Ⓑ F No cardiomegaly
Ⓒ T Prophylaxis is indicated
Ⓓ F Surgery is only indicated if right-sided pressures rise
Ⓔ T Symptomless murmur is a frequent presentation

92

Ⓐ T Right-sided pressures exceed left-sided pressures
Ⓑ F Pulmonary changes are irreversible
Ⓒ F Chest radiograph shows enlarged central pulmonary arteries
Ⓓ T Classical signs
Ⓔ F May change dramatically or disappear

93

Ⓐ F There is no aortic stenosis
Ⓑ F Cyanosis may be absent; clubbing develops later
Ⓒ F A single component to the second heart sound
Ⓓ F ECG shows right ventricular hypertrophy and chest radiograph shows small pulmonary arteries and a 'boot-shaped' heart
Ⓔ F Due to adrenergically-mediated increase in RV outflow obstruction

94

Ⓐ F An increase of 30–50% in cardiac output
Ⓑ T Masking or mimicking underlying heart disease
Ⓒ T Vascular resistance declines
Ⓓ T 'Flow' murmur
Ⓔ T

95
Ⓐ F 6 weeks post-MI
Ⓑ F Treatment indicated if total plasma cholesterol is greater than 5.0 mmol /L
Ⓒ F Dietary measures only reduce plasma cholesterol by about 10%
Ⓓ T And helps select those who may require intervention
Ⓔ T Also of benefit in asymptomatic patients with left ventricular dysfunction post-MI

96
Ⓐ T Suggesting the valve is not heavily calcified
Ⓑ F May be worsened by valvuloplasty
Ⓒ F Would not influence decision
Ⓓ F Risk of embolism
Ⓔ T Or other condition making operation more hazardous

97
Ⓐ F Rest relieves but elevation worsens pain
Ⓑ F Painless ulcers suggest underlying diabetes
Ⓒ F Anaemia or diabetes may produce claudication without loss of the pulses
Ⓓ F Exercise promotes growth of the collateral circulation
Ⓔ F Anticoagulation is unhelpful

98
Ⓐ T Unopposed α-adrenoreceptor-mediated vasospasm
Ⓑ T Immune complexes form in peripheral vessels
Ⓒ T And other connective tissue diseases
Ⓓ T
Ⓔ F

99
Ⓐ T Tissue collagen is abnormal
Ⓑ T Hypertension predisposes
Ⓒ T
Ⓓ F No association
Ⓔ T

100
Ⓐ T Type A aneurysms
Ⓑ T Due to infarction of the spinal cord
Ⓒ T The pain is often described as 'tearing'
Ⓓ T Type A aneurysms
Ⓔ T Haemothorax

4 DISEASES OF THE RESPIRATORY SYSTEM

1
- **A F** Never causes finger clubbing
- **B T** And chronic suppurative pulmonary infections
- **C T** And chronic malabsorptive diseases
- **D T** Unlike in extrinsic allergic alveolitis
- **E F** Can occur in cyanotic congenital heart disease

2
- **A F** Expansion is reduced on the affected side
- **B F** Stony dull
- **C T** Often an area of bronchial breath sounds
- **D T** As is vocal fremitus
- **E F** Sometimes heard above the effusion

3
- **A T** Particularly if there is associated pleuritic pain
- **B T** But not stony dull
- **C F** Bronchial breath sounds
- **D T** With whispering pectoriloquy
- **E F** There may be crepitations alone

4
- **A T** On the affected side
- **B F** Implies effusion
- **C F** Diminished or absent breath sounds
- **D T** As for vocal fremitus
- **E F** No specific added sounds

5
- **A F** Separates middle from upper
- **B F** Aspiration is commoner on the right
- **C T**
- **D T** To around the 6th costal cartilage
- **E F** By type II pneumocytes

6
- **A T**
- **B T**
- **C T**
- **D T**
- **E F** An increase in arterial $PaCO_2$

7
- **A F** About 7.5 L/min
- **B T** Dead space ventilation is about 2.5 L/min
- **C F** About 5 L/min
- **D T**
- **E T** ventilation/perfusion ratio varies from the base to apex

8
- **A F** Sensitivity is increased
- **B F** Also peripheral chemoreceptors
- **C F** Also sensitive to arterial $PaCO_2$
- **D F** Such patients are dependent on 'hypoxic drive'
- **E T**

9
- **A F** Hyperventilation unless embolism is massive
- **B T** With type II respiratory failure
- **C F** Hyperventilation
- **D F** Hyperventilation and type I failure
- **E T** Type II respiratory failure may ensue

10
- **A F** More than 70% is normal
- **B F** Carbon monoxide is used
- **C T** The lungs are hyperinflated
- **D T** A restrictive disorder may develop
- **E F** They measure obstructive ventilatory defects

11
A F The patient may have a metabolic acidosis
B F Also found in pericardial tamponade
C F Although subtle changes are frequently present
D T With basal pulmonary crepitations
E F Right bundle branch block or S_1, Q_3, T_3 pattern

12
A T
B F Another cause should be sought
C T May be massive
D T With associated renal disease
E T With pulmonary hypertension

13
A F Typically type II failure
B F Respiratory muscle paralysis causes type II failure
C T Arterial PCO_2 is typically normal
D T Ventilatory drive is usually maintained
E F Causes acute type II failure—asphyxia

14
A T Causes alveolar hypoventilation
B T Paralysis of respiratory muscles
C F Causes hypoxaemia alone
D F Type I respiratory failure
E F arterial $PaCO_2$ only rises in the later stages of severe attacks

15
A T PaO_2 declines with altitude
B F Indicated when PaO_2 < 7.3 breathing air
C T Also in other situations when Hb is maximally saturated
D F Occurs only in neonates
E T Such shunts may be extra- or intra-pulmonary

16
A F Controlled oxygen therapy at about 28% is best given by a Ventimask
B F a central respiratory stimulant
C F depresses respiration and can impair expectoration
D F may help relieve bronchospasm
E T but not all patients are candidates for such support

17
A F But alveolar cell carcinoma may be
B T
C T And obliterative bronchiolitis
D T And emphysema
E F But an indication for liver transplantation

18
A F Parainfluenza 1,2,3
B F Typically *Haemophilus influenzae*
C T May also cause pneumonia
D F Influenza A, B, RSV and parainfluenza
E T

19
A T May mimic coryza
B T Or *haemophilus influenzae*
C T With stridor or dyspnoea
D T
E F Crepitations suggest a lower respiratory tract disease

20
A T With headache, anorexia and myalgia
B F Early and middle adult life
C F Signs of consolidation (e.g. bronchial breath sounds dominate)
D T Bacteraemia and white cell count > 20×10^{-9}/L are associated with a poorer prognosis
E T May accompany other acute febrile illnesses

21
Ⓐ F
Ⓑ T Myocarditis is rare
Ⓒ T Septicaemic shock has a poor prognosis
Ⓓ T Consider the possibility if stony dullness develops
Ⓔ F Subphrenic abscess may cause pleural effusion or empyema

22
Ⓐ T < 60 mmHg
Ⓑ T
Ⓒ F >30/min
Ⓓ T >7 mmol/l
Ⓔ T < 4000 × 10⁹/L

23
Ⓐ T Sputum and blood cultures are therefore mandatory
Ⓑ T A form of suppurative pneumonia
Ⓒ T May be rapidly progressive in this situation
Ⓓ T Lung infection may be a secondary phenomenon
Ⓔ T Flucloxacillin or erythromycin are indicated

24
Ⓐ F Consolidation and sometimes cavitation
Ⓑ T
Ⓒ T May be blood-stained
Ⓓ F Ceftazidime and ciprofloxacin are also valuable
Ⓔ F more often associated with pre-existing ill health (e.g. alcoholics)

25
Ⓐ T Classically barracks
Ⓑ T Anaemia is rarely severe, but may suggest diagnosis
Ⓒ T In contrast to pneumococcal pneumonia
Ⓓ T In contrast to bacterial pneumonias
Ⓔ T Drugs of choice

26
Ⓐ F Transmitted in inhaled water droplets
Ⓑ T Gastrointestinal symptoms should suggest the diagnosis
Ⓒ T More frequently than in other pneumonic illnesses
Ⓓ T In contrast to 'typical' bacterial pneumonia
Ⓔ T Continue therapy for at least 14 days

27
Ⓐ F The converse is typical of such infections
Ⓑ T Chest X-ray is mandatory in a febrile patient
Ⓒ F More common in pneumococcal infection
Ⓓ T Leucopenia can occur in severe pneumococcal infection
Ⓔ T Rare in pneumococcal disease

28
Ⓐ T Used in higher dosage 120 mg/kg/day
Ⓑ T
Ⓒ T Useful but not always curative
Ⓓ T Or famciclovir
Ⓔ T

29
Ⓐ T Suggested by chronic purulent sputum and localised crackles
Ⓑ F Typically lobar or segmental
Ⓒ T As does persisting partial bronchial occlusion without collapse
Ⓓ T But it may be mimimal or absent
Ⓔ T Particularly in aspiration of gastric contents

30
Ⓐ T Bacteria secondarily infect the damaged pulmonary tissue
Ⓑ T Producing lobar collapse or impaired secretion clearance
Ⓒ T Systemic upset is marked
Ⓓ F Obstruction typically produces signs of collapse
Ⓔ T An air-fluid level may be apparent

31
Ⓐ F Older ages predominate
Ⓑ T And in other immunocompromised patients
Ⓒ T *Mycobacterium bovis* is now rare
Ⓓ T Due to immunosuppression
Ⓔ F Reactivation of dormant infection is more common

32
Ⓐ F Typically symptomless
Ⓑ T Mediastinal, cervical or mesenteric nodes are most frequently involved
Ⓒ F Suggests sarcoidosis
Ⓓ T Can also accompany pulmonary sarcoid
Ⓔ F A hypersensitivity phenomenon typically associated with positive tuberculin test

33
Ⓐ T Onset may be sudden or insidious
Ⓑ T Pancytopenia or a leukaemoid reaction
Ⓒ T But chest X-ray is usually abnormal
Ⓓ T Respiratory symptoms may also be minimal
Ⓔ T Positive urine, sputum or marrow cultures may be obtained

34
Ⓐ F Sputum is typically smear-positive
Ⓑ T But any lobe may be affected
Ⓒ T In contrast to primary disease
Ⓓ F Unusual
Ⓔ T Pathognomonic

35
Ⓐ T Superinfection of a cavity
Ⓑ T Associated with chronic immune stimulation
Ⓒ T Due to haematogenous dissemination
Ⓓ T Suggested by chronic productive cough
Ⓔ T Due to vertebral or paraspinal abscess formation

36
Ⓐ F False negatives may occur
Ⓑ T Between 2 and 4 days
Ⓒ T Implies active or previous infection
Ⓓ F Diffuse skin induration and perhaps necrosis
Ⓔ F False positives may occur

37
Ⓐ T Minimises resistance and reduces duration of treatment
Ⓑ F Patients can be regarded as non-infectious after 1 week of therapy
Ⓒ F 6 and 9 month regimes are of proven efficacy
Ⓓ F Hence their great value in the treatment of TB meningitis
Ⓔ F More often due to non-compliance

38
Ⓐ F Causes vestibular disturbance and deafness
Ⓑ F Polyneuropathy
Ⓒ F Ethambutol causes optic neuritis
Ⓓ T And rifampicin
Ⓔ F Streptomycin cause this

39
Ⓐ F Unless there is a recent contact history without previous immunisation
Ⓑ T Isoniazid for 12 months
Ⓒ T Preemptive therapy prevents the onset of refractory active tuberculosis in AIDS
Ⓓ T Reduces the risk of miliary tuberculosis or tuberculous meningitis
Ⓔ T Providing there has been no previous tuberculosis immunisation

40
Ⓐ F No association
Ⓑ T Usually in a tuberculous cavity
Ⓒ T A severe, rapidly progressive illness
Ⓓ T Typically with wheeze, pulmonary infiltrates and peripheral eosinophilia
Ⓔ F Type III and IV immune responses

41
- Ⓐ T Allergic rhinitis or eczema may coexist
- Ⓑ F Unusual but skin tests may usefully establish atopy
- Ⓒ T Sometimes without obvious precipitant
- Ⓓ T Such as asthma, allergic rhinitis or eczema
- Ⓔ F Its presence might suggest allergic bronchopulmonary aspergillosis

42
- Ⓐ F But patients are frequently smokers
- Ⓑ F Atopy is absent
- Ⓒ T As can infection
- Ⓓ T In contrast to early-onset disease
- Ⓔ T In keeping with the absence of atopy

43
- Ⓐ T But bradycardia may occur in life threatening attacks
- Ⓑ F Usually < 50% of expected PEFR
- Ⓒ T But may diminish in severe attacks
- Ⓓ F PaO_2 < 8kPa
- Ⓔ T $PaCO_2$ may remain normal until the late stages

44
- Ⓐ F High concentration, high flow should be used
- Ⓑ T Intravenous β_2-adrenoceptor agonists can also be used
- Ⓒ F Of no proven value in acute attacks
- Ⓓ T Maintain corticosteroid therapy for at least 7 days in severe attacks
- Ⓔ T Exclude pneumothorax and ventilatory failure

45
- Ⓐ T And T lymphocytes
- Ⓑ T
- Ⓒ T May contribute to development of fixed airways obstruction
- Ⓓ T A recognised feature in fatal asthma in particular
- Ⓔ T

46
- Ⓐ F A spontaneous increase is also diagnostic
- Ⓑ F May be seen in other conditions
- Ⓒ F Treat and reassess; methacholine in low concentration induces bronchoconstriction
- Ⓓ T Features of hyperinflation in acute attacks of chronic disease
- Ⓔ T

47
- Ⓐ T Typically low-dose steroids
- Ⓑ F But may be valuable in childhood
- Ⓒ T Reduces oropharyngeal and gastric deposition
- Ⓓ F Use in addition to steroids and β_2-agonist
- Ⓔ F May be valuable

48
- Ⓐ T Found in two-thirds of patients and may be associated with alcohol abuse
- Ⓑ T Increased threefold due to day time sleepiness
- Ⓒ F
- Ⓓ F Ineffective; continuous positive airway pressure (CPAP) may be effective
- Ⓔ T And also hypothyroidism

49
- Ⓐ T
- Ⓑ T And elevated total serum IgE
- Ⓒ F *Aspergillus fumigatus*
- Ⓓ T Transient pulmonary infiltrates may also be seen
- Ⓔ T Chronic low-dose steroid therapy may be necessary

50
- Ⓐ T May be associated with myasthenia gravis
- Ⓑ T Anterior superior mediastinum
- Ⓒ F Pulmonary apical mass
- Ⓓ T A retrocardiac opacity
- Ⓔ T Can be multiple

51
Ⓐ F Suggests vocal cord paralysis
Ⓑ T Obstruction may supervene
Ⓒ F A cause of hoarseness
Ⓓ T Due to left recurrent laryngeal palsy
Ⓔ T Voice may remain impaired

52
Ⓐ T And toxocara infestation
Ⓑ F Eosinophilia is necessary for the diagnosis
Ⓒ F Wheeze may be absent
Ⓓ T Or imipramine or phenylbutazone
Ⓔ T Pulmonary infiltrates and eosinophilia (PIE)

53
Ⓐ F Acute dyspnoea without wheeze is characteristic
Ⓑ T Flu-like symptoms may exist
Ⓒ T Typically bilateral
Ⓓ F Airway obstruction is absent
Ⓔ T May also be positive in healthy subjects

54
Ⓐ T Will reduce to 30 ml per year if smoking stops
Ⓑ T A diagnostic criterion
Ⓒ F < 70% to make the diagnosis
Ⓓ T
Ⓔ F Both are increased

55
Ⓐ F Immunisation should be offered yearly
Ⓑ F This encourages drug resistance
Ⓒ F Steroids may help if reversibility is objectively demonstrated
Ⓓ T PaO_2 will be < 7 kPa in such a patient at altitude
Ⓔ F Survival has been demonstrated to improve

56
Ⓐ F Most obvious in expiration
Ⓑ T Tracheal 'tug' due to mediastinal descent
Ⓒ T A sign of hyperinflation
Ⓓ T And other accessory respiratory muscles
Ⓔ F Often no added sounds

57
Ⓐ T Suggesting pulmonary hypertension
Ⓑ T A sign of hyperinflation
Ⓒ F Peripheral vessels may be attenuated
Ⓓ F Sign of left ventricular failure
Ⓔ F Signs of left ventricular failure

58
Ⓐ T Predisposes to recurrent infection
Ⓑ T Infected secretions accumulate distal to obstruction
Ⓒ T Ciliary dysfunction and recurrent infection
Ⓓ T Mucus plugging of airways
Ⓔ F

59
Ⓐ F Copious sputum production
Ⓑ T Recurrent pneumonia
Ⓒ T Secondary to inflammatory bronchial change
Ⓓ T Complicating pneumonia
Ⓔ T In the presence of large amounts of secretions

60
Ⓐ T The commonest severe autosomal recessive disorder in Caucasians
Ⓑ F Increased sweat sodium concentration
Ⓒ T Due to failure of development of the vas deferens
Ⓓ F It is normal; hence prospect for gene therapy
Ⓔ F Pseudomonas and staphylococcal sepsis

61
Ⓐ T At least twice daily
Ⓑ F Occasionally used if the affected area is confined to one lobe
Ⓒ F Only if accompanied by increased volume and signs of infection
Ⓓ T Or bronchography to demonstrate the extent of disease
Ⓔ T Respiratory reserve will be impaired

62
Ⓐ T Often termed 'obstructive emphysema'
Ⓑ F Not if there is obstructive emphysema
Ⓒ T Infection occurs with variable frequency
Ⓓ T Clinical signs may be subtle
Ⓔ F Right main bronchus is more vertically aligned

63
Ⓐ F Young males or females
Ⓑ T Extremely rare
Ⓒ T Tumours are vascular
Ⓓ T Due to bronchial obstruction
Ⓔ T Due to bronchial obstruction

64
Ⓐ F 50% of all male deaths from malignant disease
Ⓑ F Streaking of sputum with blood in a smoker is more typical
Ⓒ F Squamous 50%, adenocarcinoma 15%
Ⓓ T As is mesothelioma
Ⓔ T Smoking is the major aetiological factor

65
Ⓐ F 10% of bronchial carcinomas are surgically treatable
Ⓑ F Endobronchial lesions may be clinically silent
Ⓒ F Only applies to resected squamous carcinoma
Ⓓ F Cytology may be obtained from sputum or metastatic tissue
Ⓔ F More often absent with small-cell type

66
Ⓐ T With ataxia and nystagmus
Ⓑ T Eaton–Lambert syndrome
Ⓒ T Usually bilateral
Ⓓ T Usually distal sensorimotor
Ⓔ T Skin rash and proximal myopathy

67
Ⓐ T Also seen in chronic lymphatic leukaemia and Hodgkin's lymphoma
Ⓑ T Hyponatraemia is often the clue
Ⓒ T Hypokalaemia, pigmentation and proximal myopathy
Ⓓ F Malignant hypercalcaemia is usually caused by bony metastases not parathyroid hormone
Ⓔ F Typically peripheral squamous cell tumours

68
Ⓐ T
Ⓑ T
Ⓒ T
Ⓓ F But contralateral nodes are a contraindication
Ⓔ T

69
Ⓐ F Typically type I respiratory failure
Ⓑ T With or without evidence of connective tissue disease
Ⓒ T But not in extrinsic allergic alveolitis
Ⓓ F Dyspnoea, dry cough and crackles
Ⓔ T But this is not completely specific

70
Ⓐ F Does not progress except in progressive massive fibrosis
Ⓑ F Depends on radiological features
Ⓒ T May cavitate
Ⓓ T Usually due to smoking
Ⓔ F Frequently no specific signs

71
- **A** T Typically upper zone changes
- **B** T Specific but not highly sensitive
- **C** F Continues to progress despite reduced exposure
- **D** T Caplan's syndrome
- **E** T But now rare

72
- **A** F Often calcify
- **B** F But do raise the suspicion of malignancy
- **C** T Although cryptogenic fibrosing alveolitis is possible
- **D** F A restrictive not an obstructive ventilatory defect
- **E** F Seldom necessary

73
- **A** F Cotton dust produces byssinosis, mouldy sugar cane produces bagassosis
- **B** T Fungal antigens *Micropolyspora faenae*
- **C** F Tin produces stannosis, siderosis results from iron oxide
- **D** T Usually pigeons or budgies
- **E** F Produces malt worker's lung

74
- **A** F Caseating granulomata (e.g. TB) are associated with cavitation
- **B** F Typically negative
- **C** F Erythema nodosum is the typical skin lesion
- **D** F The normal course in stage I and stage II disease
- **E** F Due to increased vitamin D sensitivity

75
- **A** T Usually bilateral
- **B** T Typically the 7th nerve
- **C** T Or uveitis
- **D** F Non-erosive arthropathy or bone cysts
- **E** T Or lacrimal or other salivary glands

76
- **A** F Transudate in CCF
- **B** T Sometimes bloodstained or with eosinophils
- **C** T Most frequently on the right
- **D** T With polymorphonuclear leucocytes
- **E** F Severe hypoalbuminaemia produces transudates

77
- **A** T Stony dull percussion and impaired voice transmission
- **B** F An exudate is more likely to be associated with malignancy
- **C** F An effusion may be the sole X-ray finding
- **D** F May be seen in rheumatoid and systemic lupus erythematosus
- **E** T Fluid is rich in chylomicrons

78
- **A** F Typically unilateral
- **B** T Or a recent diagnostic aspiration
- **C** T Suggests lung abscess, antibiotic resistance or hypersensitivity
- **D** T Perhaps complicating subphrenic infection
- **E** F Frequently sterile post-antibiotic therapy

79
- **A** T A small pneumothorax may be asymptomatic
- **B** F Diminished or absent breath sounds
- **C** F Mediastinal shift suggests tension
- **D** T Pleurectomy may also be necessary
- **E** T Particularly if bilateral

80
- **A** F Phrenic nerve paralysis
- **B** T
- **C** T
- **D** T But underlying pathology should be sought
- **E** F May be hyperinflation

81

Ⓐ T With profound hypoxaemia
Ⓑ F Suggests pulmonary infarction
Ⓒ T Non-specific
Ⓓ T Non-specific
Ⓔ F Classical ECG pattern is S_1, Q_3, T_3

82

Ⓐ T Sometimes difficult to differentiate from pneumonia
Ⓑ T May be evanescent
Ⓒ T
Ⓓ T Cavitation of necrotic lung tissue
Ⓔ T Detectable clinically or on chest X-ray

83

Ⓐ F Unhelpful except in acute massive embolism
Ⓑ F High concentrations of oxygen are necessary
Ⓒ F May further lower the blood pressure
Ⓓ T Continue heparin until the prothrombin ratio (INR) is stable
Ⓔ F Continue for 3 months

DISTURBANCES IN WATER, ELECTROLYTE AND ACID-BASE BALANCE

5

1
- **ⓐ T** Relatively constant in health
- **ⓑ T** approx 28 litres
- **ⓒ F** 25% intravascular, 75% interstitial
- **ⓓ F** Extracellular
- **ⓔ F** Intracellular

2
- **ⓐ T** Predominantly from the oxidation of glucose
- **ⓑ F** 500–1000 ml per day
- **ⓒ T** Depends on solute load
- **ⓓ F** Usually about 100 ml
- **ⓔ T** An index of normal renal medullary function

3
- **ⓐ F** 66% of filtered water is reabsorbed
- **ⓑ T** And collecting ducts
- **ⓒ T** But only 150 mg per day is excreted in urine
- **ⓓ F** 66%
- **ⓔ F** Afferent arterioles

4
- **ⓐ F** Almost all is passively absorbed
- **ⓑ T** And the remainder is absorbed in the ascending limb of loop of Henle
- **ⓒ T** Active reabsorption process
- **ⓓ T** Coupled with sodium reabsorption
- **ⓔ F** 90% of bicarbonate is actively reabsorbed

5
- **ⓐ T** Regulated by aldosterone and atrial natriuretic peptide
- **ⓑ T** If K^+ is low, H^+ is secreted preferentially
- **ⓒ T** Via the renin angiotensin system
- **ⓓ T** ADH increases tubular permeability to water
- **ⓔ T** Permits urinary acidification

6
- **ⓐ F** Rare in isolation
- **ⓑ T** Usually with water depletion also
- **ⓒ T** An osmotic diuresis
- **ⓓ T** Mineralocorticoid insufficiency
- **ⓔ T** Loss into the 'third space'

7
- **ⓐ F** But may be seen in the syndrome of inappropriate antidiuretic hormone (ADH) secretion
- **ⓑ T** Water retention exceeds sodium retention
- **ⓒ T** Increased total body water
- **ⓓ F** But seen in adrenocortical insufficiency
- **ⓔ T** Salt loss exceeds water loss

8
- **ⓐ T**
- **ⓑ F** Can produce hyponatraemia
- **ⓒ T** Carefully monitor pulse, blood pressure and central venous pressure
- **ⓓ T** Dependent on cause of deficit
- **ⓔ T** The kidneys may be unable to excrete hydrogen ions; monitor the arterial pH

9
- **ⓐ T** Renal tubular insensitivity to antidiuretic hormone (ADH)
- **ⓑ T** Inadequate intake
- **ⓒ T** Inadequate intake
- **ⓓ T** Renal tubular insensitivity to ADH
- **ⓔ F** Combined salt and water depletion

10
- **A** F   Urine osmolality > 500 mosm/kg
- **B** F   Hypernatraemia
- **C** T   Thirst stimulated by rising plasma osmolality
- **D** T   Signs of volume depletion develop more rapidly in combined salt/water depletion
- **E** T   And confusion

11
- **A** T   Unless there is significant peripheral circulatory failure
- **B** F   Too rapid infusions produce cerebral oedema; use 4 litres over 24 hours
- **C** T
- **D** T   Hypotonic fluid therapy is rarely indicated
- **E** T   Signs develop more rapidly in combined salt/water depletion

12
- **A** T
- **B** T   Compared with extracellular concentrations of about 4 mmol/L
- **C** T
- **D** F   Increased by bicarbonate and decreased by acidaemia
- **E** T

13
- **A** T   Renal tubular cell K^+ concentration increased, excretion increased
- **B** T   Secondary hyperaldosteronism
- **C** T   Mineralocorticoid-like effect
- **D** T   Primary or secondary tubular defect; also occurs with activation of renin and angiotensin
- **E** F   Causes hyperkalaemia by an effect on the distal convoluted tubules

14
- **A** T   Tubular response to ADH is impaired
- **B** T   Lethargy and immobility in the elderly
- **C** T   QT interval is prolonged
- **D** T   Painless distension with scanty bowel sounds
- **E** F   Increased sensitivity to digoxin

15
- **A** T   Insulin promotes movement into the cells
- **B** T   Impairment of secretion in the distal nephron
- **C** T   Increased tissue breakdown
- **D** T   Especially if given with ACE inhibitor
- **E** T   Avoid concurrent supplementation

16
- **A** T   Relatively early changes
- **B** T   May be the first manifestation
- **C** T   Such symptoms are commonly overlooked
- **D** T   Occur in severe hyperkalaemia
- **E** T   Muscle weakness, loss of tendon reflexes and ileus; therefore check the plasma electrolytes

17
- **A** F   But may be necessary to prevent recurrence
- **B** F   Give parenteral dextrose and insulin
- **C** T   Cardioprotective effect
- **D** T   Also correct metabolic acidosis if present with 1.26% sodium bicarbonate i.v.
- **E** T   The resin binds potassium in exchange for calcium

18
- **A** T   Parathyroid hormone (PTH) increases urinary phosphate excretion
- **B** T   As in vitamin D deficiency due to malabsorption syndromes
- **C** T   Also common in chronic alcoholism
- **D** F   The serum calcium and phosphate concentrations are typically normal
- **E** T   And haemodialysis due to phosphate removal

19
- **A** T   And tremor and choreiform movements
- **B** T   Also from chronic diuretic therapy
- **C** T   Excess losses in the urine
- **D** T   Including secondary hyperaldosteronism
- **E** F   Very poorly absorbed orally

20

Ⓐ T

Ⓑ T Two-thirds of water absorption occurs here

Ⓒ T

Ⓓ T The absence of AVP renders the collecting ducts impermeable to water

Ⓔ T

21

Ⓐ T Dilutional hyponatraemia

Ⓑ F Typically < 250 mosm/kg

Ⓒ T Occasionally produces generalised seizures

Ⓓ F Use small volumes of hypertonic saline very cautiously

Ⓔ F ECF volume status usually appears normal

22

Ⓐ F Avoid unless there is significant volume depletion

Ⓑ F Restrict water intake to 0 5 litres or less per day

Ⓒ T Look for malignancy, infection, adverse drug effects or central nervous system disorders

Ⓓ T Its use may facilitate the co-administration of i.v. fluids

Ⓔ F The hepatorenal syndrome is characterised by an increase in urinary osmolality

23

Ⓐ T Pain and other stressors can induce ADH release

Ⓑ T And many other central nervous system disorders

Ⓒ F Water excretion is, however, impaired

Ⓓ T A rare complication

Ⓔ T And other pneumonias

24

Ⓐ F A diuretic causing sodium and water losses

Ⓑ T Inhibition of renal prostaglandin synthesis

Ⓒ T

Ⓓ F But hypothyroidism increases antidiuretic hormone (ADH) secretion

Ⓔ F inhibits aldosterone production

25

Ⓐ F Major action on thick ascending limb of loop of Henle

Ⓑ T Tubular effect inhibiting urate excretion may precipitate gout

Ⓒ F Acts on the collecting ducts

Ⓓ T Causes hyperkalaemia

Ⓔ T Due to relative water excess

26

Ⓐ T The Henderson–Hasselbach equation

Ⓑ T Note **n**mol/L not **m**mol/L

Ⓒ T Unlike $PaCO_2$ which is controlled by the respiratory centre via ventilation

Ⓓ F Excretion is predominantly renal

Ⓔ F Most is converted to H_2CO_3 by red cell carbonic anhydrase

27

Ⓐ F pH is measured directly

Ⓑ T Dissociation—equilibration formula of a weak acid

Ⓒ T Normally useful in distinguishing < 15 mmol/L and the causes of metabolic acidosis

Ⓓ T Hypoventilation causes hypercapnia

Ⓔ F Normal bicarbonate 22–28 mmol/L; normal pH = 7.35–7.45

28

Ⓐ F Plasma bicarbonate is reduced

Ⓑ T Ketoacidosis

Ⓒ F Compensatory hyperventilation

Ⓓ T Hyperchloraemic acidosis due to failure of proximal tubular bicarbonate reabsorption

Ⓔ F Acetazolamide inhibits red blood cell carbonic anhydrase and decreases production

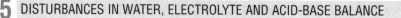
29

- **A F** Chronic respiratory alkalosis
- **B T** Diabetic ketoacidosis
- **C F** Acute respiratory acidosis due to alveolar hypoventilation
- **D T** Distal (type I) renal tubular acidosis
- **E T** Unlike chronic liver failure which typically produces metabolic alkalosis due to hyperaldosteronism

30

- **A F** This would produce a metabolic alkalosis
- **B F** This would produce a respiratory acidosis
- **C T** Mixed metabolic and respiratory acidosis
- **D T** Mixed metabolic and respiratory acidosis
- **E F** This would produce a metabolic alkalosis

DISEASES OF THE KIDNEY AND URINARY SYSTEM

6

1
- **A** T
- **B** F — 25% of the cardiac output
- **C** T
- **D** T
- **E** F — Under the control of the renin–angiotensin system

2
- **A** T — Probably in tubular cells
- **B** F — 1-hydroxycholecalciferol; 25-hydroxylation occurs in the liver
- **C** T — Vasodilators produced by mesangial cells
- **D** T — As do many other tissues
- **E** F — Produced in adrenal cortex

3
- **A** T — Due to an osmotic diuresis
- **B** T — Causes nephrogenic diabetes insipidus
- **C** F — Cranial diabetes insipidus due to antidiuretic hormone (ADH) deficiency
- **D** T — Mineralocorticoid deficiency impairs urinary concentrating ability
- **E** T — Causes nephrogenic diabetes insipidus

4
- **A** F — Immunoelectrophoresis required
- **B** T — Often with oedema and hypoalbuminaemia
- **C** F — Greater when the person is upright—'orthostatic proteinuria'
- **D** T — But no red cells on microscopy
- **E** T — Microalbuminuria is a sensitive predictor

5
- **A** F — Moderate 500 mg–2 g—rarely more
- **B** F — Usually haematuria
- **C** T
- **D** T — Commonest cause in childhood
- **E** F — No glomerular lesion

6
- **A** T
- **B** T — Risk factors include diabetes mellitus, chronic non-steroidal anti-inflammatory drug (NSAID) abuse and alcoholism
- **C** F — Typically proteinuria
- **D** T — Associated with a mesangiocapillary glomerulonephritis
- **E** T — May be frank haematuria

7
- **A** F — RTA produces an inability to acidify urine (pH > 8 suggests infection)
- **B** T — C = urine concentration/plasma concentration × urine volume
- **C** F — Glomerular disease is likely if the ratio > 3.5 mg/mmol
- **D** F — Glomerular disease is likely if the ratio > 300
- **E** F — Contraindicated if both kidneys are small (< 60% normal size)

8
- **A** T — More marked in children
- **B** T — Often with generalised oedema
- **C** T — With red blood cell casts
- **D** F — Non-selective and usually not nephrotic
- **E** F — Suggests C1q esterase inhibitor deficiency

9
- **Ⓐ F** Typically painless
- **Ⓑ T** Transudates
- **Ⓒ T** Serum albumin concentration < 30 g/L and urinary protein > 3.5 g/day
- **Ⓓ F** But may occur in chronic renal failure
- **Ⓔ F** Marked sodium retention—urinary sodium < 10 mmol/L

10
- **Ⓐ F** Tubulointerstitial damage only
- **Ⓑ T** Also a feature of HIV infection
- **Ⓒ T** Typical of small vessel vasculitis
- **Ⓓ T** Presents with recurrent macroscopic haematuria
- **Ⓔ F** Immunoglobulin light chain deposits

11
- **Ⓐ T**
- **Ⓑ T** Especially haemolytic streptococci; rare in the UK
- **Ⓒ T**
- **Ⓓ F** Suggests Goodpasture's disease
- **Ⓔ F** Usually resolves spontaneously, especially in children

12
- **Ⓐ T**
- **Ⓑ F** Typically normal
- **Ⓒ T** 'Classical' pathway activation
- **Ⓓ T** Oedema and oliguria are typical
- **Ⓔ T** 'Smoky urine' with red cell casts on microscopy

13
- **Ⓐ T** Occurs at any age but common in young adult males
- **Ⓑ F** Usually < 7 days
- **Ⓒ T** Minor proteinuria in the remainder
- **Ⓓ T** Hypertension is common
- **Ⓔ T** Or focal segmental glomerulonephritis in acute disease

14
- **Ⓐ T** More common in females
- **Ⓑ T**
- **Ⓒ T** Occurs in type II MCGN (dense deposit disease)
- **Ⓓ T** The majority progress to renal failure
- **Ⓔ F** Hypocomplementaemia

15
- **Ⓐ T** Causes a variety of histological types of glomerulonephritis
- **Ⓑ T**
- **Ⓒ T**
- **Ⓓ T**
- **Ⓔ T**

16
- **Ⓐ T** Removable by plasmapheresis
- **Ⓑ T** With linear IgG deposition
- **Ⓒ T**
- **Ⓓ T** Antibodies have pulmonary basement membrane cross-reactivity
- **Ⓔ T** Previously termed HLA-DR2; autoimmunity to type IV collagen

17
- **Ⓐ T** Uniform basement membrane thickening
- **Ⓑ T** Commonest cause of the nephrotic syndrome in adults
- **Ⓒ T** Hypertension and/or renal failure are common
- **Ⓓ T** Remains static in one-third of patients
- **Ⓔ F** Best reserved for rapidly progressive or severe disease

18
- **Ⓐ T**
- **Ⓑ T** Causes focal necrotising glomerulonephritis
- **Ⓒ T**
- **Ⓓ T** Including Henoch–Schönlein purpura
- **Ⓔ F**

19
- **Ⓐ F** Usually children; accounts for 25% of nephrotic syndrome in adults
- **Ⓑ F** Minor or absent
- **Ⓒ F** Selective proteinuria
- **Ⓓ F** Suggests an alternative cause
- **Ⓔ F** Renal function is otherwise unimpaired

20
- **Ⓐ F** Diagnosis in children rarely requires histological confirmation
- **Ⓑ F** Useful in management of oedema
- **Ⓒ T** Longer term steroids may be helpful
- **Ⓓ T** E.g. cyclophosphamide
- **Ⓔ F** Rarely, even in relapsing disease

21
- **Ⓐ T** Anion gap = plasma $(Na^+ + K^+) - (Cl^- + HCO_3^-)$ normally < 15 mmol/L
- **Ⓑ T** increased chloride preserves anion gap
- **Ⓒ T** Even in presence of systemic acidosis
- **Ⓓ F** GFR is normal
- **Ⓔ F** No features of uraemia

22
- **Ⓐ T** And amphotericin
- **Ⓑ T** And vitamin D intoxication
- **Ⓒ T** And systemic lupus erythematosus
- **Ⓓ T** Also causes proximal type 2 RTA
- **Ⓔ T** And hydronephrosis

23
- **Ⓐ F** Less than 30% of drug-induced AIN have features of generalised hypersensitivity
- **Ⓑ F** Eosinophilia occurs in 30% in the peripheral blood and 70% in the urine
- **Ⓒ T** And neutrophil or monocytic infiltrate
- **Ⓓ F** Typically resolves
- **Ⓔ T** E.g. penicillin or naproxen

24
- **Ⓐ T** Also associated with allopurinol and frusemide
- **Ⓑ T** Recorded with most of the non-steroidal anti-inflammatory agents
- **Ⓒ T**
- **Ⓓ T**
- **Ⓔ T**

25
- **Ⓐ T** Also associated with sarcoidosis and systemic lupus erythematosus
- **Ⓑ T** And other heavy metal poisoning
- **Ⓒ T**
- **Ⓓ T**
- **Ⓔ T** Resulting in medullary ischaemia

26
- **Ⓐ F** 20% of acute renal failure is non-oliguric
- **Ⓑ T** Indicating preservation of renal medullary function
- **Ⓒ T** Indicating preservation of renal medullary function
- **Ⓓ T** Indicating preservation of renal medullary function
- **Ⓔ F** Suggests primary renal disease

27
- **Ⓐ F** Suggests acute pyelonephritis
- **Ⓑ T** And urinary frequency
- **Ⓒ F** Suggests an abnormality of the urinary tract
- **Ⓓ T** *E. coli* causes 75% of UTIs in the community
- **Ⓔ F** Trimethoprim or co-amoxiclav pending the results of bacterial sensitivities

28
- **Ⓐ T** But ureteric obstruction may be a predisposing factor
- **Ⓑ T** With loin or epigastric pain
- **Ⓒ F** Typically unilateral but can be bilateral
- **Ⓓ F** Commonly found in chilren but not adults
- **Ⓔ F** Suggests perinephric abscess

29
- **Ⓐ F** 5% (compare 40% in elderly women)
- **Ⓑ T** And ureteric dilatation
- **Ⓒ T** 40% develop symptoms if untreated
- **Ⓓ F** Contraindicated in early pregnancy
- **Ⓔ F** Teratogenic risk (a folate antagonist)

30
Ⓐ T Chronic infection predisposes to phosphate stone formation
Ⓑ F Usually asymptomatic and presents with uraemia or hypertension
Ⓒ T Recurrent infections can be difficult to prevent
Ⓓ F Usually presents before the age of 30 years
Ⓔ T 'Salt-losing nephropathy'

31
Ⓐ F 14% of patients with CRF
Ⓑ T Other aetiological factors may also be important
Ⓒ F Similar to chronic interstitial nephritis
Ⓓ F Reflux is often no longer demonstrable in adulthood
Ⓔ T As a result of a 'salt-losing' nephropathy

32
Ⓐ F Typically normocytic or microcytic
Ⓑ T Can improve with haemodialysis
Ⓒ T Renal osteodystrophy with osteomalacia
Ⓓ T Even haemorrhagic pericarditis with tamponade
Ⓔ F Chronic metabolic acidosis

33
Ⓐ T Hence polyuria; urinary diluting ability also impaired
Ⓑ F Hyperphosphataemia
Ⓒ F Hypocalcaemia
Ⓓ T Resulting in hyperpnoea
Ⓔ F Severe proteinuria diminishes as renal failure progresses

34
Ⓐ T Urine stasis and infection
Ⓑ T Or radiotherapy for such cancer
Ⓒ F Haematuria is common in either
Ⓓ T Thought to be the result of a neuromuscular defect
Ⓔ F Typically painful

35
Ⓐ T Typically phosphate stones
Ⓑ T Produces osteoporosis and hypercalciuria
Ⓒ F Hyperparathyroidism
Ⓓ T Normocalcaemic hypercalciuria
Ⓔ T Hypercalciuria with or without hypercalcaemia

36
Ⓐ T Suggests total obstruction
Ⓑ F Acidification with ammonium chloride may benefit
Ⓒ F Decreases urinary calcium excretion by 30% in hypercalciuric patients
Ⓓ F Decreases urinary urate and may reduce oxalate stone formation
Ⓔ F Fragmentation by lithotripsy and endoscopic removal is possible

37
Ⓐ F Autosomal dominant
Ⓑ T But liver function tests normal
Ⓒ T And hypertension and urinary tract infection
Ⓓ T Common but rarely severe
Ⓔ T 10% will have a subarachnoid haemorrhage

38
Ⓐ F Autosomal recessive and X-linked modes
Ⓑ T
Ⓒ T Located at Xq22
Ⓓ T Second most common inherited form of chronic renal failure
Ⓔ T Characteristic feature preceding severe sensorineural deafness

39
Ⓐ T Occurs in 20% and is due to increased interleukin release
Ⓑ T Typically osteolytic metastases
Ⓒ T Due to blood clot or direct tumour obstruction of ureter
Ⓓ T Erythropoietin secretion
Ⓔ F Suggests hepatoma

40
Ⓐ T Renin production
Ⓑ T May resolve after nephrectomy
Ⓒ T Due to tumour-associated neural antibodies
Ⓓ T Due to parathyroid hormone-like activity
Ⓔ F

41
Ⓐ F Typically transitional cell
Ⓑ F Painless haematuria is typical
Ⓒ F Radiotherapy is of palliative benefit
Ⓓ F Local spread occurs early and metastases late
Ⓔ T Also associated with chronic schistosomiasis

42
Ⓐ T As also benign prostatic disease
Ⓑ T Or haematuria
Ⓒ F Hard with obliteration of median furrow
Ⓓ T And may involve ureters
Ⓔ F Osteosclerotic metastases

43
Ⓐ F Aged over 60 years
Ⓑ T Sometimes precipitated by urinary tract infection
Ⓒ F Associated with diminished androgen secretion
Ⓓ T Even modest changes may herald prostatic carcinoma
Ⓔ F Typically symmetrical

44
Ⓐ F Typically painless
Ⓑ T Helps in the assessment of treatment response
Ⓒ F Haematogenous spread may occur
Ⓓ F Peak incidence aged 25–34 years
Ⓔ T Chemotherapy is given if disease is widespread

7 DIABETES MELLITUS, AND NUTRITIONAL AND METABOLIC DISORDERS

1
- **Ⓐ T** 50% of NIDDM is undetected
- **Ⓑ F** Converse applies, particularly if obese
- **Ⓒ F** Inheritance is polygenic
- **Ⓓ T** 70% aged over 50 years
- **Ⓔ F** 90% of islet cell mass must be destroyed

2
- **Ⓐ T** Patchy distribution in pancreas
- **Ⓑ T** Cross-reactivity of antibodies to bovine serum albumin
- **Ⓒ T** And anti-insulin antibodies
- **Ⓓ T** Indicating the importance of environmental factors
- **Ⓔ T** Encoded on the short arm of chromosome 6

3
- **Ⓐ F** In contrast to IDDM
- **Ⓑ T** Compare 35% concordance in monozygotic twins with IDDM
- **Ⓒ F** Variable insulin resistance
- **Ⓓ T** Especially if combined with underactivity
- **Ⓔ T** In contrast to IDDM

4
- **Ⓐ T** Hypokalaemic alkalosis impairs insulin secretion
- **Ⓑ T** Pancreatic fibrosis
- **Ⓒ T** Conn's syndrome produces an hypokalaemic alkalosis
- **Ⓓ T** Islet cell destruction
- **Ⓔ T** Also occurs in phaeochromocytoma and acromegaly

5
- **Ⓐ T**
- **Ⓑ T**
- **Ⓒ F** Decreased lipolysis and enhanced ketogenesis
- **Ⓓ F** Decreased gluconeogenesis
- **Ⓔ F** Decreased protein catabolism

6
- **Ⓐ T** And produces an increase in plasma osmolality
- **Ⓑ T** Resulting in a metabolic acidosis
- **Ⓒ T** Insulin deficiency increases protein degradation
- **Ⓓ T** More profound ketogenesis occurs in IDDM
- **Ⓔ F** Insulin deficiency increases ketoacid production

7
- **Ⓐ F** Too insensitive to detect all cases
- **Ⓑ F** Renal threshold may be high
- **Ⓒ T** But it should never be assumed to be so
- **Ⓓ F** 20% have significant diabetic complications
- **Ⓔ T** Red cells contain less glucose

8
- **Ⓐ T**
- **Ⓑ T**
- **Ⓒ F** Prolonged carbohydrate restriction impairs glucose tolerance
- **Ⓓ T** WHO standard test
- **Ⓔ F** Higher concentrations may occur normally if gastric emptying is rapid (lag storage)

9

A T Catabolism and osmotic diuresis

B T Predisposition to monilial infection

C T Particularly in ketosis

D T Small vessel disease and neuropathy

E T Often detected on routine urine testing

10

A F 50% of new diabetics can be controlled on diet alone

B T Higher than that in average UK diet

C F Consume within dietary guidelines

D T UK national diet tends to higher proportion of fat

E F Calorie restriction to < 1500 kcal per day cannot be sustained for long

11

A F Combined treatment may limit weight gain

B F Stimulates pancreatic insulin secretion

C F Such an action would produce insulin resistance

D T Also decreases hepatic gluconeogenesis to reduce hyperglycaemia

E T Disulfiram-like reaction

12

A T Sometimes a useful adjunct to calorie-restricted diets

B F Hence does not cause hypoglycaemia in non-diabetics

C F Increases the sensitivity of peripheral insulin receptors

D T Thus limiting hyperglycaemia

E F Causes diarrhoea which may limit drug compliance

13

A T Onset of effect 15–30 minutes after injection

B T Isophane insulin action peaks at 3–8 hours and lasts 7–14 hours

C F Often relative insulin resistance

D T Varies in other countries

E F Conversion from animal-derived to human insulin may cause hypoglycaemia

14

A T Causes and effects of hypoglycaemia should be familiar to patients

B T Insulin resistance declines as glycaemic control improves

C F Unlikely to achieve good glycaemic control

D F Check every 3–6 months (RBC lifespan = 120 days)

E F Patients need to check blood glucose concentrations regularly

15

A T But 50% of long.term IDDM patients have no symptoms

B T Sympathetic nervous system activation

C T Neuroglycopenia

D F But plasma glucose concentration does not mirror CSF glucose perfectly

E T Nocturnal hypoglycaemia may be difficult to recognise

16

A T 25 g of glucose and/or intramuscular glucagon

B T Because glucagon increases insulin secretion

C T Hypoglycaemia does not occur with biguanides

D F Can recur following initial treatment

E F Long-acting hypoglycaemics cause prolonged hypoglycaemia

17
- **A** T Or inadequate size of meal
- **B** T Often unanticipated
- **C** T A problem with patients on sulphonylurea drugs
- **D** T Increased sensitivity to insulin; weight loss and nocturia should signal the possibility
- **E** T Inadvertent and even occasionally deliberate

18
- **A** F Volume depletion in ketoacidosis
- **B** T Diminished in ketoacidosis
- **C** F Suggests metabolic acidosis
- **D** T Dehydration in ketoacidosis
- **E** F An insensitive indicator of ketoacidosis

19
- **A** T Hypertension is an important comorbid risk factor for macrovascular disease
- **B** T Check feet (nails and skin) for evidence of neuropathy
- **C** T To assess drug and dietary compliance
- **D** T Including assessment of albumin: creatinine ratio
- **E** T Retinopathy is potentially preventable

20
- **A** T Due to ketoacidosis
- **B** T Due to dehydration
- **C** F Skin is typically dry
- **D** T Due to ketosis and dehydration
- **E** F Suggests severe hypoglycaemia

21
- **A** T Average deficit = 6 L (50% intracellular + 50% extracellular)
- **B** T Chloride deficit similar
- **C** F Picture should be that of an acute metabolic not respiratory acidosis
- **D** F Typically normal or high
- **E** T Even in absence of infection

22
- **A** F Use isotonic solutions; change to 5% dextrose when blood glucose is near normal
- **B** F Avoid if $K^+ > 5.5$ mmol/L
- **C** T Or in severe acidosis—pH < 7.0
- **D** F Dextrose is used to correct intracellular fluid depletion and if blood glucose < 15 mmol/L
- **E** T Give plasma expander if blood pressure does not improve rapidly; monitor urine output + central venous pressure

23
- **A** F Photocoagulation is indicated
- **B** F Often the first sign of retinopathy detected at ophthalmoscopy
- **C** F Regular examination is mandatory
- **D** F Suggests glomerular dysfunction and is a sensitive indicator of microangiopathy
- **E** T 30–50% mortality over 10 years

24
- **A** T Due to intrauterine death, prematurity and congenital malformation
- **B** F Typically larger than expected
- **C** F Defer delivery to 38–39 weeks or later if possible
- **D** F Insulin is necessary to achieve optimal control
- **E** F Insulin requirements increase from the second trimester onwards

25
- **A** T Minimise risk of intraoperative hypoglycaemia
- **B** F Usual insulin should be substituted with glucose, potassium and insulin (GKI) infusion
- **C** T Observation alone in minor surgery
- **D** F Often higher
- **E** T With 2–4 hourly measurement of capillary glucose concentrations

26
- **Ⓐ T**
- **Ⓑ T** Also increased plasminogen activator inhibitor
- **Ⓒ T** Associated with high mortality
- **Ⓓ T** 'Insulin resistance syndrome'
- **Ⓔ T** Major risk factor for macrovascular disease

27
- **Ⓐ F**
- **Ⓑ T** Sausage-like venous 'beading'
- **Ⓒ T** Soft exudates indicate retinal ischaemia; hard exudates indicate plasma leakage
- **Ⓓ T** Appearance reflects their depth in the retina
- **Ⓔ T** Major risk factor for macrovascular disease

28
- **Ⓐ T** A pancytopenia is common
- **Ⓑ T** Predisposition to tuberculosis
- **Ⓒ T** Increased susceptibility to infection
- **Ⓓ T** Skin ulcers, bed sores and delayed wound healing
- **Ⓔ T** Loss of gut secretions and increased risk of gastroenteritis

29
- **Ⓐ F** 2–10 µg per day
- **Ⓑ T** 1 litre
- **Ⓒ T** Optimally 10% of total calories
- **Ⓓ T** Highest level for a specific vitamin
- **Ⓔ F** Approximately 500–1000 mg

30
- **Ⓐ T** Or 16 kJ/g
- **Ⓑ F** About 9 kcal (36 kJ) per g
- **Ⓒ F** 2800 kcal (i.e. alcohol has a calorific value of 7 kcal/g)
- **Ⓓ T** And arachidonic acid
- **Ⓔ T** Arginine is an additional essential amino acid in infants

31
- **Ⓐ F** About 2700 kcal (11 3 MJ)
- **Ⓑ F** CHO should provide 50% of calories = 340 g (ketosis occurs if < 100 g a day)
- **Ⓒ T** And niacin and vitamin E
- **Ⓓ T** Minimum around 40 g
- **Ⓔ F** 200 µg of folate per day

32
- **Ⓐ F** BMI < 16. The normal BMI is calculated from the formula Weight (kg) ÷ height(m)^2
- **Ⓑ T** 'Famine oedema'
- **Ⓒ T** And weakness, amenorrhoea or impotence
- **Ⓓ T** Adolescents may maintain hair growth
- **Ⓔ F** Brain weight is preserved; bradycardia is the rule

33
- **Ⓐ F** Increased plasma FFA concentrations
- **Ⓑ T** Plasma glucagon concentration also rises
- **Ⓒ T** False-negative Mantoux may occur
- **Ⓓ T** And occasionally a metabolic acidosis
- **Ⓔ T** Also pancytopenia

34
- **Ⓐ F** Predominantly protein deficiency with a normal total energy intake
- **Ⓑ F** Protein and energy malnutrition in infancy
- **Ⓒ F** BMI is normal or low normal
- **Ⓓ T** Compromised humoral and cell mediated immunity
- **Ⓔ T** Exacerbated by diarrhoeal illness

35
- **Ⓐ T** And absence of oedema
- **Ⓑ T** Weight < 60% standard for age
- **Ⓒ T** With low plasma lipids
- **Ⓓ F** Features of kwashiorkor
- **Ⓔ T** Contributing to dermatosis

36
- **A** **T** Dehydration and infection
- **B** **T** Especially hypokalaemia and hypomagnesaemia
- **C** **F** Isolated calorie replacement may do so
- **D** **F** And resolves on refeeding
- **E** **T**

37
- **A** **T** Chiefly as calcium hydroxyapatite
- **B** **T** 350–550 mg daily for children
- **C** **T**
- **D** **F** Impair absorption (e.g. whole grain cereals and spinach)
- **E** **F** Correlates poorly

38
- **A** **T** 8 mg per day for men
- **B** **F** 15% is absorbed
- **C** **T** E.g. red muscle meat or organ meat
- **D** **F** Average loss 2 mg/day due to menstruation
- **E** **F** Contains 250 mg of iron

39
- **A** **F** Goitre alone or with hypothyroidism
- **B** **F** Hard water contains more fluoride
- **C** **T** Acrodermatitis enteropathica
- **D** **T** And skeletal rarefaction
- **E** **F** More likely in breast-fed infants

40
- **A** **T** A, D, E, K are the fat-soluble vitamins
- **B** **F** Occurs as retinol in animal produce and as carotene in plants
- **C** **T** Both conditions are the result of vitamin A deficiency and lead to blindness
- **D** **F** Minimum recommended daily intake = 1–2 mg
- **E** **T** Present as retinol

41
- **A** **F** Some margarines are fortified
- **B** **T** But less efficiently produced in old age
- **C** **F** But metabolism partly occurs in the liver
- **D** **T** 1-alpha hydroxylation occurs in the kidney and 25-hydroxylation in the liver
- **E** **T** And stimulates osteoclast proliferation

42
- **A** **T** And also found in liver
- **B** **F** Absorbed as vitamin K_1
- **C** **T** All contain γ-carboxyglutamic acid
- **D** **T** Breast milk contains little vitamin K and placental transfer is poor
- **E** **F** Warfarin blocks synthesis of vitamin K-dependent synthesis of coagulation factors

43
- **A** **T** Ascorbic acid deficiency prevents the conversion of proline to hydroxyproline
- **B** **T** Recommended intake 30–75 mg
- **C** **F** Gingivitis only occurs in presence of teeth
- **D** **T** Then petechial haemorrhage and ecchymoses
- **E** **T** With subperiosteal haemorrhage

44
- **A** **F** Aerobic metabolism of glucose is impaired
- **B** **F** Wheat, yeast and legumes are rich in vitamin B_1
- **C** **F** Vasodilatation and high output failure
- **D** **T** A mixed sensorimotor neuropathy
- **E** **T** And gaze palsies and confusion

45

Ⓐ T Dermatitis, diarrhoea and dementia

Ⓑ T Add to anti-TB regimens using isoniazid

Ⓒ F Sideroblastic anaemia may respond

Ⓓ T And also nasolabial seborrhoea

Ⓔ T Also seen in niacin deficiency

46

Ⓐ T But deficiency may take years to manifest

Ⓑ T Vital to tetrahydrofolate metabolism

Ⓒ T Mainly in animal foodstuffs

Ⓓ F Recommended intake 100 μg daily

Ⓔ T And megaloblastic anaemia

47

Ⓐ T If colonic flora are reduced

Ⓑ T

Ⓒ T 1 g glucose = 40 kcal

Ⓓ F Use of > 10% dextrose solutions causes local phlebitis

Ⓔ T Due to elevated insulin levels

48

Ⓐ F Nutritional deficiency should be suspected in all ill patients

Ⓑ T Less if mainly protein loss

Ⓒ T But not specific

Ⓓ T And macrocytosis

Ⓔ F Lymphopenia

49

Ⓐ T Gross obesity > 40

Ⓑ T Hyperinsulinaemia is common

Ⓒ T But no single gene defect identified

Ⓓ T But precise endocrine mechanisms unclear

Ⓔ T After correction for total body mass

50

Ⓐ T And clinical gout

Ⓑ T And anxiety disorders

Ⓒ T Often asymptomatic

Ⓓ T With insulin resistance

Ⓔ T And coronary artery disease

51

Ⓐ T

Ⓑ T And sodium valproate

Ⓒ T

Ⓓ F Stimulates satiety and can help some patients lose weight

Ⓔ T Increases insulin secretion

52

Ⓐ F Aim to reduce intake by no more than 600 kcal per day

Ⓑ F 1.5 lb per week (600 kcal deficit /day = 4200 kcal /week = 0.6 kg human tissue)

Ⓒ T Sufficient to achieve a significant improvement in heath

Ⓓ F 40 g minimum recommended protein intake

Ⓔ F Fat restriction < 50 g/day (calorific values fat = 9 kcal/g, CHO = 4 kcal/g)

53

Ⓐ T In females, the risk is increased with waist > 32 inches (80 cm)

Ⓑ T Walking expends 5 kcal/min (includes BMR = 1 kcal/min)

Ⓒ F Even a small intake of carbohydrate prevents significant ketosis

Ⓓ T Calorific value of alcohol = 7 kcal per gram

Ⓔ T Effect of anti-obesity drugs plateaus at about 12 weeks

54

Ⓐ T

Ⓑ T

Ⓒ T In patients with diabetes, HbA_{1c} concentrations fall by 15%

Ⓓ F Reduction in total cholesterol by 10%

Ⓔ F Improves by 90%; 33% increase in exercise tolerance

55

Ⓐ F Mainly triglycerides; not present in the normal fasting plasma

Ⓑ T VLDL is synthesised in the liver and is the precursor of LDL

Ⓒ T Generated from VLDL in the bloodstream

Ⓓ T

Ⓔ F HDL aids cholesterol excretion and is cardioprotective

56

Ⓐ T Risk of pancreatitis with both types I and V but no atherogenic risk

Ⓑ T Triglycerides variably abnormal in all except type IIa

Ⓒ T And all are associated with increased atherosclerosis

Ⓓ T And premature coronary atherosclerosis

Ⓔ F Defective LDL receptor gene is typical of type II familial hypercholesterolaemia

57

Ⓐ T Increases triglycerides and very low density lipoprotein (VLDL) but decreases high density lipoprotein (HDL)

Ⓑ T Increases triglycerides and VLDL but decreases HDL

Ⓒ F Hypothyroidism increases cholesterol and low density lipoprotein (LDL)

Ⓓ T Increases triglycerides, VLDL and HDL

Ⓔ T Increases triglycerides and HDL

58

Ⓐ T Increase LDL catabolism

Ⓑ F Decrease plasma LDL and cholesterol

Ⓒ F Decrease lipolysis and plasma triglycerides but increase plasma HDL

Ⓓ T Decrease plasma triglycerides and plasma LDL and increase plasma HDL

Ⓔ T Like cholestyramine, it blocks bile acid reabsorption in the gut

59

Ⓐ T And aim for weight reduction to body mass index < 25

Ⓑ F Aim to reduce cholesterol if > 4.5 mmol/L in patients with coronary artery disease

Ⓒ T Especially if refractory to dietary measures

Ⓓ F Suggests better risk profile

Ⓔ F Statins not fibrates have this specific effect

60

Ⓐ T By definition, plasma glucose < 2.4 mmol/L

Ⓑ T Reduces hepatic glycogen and decreases hepatic gluconeogenesis

Ⓒ F An overnight or 12-hour fast is usually sufficient

Ⓓ F Late dumping; early dumping is due to the release of gut neuropeptides

Ⓔ T Whipple's triad—symptoms induced by fasting, relieved by glucose and associated with a subnormal blood glucose concentration

61

Ⓐ T Also haemangiopericytoma

Ⓑ T Also anti-insulin receptor antibody syndrome

Ⓒ T Also severe renal failure

Ⓓ T Decreased insulin antagonism

Ⓔ T

62

Ⓐ T Rate-limiting step in biosynthesis of haem

Ⓑ T Porphobilinogen accumulates

Ⓒ F Typical of acute porphyria

Ⓓ F Typical of the non-acute porphyrias

Ⓔ T Both are hepatic porphyrias

63

A F Decreased porphobilinogen deaminase enzyme activity levels

B T Until precipitated by drugs or alcohol in some

C T Pain may mimic acute abdomen

D T Marked systemic upset

E F Barbiturates and oral contraceptives typically induce exacerbations

64

A T Reactive (AA) amyloidosis

B T Primary (AL) amyloidosis

C F Type 1 diabetes mellitus

D T Also the spongiform encephalitides

E T Reactive (AA) amyloidosis

8 ENDOCRINE DISEASE

1
Ⓐ F Dopamine inhibits prolactin release
Ⓑ F Somatostatin inhibits growth hormone release
Ⓒ T In vivo significance of effect on prolactin is uncertain
Ⓓ T Gonadal steroids and inhibin modify GnRH effects
Ⓔ T Arginine vasopressin also effects ACTH release

2
Ⓐ F Prolactin-secreting tumours may be chromophobe macroadenomas
Ⓑ T May be confirmed on MR scanning
Ⓒ F Usually basophil microadenoma
Ⓓ F Usually acidophil macroadenoma
Ⓔ T Other visual field losses may occur

3
Ⓐ T And pregnancy
Ⓑ T Dopamine antagonist like metoclopramide
Ⓒ T High plasma TRH
Ⓓ T High plasma ACTH
Ⓔ T High plasma ACTH

4
Ⓐ T Unilateral galactorrhoea suggests a breast tumour
Ⓑ T Typical
Ⓒ T
Ⓓ T Pressure effects are only associated with macroadenomas
Ⓔ T E.g. cabergoline and quinogolide

5
Ⓐ T Also carpal tunnel syndrome
Ⓑ T Both occur in 25%
Ⓒ T Visceromegaly and hepatomegaly
Ⓓ T The commonest of all the symptoms
Ⓔ F The skin is thickened with increased sebum production

6
Ⓐ F Failure to suppress plasma GH—may even rise; GH normally falls during the GTT
Ⓑ F Increased serum prolactin occurs in 30%
Ⓒ T
Ⓓ F Rarely abnormal—MR scanning is used for preoperative assessment
Ⓔ F Somatostatin analogues reduce GH secretion but not tumour size

7
Ⓐ T Then loss of ACTH and finally loss of TSH
Ⓑ F Hypotension due to the effects of cortisol deficiency on the vascular bed and kidneys
Ⓒ F Striking pallor due to the effects of ß-LPH deficiency on melanocytes
Ⓓ F Unlike primary hypothyroidism, the skin changes do not occur
Ⓔ T Due to increased ADH release and ADH sensitivity induced by hypotension and cortisol deficiency—ADH deficiency occurs if there is posterior pituitary damage

8

Ⓐ T GnRH deficiency associated with hypogonadotrophic hypogonadism and anosmia

Ⓑ T Any tumour close to the pituitary fossa including meningiomas

Ⓒ T Including radiotherapy

Ⓓ T Post-partum necrosis of the pituitary gland

Ⓔ T Also tuberculosis causing chronic basal meningitis

9

Ⓐ T Nephrogenic diabetes insipidus (DI); also congenital cranial DI—autosomal dominant

Ⓑ T Any tumour or radiotherapy close to the pituitary fossa

Ⓒ T DI, diabetes mellitus, optic atrophy and deafness

Ⓓ F Severe hypokalaemia and hypercalcaemia

Ⓔ T Also tuberculosis causing chronic basal meningitis

10

Ⓐ F Severe hypernatraemia only when water access denied

Ⓑ T Glucocorticoid insufficiency may mask diabetes insipidus

Ⓒ T Or secondary to pituitary tumours or sarcoid

Ⓓ F Carbamazepine stimulates ADH release

Ⓔ T An effect of long-term overhydration in psychogenic polydipsia

11

Ⓐ T Used in manic depressive states

Ⓑ T Rarely encountered in clinical practice

Ⓒ T Also inherited in cystinosis

Ⓓ F Chlorpropramide increases renal sensitivity to vasopressin

Ⓔ T

12

Ⓐ T And encephalitis

Ⓑ T Even apparently minor injury

Ⓒ T And pulmonary tuberculosis

Ⓓ T And pancreas, ureter, bladder, prostatic and other malignancies

Ⓔ T As well as carbamazepine, chlorpropamide and others

13

Ⓐ F An ACTH stimulation test is often the more appropriate test

Ⓑ T Or if severe hypoglycaemic symptoms develop

Ⓒ F Needs an adequate hypoglycaemic stimulus but runs the risk of hypoglycaemia

Ⓓ T Plasma cortisol at 0800 hrs < 180 nmol/l

Ⓔ F Test of hypothalamic–pituitary–adrenal axis

14

Ⓐ F Usually isolated growth hormone secretory failure

Ⓑ F Affects the minority

Ⓒ T As an isolated abnormality

Ⓓ T With consequent short stature

Ⓔ F Puberty not affected

15

Ⓐ F May cause gigantism

Ⓑ T And other chromosomal abnormalities

Ⓒ T And malnutrition

Ⓓ T Usually with obesity

Ⓔ F Primary hypothyroidism

16

Ⓐ T Thyroglobulin in synthesised within thyroid cells

Ⓑ F T_4 should be regarded as a pro-hormone

Ⓒ F Bound to thyroxine-binding globulin and also to pre-albumin

Ⓓ T T_4 is deiodinated in liver, muscle and kidney

Ⓔ T Production of reverse T_3 may increase

17
- **A** T With secondary hypothyroidism
- **B** F Serum TSH would be elevated
- **C** F Free T_4 is normal but total T_4 is often increased (high thyroxine-binding globulin (TBG) concentrations)
- **D** T Sick euthyroid syndrome—total and free T_4 may be reduced
- **E** F Free T_4 and TSH are normal; total T_4 is often increased (high TBG concentrations)

18
- **A** T 75% of cases
- **B** T 15% multinodular, 5% single nodule
- **C** T May also cause hypothyroidism
- **D** T A goitre is therefore usually present
- **E** T And HLA-B8 and DR2

19
- **A** T Or persisting resting sinus tachycardia
- **B** T Appetite is maintained
- **C** F Muscular weakness may occur
- **D** T Occasionally with ophthalmoplegia
- **E** F Insulin requirements may increase

20
- **A** F Controls ventricular response rate
- **B** F Inhibits the iodination of tyrosine
- **C** F TSH measurement alone should not guide therapy
- **D** F But titres correlate poorly with disease activity
- **E** T Especially patients with large goitres

21
- **A** F Suggests treatment-induced hypothyroidism
- **B** T 40% in first year—long-term follow-up necessary
- **C** F Relapse is uncommon
- **D** T In 75% if given a standard dose
- **E** F In 25% if given a standard dose

22
- **A** F Radioiodine is better avoided in patients < 40 years of age
- **B** F Potassium perchlorate is now avoided—high toxicity
- **C** T β-blockers are useful for symptomatic treatment
- **D** T Particularly if a recurrent episode
- **E** T Steroids are used in thyroid crisis and severe eye complications

23
- **A** T 15% are rendered permanently hypothyroid at 1 year
- **B** T Producing dysphonia
- **C** T 5–10% develop postoperative hypocalcaemia
- **D** T 5% at one year
- **E** F No known association

24
- **A** F Excessive lacrimation and conjunctivitis are more common
- **B** F Ophthalmopathy may precede hyperthyroidism or even follow treatment
- **C** F No such test available unfortunately
- **D** T Steroids or surgery may be needed in other cases
- **E** T Therefore avoid over-treatment of hyperthyroidism if possible

25
- **A** T Both however, are non-specific
- **B** T And infertility and impotence
- **C** T Perhaps due to oedema of the middle ear
- **D** T And rarely alopecia, vitiligo and dry hair
- **E** F Reflexes preserved with delayed relaxation

26
Ⓐ F Decreased serum free T_4 and increased serum TSH concentration
Ⓑ T Rarely causing galactorrhoea
Ⓒ T Producing hyponatraemia
Ⓓ F Serum lactate dehydrogenase and creatine kinase may be elevated
Ⓔ T And serum triglyceride levels

27
Ⓐ F There may be constipation
Ⓑ T But puberty is usually delayed
Ⓒ T May present with short stature
Ⓓ T Epiphyseal closure is delayed
Ⓔ T But a rare occurrence

28
Ⓐ T Generalised visceromegaly can occur
Ⓑ T Usually with hypothyroidism
Ⓒ T Often associated with hypothyroidism
Ⓓ T Usually no treatment required
Ⓔ T With nerve deafness; autosomal recessive

29
Ⓐ F Goitre may occur at any age
Ⓑ T The most common cause of goitrous hypothyroidism
Ⓒ T Typically deficiency of intrathyroidal peroxidase
Ⓓ F Should suppress the serum TSH
Ⓔ F May be seen in Hashimoto's disease

30
Ⓐ F The thyroid is typically painful
Ⓑ T Virus induced thyroid inflammation
Ⓒ F But biochemical evidence of hyperthyroidism is common
Ⓓ T Antibodies in low titre transiently
Ⓔ F Transient hypothyroidism with thyroidal recovery usually

31
Ⓐ F May cause painful thyroiditis with transient hypothyroidism
Ⓑ T Hypothyroidism if iodine deficiency is severe
Ⓒ F No association
Ⓓ T Secondary hypothyroidism
Ⓔ T E.g. cassava root

32
Ⓐ F 'Hot' nodules are almost always benign
Ⓑ F Radiotherapy provides brief symptomatic relief only
Ⓒ F Total thyroidectomy, radioiodine and longterm thyroxine
Ⓓ T Papillary tumours are the most common cell type
Ⓔ F Rare despite high calcitonin levels; carcinoid syndrome can occur

33
Ⓐ F 40% of calcium is protein-bound; normal after correction for serum albumin
Ⓑ F But metabolic alkalosis decreases the level of ionised calcium
Ⓒ T Due to bone metastases (often microscopic)
Ⓓ F Decreases serum calcium levels
Ⓔ T Increased vitamin D synthesis with decreased PTH concentration

34
Ⓐ T But 50% are asymptomatic
Ⓑ F Solitary parathyroid adenoma in 90%
Ⓒ F A relatively late feature
Ⓓ T And peptic ulceration and myopathy
Ⓔ T With characteristic polyuria

35
Ⓐ F Phosphate is usually low
Ⓑ F Increased 1,25-dihydroxycholecalciferol concentration
Ⓒ T Predisposing to stone formation
Ⓓ T indicating osteoblastic activity
Ⓔ T Serum chloride concentration is usually elevated

36

Ⓐ F Feature of idiopathic hypoparathyroidism

Ⓑ T Secondary to hyperphosphataemia, hypocalcaemia and low vitamin D concentration

Ⓒ F Diffuse hypertrophy of small glands

Ⓓ T Tertiary hyperparathyroidism

Ⓔ T Failure of vitamin D absorption

37

Ⓐ T Often via production of osteoclast activating factors

Ⓑ T Undetectable using standard PTH assays

Ⓒ T Increased vitamin D synthesis with low PTH concentration

Ⓓ F Hyperthyroidism is a rare cause

Ⓔ T Increased vitamin D levels production with low PTH concentration

38

Ⓐ T Features of tetany

Ⓑ T And mouth and oesophagus

Ⓒ F Features of hypercalcaemia

Ⓓ T Basal ganglia calcification is typical

Ⓔ T In prolonged hypocalcaemia

39

Ⓐ T Adrenal, thyroid and ovary

Ⓑ T Presents in infancy

Ⓒ T Occurs in 1%

Ⓓ F Increased serum calcitonin may cause hypocalcaemia

Ⓔ F

40

Ⓐ T Producing tissue resistance to PTH

Ⓑ F PTH concentrations rise (compare with true hypoparathyroidism)

Ⓒ F Serum phosphate is high

Ⓓ T And occasionally mental retardation

Ⓔ F 1-α-hydroxycholecalciferol treatment

41

Ⓐ F Alkalosis reduces the ionised calcium concentration

Ⓑ F Alkalosis reduces the ionised calcium concentration

Ⓒ F Alkalosis reduces the ionised calcium concentration

Ⓓ T Due to sequestration in areas of pancreatic and fat necrosis

Ⓔ T Vitamin D malabsorption

42

Ⓐ T Usually 20 ml of a 10% solution

Ⓑ T Given by slow i.v. infusion

Ⓒ F Calcitonin may worsen hypocalcaemia

Ⓓ T But serum calcium must be monitored

Ⓔ F But indicated in tetany associated with an alkalosis (e.g. hyperventilation)

43

Ⓐ F Principally under control of angiotensin II

Ⓑ T In the zona reticularis and fasciculata respectively

Ⓒ F Cortisol levels fall to a nadir at around midnight

Ⓓ F Hypoglycaemia stimulates cortisol release

Ⓔ T Anti-insulin effects

44

Ⓐ T 'Pseudo-Cushing's' syndrome due to stress responses

Ⓑ F Pituitary microadenoma or hyperplasia

Ⓒ F Weight loss, pigmentation and metabolic alkalosis

Ⓓ T Non-ACTH dependent Cushing's

Ⓔ F Mineralocorticoid effects

45

Ⓐ T Protein catabolism in bone

Ⓑ F Hypertension may occur

Ⓒ T Impotence in men

Ⓓ T Muscle protein catabolism

Ⓔ F Impaired glucose tolerance

46
- **A** F   Rarely apparent on plain skull X-ray
- **B** T   Impotence in men
- **C** T   Impaired glucose tolerance
- **D** F   Plasma cortisol is not suppressed
- **E** F   Hypertension and hypokalaemia

47
- **A** F   Diurnal pattern of secretion is lost
- **B** F   Plasma cortisol fails to suppress with dexamethasone
- **C** T   Sometimes used as a screening test
- **D** T   Particularly in virilising tumours
- **E** F   ACTH is undetectable at all times

48
- **A** T   Decreases mucosal resistance
- **B** T   Increased renal sodium reabsorption
- **C** T   Particularly likely to affect the femoral heads
- **D** F   Sometimes used to treat severe pseudogout
- **E** T   Typical; causes day–night reversal of biorhythms

49
- **A** F   Compare oedema in patients with secondary hyperaldosteronism
- **B** T   Rarely hypokalaemic paralysis
- **C** T   Hypertension and hypokalaemia are characteristic
- **D** F   NIDDM is however associated with primary hypoadrenalism
- **E** F   Associated with renin suppression

50
- **A** T   Rare cause
- **B** T   Commonest cause
- **C** T   Rare
- **D** F   Both may cause hypercalcaemia
- **E** T   Now a rare cause

51
- **A** T   All features of glucocorticoid insufficiency
- **B** F   Only new scars become pigmented
- **C** T   Vitiligo is seen in 10–20%
- **D** F   Increased insulin sensitivity with hypoglycaemia
- **E** T   Loss of adrenal androgen

52
- **A** T   Especially if caused by an expanding pituitary lesion
- **B** T   ACTH stimulation cannot distinguish primary from secondary failure
- **C** F   ACTH levels are not elevated and no autoimmune association
- **D** F   No mineralocorticoid deficiency
- **E** F   Replacement therapy should mimic the diurnal rhythm

53
- **A** T   Cortisol acetate requires initial hepatic metabolism
- **B** F   Mineralocorticoid is invariably required
- **C** F   Patients must increase dose with intercurrent illness
- **D** T   Pay attention to the underlying precipitant
- **E** F   30–40 mg per day usually

54
- **A** T   With defective cortisol production; 20% are due to 11-hydroxylase deficiency
- **B** T   But mineralocorticoids preserved in two-thirds
- **C** T   Unlike females, appear normally virilised and recognition can be delayed
- **D** T   High levels of androgens
- **E** T   Increased ACTH secretion

55
- **A** F   Noradrenaline is a precursor of adrenaline
- **B** T   Catecholamine secretion
- **C** F   90% are benign
- **D** T   Occurs in MEN type II syndrome
- **E** F   Symptoms worsen due to unopposed α-adrenoreceptor activity

56
Ⓐ T Hyperprolactinaemia and testicular dysfunction
Ⓑ T Psychogenic impotence
Ⓒ T Involving internal pudendal artery
Ⓓ T Vascular disease and autonomic neuropathy
Ⓔ T Spinal cord demyelination

57
Ⓐ T E.g. following severe orchitis
Ⓑ F Maldescended testes in an adult should be removed
Ⓒ T Antisperm antibodies may subsequently destroy sperm
Ⓓ F No treatment is widely effective
Ⓔ F Suggests pituitary/hypothalamic cause

58
Ⓐ T E.g. hypogonadism or chronic liver failure
Ⓑ T Inhibition of LH/FSH secretion caused by prolactin
Ⓒ T Also spironolactone and anti-androgen therapy (e.g. cyproterone + GnRH analogues)
Ⓓ T Hypergonadotrophic hypogonadism
Ⓔ T Rare cause of excessive oestrogen production

59
Ⓐ F Serum LH concentration is elevated
Ⓑ F Serum FSH concentration is elevated
Ⓒ T Also characterised by anosmia due to maldevelopment of the amygdala
Ⓓ F Testicular damage—hypergonadotrophic
Ⓔ F Altered metabolism of testosterone—hypergonadotrophic

60
Ⓐ F Adrenal androgen production is spared
Ⓑ F Height is excessive due to failure of epiphyseal fusion
Ⓒ T Testicular atrophy in particular
Ⓓ T Androgen deficiency
Ⓔ T Testosterone withdrawal

61
Ⓐ T Usually 47, XXY chromosomal composition
Ⓑ T Usually 45, XO
Ⓒ T May present with secondary amenorrhoea or premature menopause
Ⓓ T Affects 15% of males with leprosy
Ⓔ T May also be associated with reduced serum gonadotrophins

62
Ⓐ T Chromosomal abnormalities are rare
Ⓑ T Occurs in the minority
Ⓒ F Sterility follows if bilateral
Ⓓ T Secondary sexual characteristics are preserved
Ⓔ F Testicular descent ensues in 40%

63
Ⓐ F May cause dysmenorrhoea
Ⓑ T Elevated adrenal androgens
Ⓒ T Distinctive morphological features
Ⓓ T Or other severe systemic disease
Ⓔ T Or other hypothalamic or pituitary problem

64
Ⓐ T Suppression of LH and FSH secretion by prolactin
Ⓑ T Failure of gonadotrophin secretion
Ⓒ T Associated with hyperprolactinaemia
Ⓓ T Or other severe systemic disease
Ⓔ T Polycystic ovary disease

65
Ⓐ F Gonadotrophins elevated
Ⓑ F Features of androgen excess
Ⓒ F Osteoporosis develops prematurely
Ⓓ T Due to oestrogen deficiency
Ⓔ F Normal menopause occurs at this age

66

Ⓐ T Commonest cause and treated with anti-androgens (e.g. cyproterone)

Ⓑ T PCO is associated with obesity and infertility; plasma LH:FSH ratio > 2 5

Ⓒ T Modest increase in adrenal androgen synthesis

Ⓓ F Primary adrenal, thyroid, parathyroid, gastric parietal and gonadal failure syndromes

Ⓔ T Ectopic androgen production does not suppress with dexamethasone (unlike excessive androgen production in congenital adrenal hyperplasia)

67

Ⓐ F Autosomal dominant

Ⓑ T E.g. acromegaly

Ⓒ F MEN type II

Ⓓ T Zollinger–Ellison syndrome

Ⓔ T

68

Ⓐ F Autosomal dominant like MEN type I

Ⓑ T Associated with parathyroid adenoma and similar to MEN type I

Ⓒ T High plasma calcitonin concentration

Ⓓ T Multiple mucosal neurofibromata and marfanoid appearance in MEN type IIb

Ⓔ F

9 DISEASES OF THE ALIMENTARY TRACT AND PANCREAS

1
- **Ⓐ T** Vasoactive intestinal peptide and substance P
- **Ⓑ F** The thought or smell of food induces a vagally-mediated response
- **Ⓒ T** And thence to the myenteric and submucous plexuses
- **Ⓓ F** Vagal stimulation
- **Ⓔ F** Inhibits secretion of many of the GI hormones

2
- **Ⓐ T** An important defence mechanism
- **Ⓑ T** Synthesised by B lymphocytes
- **Ⓒ T** Together with chylomicrons and lipoproteins
- **Ⓓ F** Actively absorbed throughout the entire small intestine
- **Ⓔ T** Autonomic nervous system is also involved

3
- **Ⓐ F** Migrating motor complexes (MMC) traverse the small bowel every 1–2 hours
- **Ⓑ F** Lipase and colipase; secretin induces pancreatic secretion of bicarbonate
- **Ⓒ F** Digested by the mucosal disaccharidase enzymes lactase, sucrase and maltase
- **Ⓓ T** Trypsinogen is activated to trypsin by duodenal enterokinase
- **Ⓔ F** The autonomic nervous system, neuropeptides and other hormones

4
- **Ⓐ T** And systemic lupus erythematosus, Behçet's syndrome, Reiter's syndrome
- **Ⓑ T** And ulcerative colitis
- **Ⓒ T** And pemphigoid and pemphigus
- **Ⓓ T** Stevens–Johnson syndrome due either to drugs or infections
- **Ⓔ T** Aphthous mouth ulcers are usually idiopathic rather than viral-induced

5
- **Ⓐ T** Also associated with malnutrition and autoimmune hepatitis
- **Ⓑ T** Associated with dry mouth and kerotoconjunctivitis sicca (dry eyes)
- **Ⓒ T** May be associated with calculi in the parotid duct
- **Ⓓ T** Uveoparotid fever (Heerdfordt's syndrome)
- **Ⓔ F** Associated with mumps

6
- **Ⓐ T** Via formation of an oesophageal web—'sideropenic dysphagia'
- **Ⓑ T** May also be associated with regurgitation and recurrent aspiration
- **Ⓒ F** Asymptomatic unless complicated by malignancy
- **Ⓓ T** More commonly caused by stroke; typically worse with fluids rather than solids
- **Ⓔ T** Best diagnosed on oesophageal manometry

7

Ⓐ F May be hazardous due to inadvertent perforation

Ⓑ T Characteristic and may be associated with regurgitation

Ⓒ F Typically presents in later life

Ⓓ T Due to recurrent aspiration

Ⓔ F Dysphagia only progresses very slowly

8

Ⓐ T Due to regurgitation and aspiration

Ⓑ F Failure to relax the LOS with loss of ganglion cells in Auerbach's plexus on histology

Ⓒ F Acid reflux is prevented by the non-relaxing lower oesophageal sphincter

Ⓓ T Even if the obstruction is treated

Ⓔ T If this fails, Heller's myotomy may be indicated

9

Ⓐ T Oesophageal muscular hypertrophy and degenerative vagal nerve changes

Ⓑ T But presentation can be at any age

Ⓒ T Emotion may precipitate contraction

Ⓓ F Uncoordinated contractions per se may cause dysphagia

Ⓔ F Only if the contractions are associated with acid reflux

10

Ⓐ F Associated with increased intra-abdominal pressure (e.g. pregnancy)

Ⓑ T

Ⓒ T Delayed oesophageal clearance is more common in the elderly

Ⓓ F Associated with decreased lower oesophageal sphincter tone

Ⓔ T

11

Ⓐ T Produces slowly progressive dysphagia for solids

Ⓑ T

Ⓒ T Extrinsic oesophageal compression

Ⓓ T Also associated with ingestion of corrosives (e.g. dental cleansing tablets)

Ⓔ F Often asymptomatic

12

Ⓐ T Squamous rather than adenocarcinoma

Ⓑ F 80–90% are squamous cell

Ⓒ T Adenocarcinoma is associated with chronic oesophagitis

Ⓓ F 90% are in the lower two-thirds

Ⓔ T And betel nut chewing in the East

13

Ⓐ F More suggestive of reflux with oesophagitis and stricture formation

Ⓑ T Painless due to destruction of the mucosal innervation

Ⓒ T Weight loss relates to poor food intake

Ⓓ T 75% have lymph node, liver and/or mediastinal spread

Ⓔ F 5 year survival is about 5%

14

Ⓐ F

Ⓑ T Plays a role in gastric ulcer

Ⓒ F Associated with achlorhydria 'no acid, no ulcer'

Ⓓ T Implicated in > 90% of instances

Ⓔ T Associated with both gastric and duodenal ulcer recurrence rates

15

Ⓐ T Hunger pain

Ⓑ T Perhaps with the 'pointing sign'

Ⓒ T Pain is characteristically periodic

Ⓓ F More suggestive of biliary colic; pain rarely lasts > 2 hours

Ⓔ T Relieved by antacid or food

16
Ⓐ F
Ⓑ F Tobacco also has an aetiological role
Ⓒ T Prevents ulcer recurrence
Ⓓ T Prevents ulcer recurrence
Ⓔ T MALTomas often regress with *H. pylori* eradication

17
Ⓐ F Only about 20%; most have reflux dyspepsia or functional dyspepsia
Ⓑ F 85% relapse if *H. pylori* has not been eradicated
Ⓒ F Cause diarrhoea; aluminium-containing antacids cause constipation
Ⓓ T Due to potential accumulation of bismuth, acid-lowering drugs are preferable
Ⓔ T 30% of gastric ulcers are not associated with *H. pylori* (NSAID-induced ulcers)

18
Ⓐ T Peptic ulcer 35%–50%, varices < 5%
Ⓑ T Higher mortality in the elderly and especially in patients who rebleed
Ⓒ T Cushing's stress ulcers
Ⓓ T Diagnostic yield reduces with time post-admission
Ⓔ T 75% of patients with gastrointestinal bleed have recently taken NSAIDs (only 50% of 'controls')

19
Ⓐ F Typically pain free
Ⓑ T Sympathetic activation
Ⓒ T Particularly in older patients
Ⓓ F Blood urea not creatinine rises due to digestion of the blood in the gut
Ⓔ F Only present if preceding iron deficiency

20
Ⓐ F A sign of hypovolaemia
Ⓑ F Bradycardia may occur in profound blood loss
Ⓒ F Haemoglobin concentration remains unaltered until haemodilution occurs
Ⓓ F Monitoring the urine output as a measure of perfusion is important
Ⓔ T Patients should first be haemodynamically stable if possible

21
Ⓐ T Especially in patients with shock
Ⓑ F Colloid infusion and packed red cells are adequate for volume replacement
Ⓒ T Crystalloids rapidly redistribute to the extravascular space
Ⓓ T Facilitates restoration of optimal circulating volume
Ⓔ T Consider surgical options in all patients with continuing bleeding

22
Ⓐ F 25% occur in acute ulcers
Ⓑ T Especially anterior wall ulcers
Ⓒ T Diaphragmatic pain referred to one or both shoulder tips
Ⓓ F Vomiting is common
Ⓔ T But abdominal rigidity typically persists

23
Ⓐ F Hypokalaemic metabolic alkalosis
Ⓑ F Suggests more distal obstruction
Ⓒ T Paradoxical aciduria due to renal tubular mechanisms
Ⓓ T Unusually, patients may feel like eating immediately after vomiting
Ⓔ F Often prominent gastric peristalsis and a succussion splash

24
A F Tumour is usually in the pancreas or duodenum
B T 50% of tumours have metastasised at presentation
C T Occur in 30–60% (multiple endocrine neoplasia MEN type I)
D F 40% of patients with the Zollinger–Ellison syndrome have diarrhoea
E T Acid secretion is already maximally stimulated

25
A T May also cause peptic ulceration
B T Any severe stress (e.g. burns)
C T Acute mucosal injury
D T And other drugs (e.g. theophylline)
E T Protection with proton pump inhibitors is occasionally necessary

26
A T Causes both acute and chronic gastritis
B T Autoimmune atrophic gastritis
C T And sarcoidosis
D T Due to reflux of duodenal contents
E F No pathognomonic changes

27
A T Smaller stomach and loss of vagally-mediated gastric relaxation
B T Malabsorption is common and can produce folate, B_{12} and vitamin D deficiency
C T Most patients will lose at least 5 kg
D T Late dumping syndrome with exaggerated insulin release
E T Early dumping syndrome with the exaggerated release of upper gastrointestinal hormones

28
A T Women are more commonly affected than men
B T Dysmotility state
C F Features suggesting serious underlying disease
D T Often associated with an irritable bowel syndrome
E T Often associated with stressful life events and difficulties

29
A T
B T Pernicious anaemia and partial gastrectomy
C T *H. pylori* may account for 60% of gastric carcinoma
D T Hypertrophic gastritis with protein-losing enteropathy
E T

30
A F Extraordinary but true
B F But may present as a malignant ulcer
C F 10% 5-year survival
D F Iron deficiency anaemia is typical
E T Virchow's node

31
A F Peak incidence in the age groups 1–5 years and 20–39 years
B T Symptoms return without dietary indiscretion
C T A component of the gluten protein
D F Villous atrophy should resolve
E T Also antigliadin IgA antibody titres

32
A T Most patients have an associated gluten enteropathy
B T Rare infection with Gram-positive bacilli *Tropheryma whippelli*
C T
D T Reduced serum IgA and IgM; often associated with giardiasis
E T Small bowel infection in West Indies and Asia particularly

33
- **A** T Reduced small intestinal motility
- **B** T E.g. long-term proton pump inhibitor therapy and pernicious anaemia
- **C** T Best demonstrated by barium meal
- **D** T Reduced small intestinal motility
- **E** T E.g. Crohn's disease

34
- **A** F 10^8 coliform organisms per ml would be diagnostic
- **B** F Usually vitamin B_{12} deficiency due to bacterial consumption
- **C** F Bacterial deconjugation of the bile acids impairs fat absorption
- **D** F Best confirmed using the ^{14}C-glycocholic acid breath test
- **E** T Hypogammaglobulinaemia predisposes to giardiasis—treat with metronidazole

35
- **A** F Predominantly affects middle aged men
- **B** F Usually peripheral joints, occasionally the sacroiliac joints
- **C** T Also fever and lymphadenopathy
- **D** T Produces characteristic disorder of ocular movements
- **E** T Gram-positive bacilli *Tropheryma whippelli* found in macrophages on duodenal biopsy

36
- **A** T Often resolves spontaneously
- **B** T Usually due to terminal ileal irradiation
- **C** T Also colovesical and rectovaginal fistulas
- **D** T May produce a blind loop syndrome
- **E** F

37
- **A** T And ulcerative colitis
- **B** T
- **C** T And gluten enteropathy
- **D** T
- **E** T And constrictive pericarditis

38
- **A** T May also affect the colon
- **B** T *Yersinia enterocolitica* may mimic appendicitis
- **C** F Unlike Crohn's disease
- **D** T Locally corrosive effect
- **E** F

39
- **A** F Predominantly affects the ileocaecal region
- **B** T Characteristic
- **C** T Often with pain and fever associated with tuberculous peritonitis
- **D** T Identified on liver biopsy
- **E** F Typically pain without alteration in bowel habit

40
- **A** F Facial telangiectasia, flushing and wheezing
- **B** F Diarrhoea is characteristic
- **C** T Due to mesenteric infiltration and/or vasospasm
- **D** T Identified on liver biopsy
- **E** F Typically associated with widespread liver metastases

41
- **A** F Mumps and Coxsackie B viral infections
- **B** T And hyperlipidaemia
- **C** T 50% are associated with biliary tract disease
- **D** T And thiazides and corticosteroids
- **E** T Common cause in the UK

42
- **A** F Guarding occurs relatively late
- **B** F Serum amylase rises and falls rapidly
- **C** T Or pancreatic abscess or non-pancreatic cause
- **D** F Hypocalcaemia
- **E** F Bowel sounds usually absent or diminished due to paralytic ileus

43
- **A** T Administer high flow oxygen therapy
- **B** F Poorer prognosis indicated by white blood cell count > 15×10^9/L
- **C** T Reflects extent of peritoneal reaction
- **D** F Hyperglycaemia > 10 mmol/L
- **E** T

44
- **A** F Diagnostic laparotomy is rarely required
- **B** F Effective pain relief is important
- **C** F Heart rate alone is a poor guide to volume losses
- **D** T Shock and respiratory failure are serious complications
- **E** T Resulting in pancreatic pseudocyst

45
- **A** F Typically impaired GTT
- **B** F Occurs in acute pancreatitis
- **C** F Pancreatic visualisation is superior with CT
- **D** F Surgery may be necessary
- **E** T Biliary tract disease is rarely the cause

46
- **A** T Sometimes relieved by crouching or leaning forward
- **B** T Pancreatic proteases assist vitamin B_{12} absorption
- **C** F Occasionally in cystic fibrosis
- **D** T May persist for days or weeks
- **E** T But insensitive diagnostic tests

47
- **A** F Associated with pancreas divisum
- **B** T Accounts for 70–80% of instances
- **C** F Common but not the cause of chronic pancreatitis
- **D** T
- **E** F

48
- **A** T Also associated with acute pancreatitis
- **B** T Due to stricture of the common bile duct as it passes the head of the pancreas
- **C** T And splenic vein thrombosis leading to gastric varices
- **D** T Occurs in 30% overall
- **E** T May occur in up to 20% of patients

49
- **A** F Prevalence rate 7–10%
- **B** T Pancreatic drainage is via the smaller accessory ampulla
- **C** T
- **D** F This can occur in annular pancreas
- **E** F This and gut atresias are associated with annular pancreas

50
- **A** T Large volume stools may result in rectal prolapse
- **B** T Diabetes occurs in about 40% of cases
- **C** T As a result of impaired pancreatic bicarbonate secretion
- **D** F Most patients survive well into adulthood
- **E** T As a result of viscid secretions

51
- **A** T The vast majority
- **B** F Head of pancreas is the origin in 60% of patients
- **C** F Obstructive jaundice
- **D** T Even in the absence of metastatic spread
- **E** T Usually due to a tumour in the head of pancreas

52
- **A** T Proctitis is a typical finding
- **B** F Suggests Crohn's disease
- **C** T Due to oedema and hyperplasia
- **D** F Affects mucosa and submucosa only
- **E** F Suggest Crohn's disease

53
Ⓐ F Both have a peak incidence at about the age of 20 years
Ⓑ T Smoking exacerbates Crohn's disease but not ulcerative colitis
Ⓒ F Also occurs in severe Crohn's colitis
Ⓓ F Occurs in both
Ⓔ T

54
Ⓐ T Also occurs in Crohn's disease and rheumatoid arthritis
Ⓑ T Suggested by abnormal liver function tests
Ⓒ T Induced by many chronic inflammatory diseases
Ⓓ T Long standing disease (>10 years)
Ⓔ T Large joints especially, or spondyloarthritis

55
Ⓐ F Pyrexia results from the inflammatory process
Ⓑ T E.g. loperamide and codeine phosphate
Ⓒ T Minority require surgery
Ⓓ F Improves as the disease improves; indication for nutritional support
Ⓔ T Or if there is progressive colonic dilatation or perforation

56
Ⓐ F Oral steroids are reserved for more active disease
Ⓑ F Reduces the rate of relapse
Ⓒ T 'Steroid-sparing' effect helps minimise adverse effects
Ⓓ T Causes interstitial nephritis; monitoring renal function is advisable
Ⓔ F Effective given orally or rectally

57
Ⓐ T And vice versa
Ⓑ F Early adult life most commonly
Ⓒ F Affects any part of the alimentary tract
Ⓓ T Bile acid malabsorption and hyperoxaluria
Ⓔ T Crohn's granulomata are non-caseating unlike tuberculosis

58
Ⓐ T In contrast to ulcerative colitis
Ⓑ F The principal symptom is usually pain rather than diarrhoea
Ⓒ T With episodes of colicky pain
Ⓓ T In contrast to ulcerative colitis
Ⓔ F Inflammation is transmural

59
Ⓐ F Vitamin B_{12} deficiency occurs but is not due to pernicious anaemia
Ⓑ T Also amyloidosis
Ⓒ T Seronegative spondyloarthritis
Ⓓ T Can be severe
Ⓔ F But colonic cancer may occur

60
Ⓐ F Strictureplasty helps to limit the length of gut resected
Ⓑ T And reduces the likelihood of further surgery
Ⓒ F Intravenous hydrocortisone in severe active disease
Ⓓ T Binds bile salts and impairs fat absorption
Ⓔ F Major role is in colonic disease

61
Ⓐ T And femoral hernia
Ⓑ T Diffuse mesenteric ischaemia
Ⓒ F Paralytic ileus occurs
Ⓓ F Strangulation impairs blood supply and leads to paralytic obstruction
Ⓔ F But the converse may occur

62
Ⓐ F Late or absent in colonic obstruction
Ⓑ T
Ⓒ T Absent bowel sounds suggest paralytic ileus
Ⓓ F Fluid stools can occur—'spurious' diarrhoea
Ⓔ T Usually with constant severe pain

63

Ⓐ F Such symptoms suggest organic pathology

Ⓑ F Typically affects females aged 16–45 years

Ⓒ T Many also have dyspeptic and urinary symptoms

Ⓓ T Pain may be relieved by defaecation

Ⓔ T May be tenesmus, mucus PR and diarrhoea

64

Ⓐ T Probably the most important therapeutic tools

Ⓑ F Investigations are important in older patients

Ⓒ T Anxiety and or depression is often associated with refractory symptoms

Ⓓ F Although occasionally psychiatric intervention may be necessary

Ⓔ F Use loperamide, a safer opioid that does not cross the blood–brain barrier

65

Ⓐ F Sigmoid colon is most commonly involved

Ⓑ F No causative association

Ⓒ T Especially bleeding and perforation

Ⓓ F But symptoms may be improved

Ⓔ T Such as acute diverticulitis

66

Ⓐ T Exclusion of malignancy may be necessary

Ⓑ F But this may be a feature of chronic diverticulosis

Ⓒ T With or without perforation

Ⓓ F Left iliac fossa or hypogastric pain is typical

Ⓔ T Or enterocolic or colovaginal

67

Ⓐ F Superior mesenteric artery supplies the mid gut

Ⓑ T Predisposing to cardiogenic embolism

Ⓒ T May be bloody diarrhoea

Ⓓ T Progression may be rapid

Ⓔ F Usually fluid-filled loops with little air seen

68

Ⓐ F Diarrhoea without rigors would be typical

Ⓑ F Occlusion of the inferior mesenteric artery, usually with a diseased SMA

Ⓒ T May be a history of intermittent abdominal pain previously

Ⓓ T May be visible on a plain abdominal film

Ⓔ T But 10% progress to gangrene and peritonitis

69

Ⓐ T Occurs from 4 days to 6 weeks post-antibiotics

Ⓑ F Usually appears as a non-specific proctitis

Ⓒ T

Ⓓ T And even bloody diarrhoea

Ⓔ T Treated with metronidazole or vancomycin

70

Ⓐ F Family history in 30% of cases

Ⓑ F Symptoms usually date from birth

Ⓒ T In the pelvic colon and rectum

Ⓓ F Rectum is empty

Ⓔ F Excision of the abnormal segment with colorectal anastomosis

71

Ⓐ F Most occur in the left hemicolon

Ⓑ T And tubulovillous and villous adenomata

Ⓒ T > 50% are malignant if > 2 cm in size

Ⓓ T Causing mechanical bowel obstruction

Ⓔ F Bleeding or mucus discharge are common

72
- **Ⓐ F** Autosomal dominant with a prevalence of 1 in 14 000
- **Ⓑ F** Typically presents in the age group 20–40 years
- **Ⓒ T** Carcinoma is usually present when symptoms commence
- **Ⓓ T** Also with lipomas, epidermoid cysts, osteomas and desmoid tumours
- **Ⓔ F** Immunosuppressives have no role; prophylactic colectomy is warranted

73
- **Ⓐ T** In Western communities
- **Ⓑ F** 75% occur in the left hemicolon
- **Ⓒ T** Particularly in the presence of colonic polyps
- **Ⓓ F** Spread not beyond muscularis
- **Ⓔ F** Majority are palpable hence the need to do a PR examination

74
- **Ⓐ T** Non-specific presentation leads to diagnostic delay
- **Ⓑ T** Late event in right-sided tumours
- **Ⓒ F** Portal venous dissemination to the liver is typical
- **Ⓓ F** Synchronous tumours occur in 2%
- **Ⓔ T** But too insensitive for initial routine diagnostic purposes

DISEASES OF THE LIVER AND BILIARY SYSTEM

10

1

ⓐ T   Accessed via fenestrations in the endothelium

ⓑ T   But only 25% of hepatic blood flow

ⓒ T   Account for 80% of the body's phagocytic capacity

ⓓ T   Stellate cells also produce cytokines and collagenases

ⓔ F   Eight segments associated with the subdivisions of the hepatic and portal veins

2

ⓐ F   Also from catabolism of other haem-containing proteins (e.g. myoglobin)

ⓑ F   Bound to albumin

ⓒ T   By enzymes of the smooth endoplasmic reticulum

ⓓ F   Only reabsorbed after metabolism to stercobilinogen

ⓔ T   And as the oxidation products stercobilin and urobilin

3

ⓐ F   Unconjugated hyperbilirubinaemia

ⓑ T   As almost all bilirubin is unconjugated and albumin bound

ⓒ F   Most of the serum bilirubin is unconjugated

ⓓ F   Unconjugated bilirubin is increased

ⓔ F   Urobilinogen is an unreliable indicator of hepatobiliary disease

4

ⓐ F   Neither ALT nor AST are specific to the liver

ⓑ F   Rarely more than three times normal

ⓒ F   May be elevated in either

ⓓ F   Changes in serum ALT precede changes in the serum bilirubin

ⓔ F   Only the gamma-glutamyl transferase levels increase

5

ⓐ T   Therefore not specific to liver disease

ⓑ F   Not usually > 2.5 times normal

ⓒ T   Excess synthesis in cholestasis

ⓓ F   No prognostic value

ⓔ F   No site-specific pattern

6

ⓐ F   The half-life of serum albumin is about 20–26 days

ⓑ F   May reflect bypass of hepatic immune mechanisms

ⓒ T   But not completely specific

ⓓ T   Half-lives of clotting factors 2, 7, 9 and 10 are short (5–72 hours)

ⓔ F   Typically an increased IgM level

7

ⓐ T

ⓑ F   May appear normal in disease

ⓒ F   May be normal in 10–15% of patients with cirrhosis

ⓓ F   Approximately 0.05%

ⓔ T   And tuberculosis and hepatic vein obstruction; protein concentration < 30 g/L = transudate

8

ⓐ F

ⓑ T   Hence the increase in the serum gamma-glutamyl transferase

ⓒ T

ⓓ T   May also cause chemical hepatitis

ⓔ F

9

Ⓐ F Typically autosomal dominant
Ⓑ T Causing failure of bilirubin conjugation
Ⓒ T And no abnormality of other liver function tests
Ⓓ T Sometimes used as a diagnostic test
Ⓔ F Unconjugated hyperbilirubinaemia is the sole abnormality

10

Ⓐ F Typically pale—steatorrhoea
Ⓑ T Due to conjugated bilirubinuria
Ⓒ F Conjugated hyperbilirubinaemia
Ⓓ T Diagnostic feature
Ⓔ T

11

Ⓐ F Intrahepatic
Ⓑ F Intrahepatic
Ⓒ T CBD obstruction from chronic pancreatitis
Ⓓ F Intrahepatic
Ⓔ T

12

Ⓐ T E.g. pancreatic carcinoma
Ⓑ F Also common in acute hepatitis
Ⓒ T
Ⓓ T Suggests obstruction with cholangitis
Ⓔ T Sometimes relative lymphocytosis in viral hepatitis

13

Ⓐ F Mononuclear cell infiltrate 'lobulitis'
Ⓑ F These areas tend to be more affected
Ⓒ T Mononuclear cell infiltrate 'triaditis'
Ⓓ T Councilman bodies
Ⓔ F Seen in alcohol abuse and with other hepatotoxins

14

Ⓐ F Lymphocyte invasion of the portal–periportal interface
Ⓑ T Classical
Ⓒ T
Ⓓ T The hallmark of early cirrhosis
Ⓔ F Hepatitis A virus does not cause severe chronic hepatitis

15

Ⓐ T Often asymptomatic
Ⓑ F Microvesicular steatosis
Ⓒ F Microvesicular steatosis
Ⓓ T Steatohepatitis (macrovesicular steatosis with hepatocyte necrosis) can be serious
Ⓔ T Common and benign

16

Ⓐ T Faecal-oral spread of a picornavirus
Ⓑ F 2–4 weeks
Ⓒ F But children are more frequently infected
Ⓓ T Non-specific findings of acute hepatitis
Ⓔ F Chronic hepatitis does not occur

17

Ⓐ F Viraemia is only transient in hepatitis A
Ⓑ F Spontaneous recovery is the typical outcome
Ⓒ T But a recognised rarity
Ⓓ T Serological investigations should help distinguish
Ⓔ T Some will have natural endogenous protection

18

Ⓐ T A reliable marker of hepatitis B infection
Ⓑ T A DNA hepadna virus
Ⓒ F Chronic carriage occurs in 5–10% of adults
Ⓓ F Alternative serological evidence of infection should be sought
Ⓔ F Carriage rates are highest in the Middle East and Far East

19

Ⓐ F Average incubation 3 months
Ⓑ T Or other exposure to blood or blood products
Ⓒ T May cause serum sickness
Ⓓ T Hepatitis A is usually a mild illness
Ⓔ F And hepatic cirrhosis also occurs

20
ⓐ **T** With varying degrees of severity
ⓑ **T**
ⓒ **F** Hepatitis C may progress to chronic disease
ⓓ **F** Most patients are asymptomatic; incubation period is 2–26 weeks
ⓔ **T** Although serological screening methods have greatly reduced this

21
ⓐ **F** An incomplete RNA virus
ⓑ **F** Transmitted with hepatitis B parenterally
ⓒ **T** Incapable of replication alone; incubation is 6–9 weeks
ⓓ **T** Often limited by resolution of hepatitis B
ⓔ **T** Hepatitis B may then resolve

22
ⓐ **T** An RNA virus
ⓑ **T**
ⓒ **T** Incubation period is 3–8 weeks
ⓓ **T**
ⓔ **T** Chronic hepatitis does not develop

23
ⓐ **T** Without evidence of pre-existing liver disease
ⓑ **F** Suggest chronic liver disease
ⓒ **T** With confusion and asterixis (liver flap)
ⓓ **T** Renal failure is an ominous development
ⓔ **T** Occurs late, if at all

24
ⓐ **F** Serum albumin has a long half-life
ⓑ **T** Impaired hepatic gluconeogenesis
ⓒ **T** Useful in determining prognosis
ⓓ **F** Typically not so elevated, unlike the serum transaminases
ⓔ **F** May be a polymorphonuclear leucocytosis

25
ⓐ **T** To minimise encephalopathy
ⓑ **T** Stress ulceration is common
ⓒ **T** Disseminated intravascular coagulation may also be present
ⓓ **T** Frequent blood glucose monitoring is vital
ⓔ **T**

26
ⓐ **T** Due to autoimmune liver disease
ⓑ **T** But symptoms persist
ⓒ **T** And fatigue, anorexia and jaundice
ⓓ **T** And other signs of chronic liver disease
ⓔ **T** Altered steroid hormone metabolism

27
ⓐ **T** In contrast to autoimmune hepatitis
ⓑ **F** A chronically progressive course is more typical
ⓒ **F** Signs are sparse; hepatomegaly is common
ⓓ **T** Particularly if HBeAg present
ⓔ **F** Hepatoma is more common

28
ⓐ **T** Coomb's positive anaemia
ⓑ **T** Thyrotoxicosis or myxoedema
ⓒ **T** Less commonly
ⓓ **T** And glomerulonephritis
ⓔ **T** More commonly transient arthralgia

29
ⓐ **T** Found in 50–66% of patients with autoimmune hepatitis (AIH)
ⓑ **T** Type II AIH with microsomal antibodies to liver and kidney
ⓒ **T** In presence of elevated serum ALT levels
ⓓ **F** Suggests Wilson's disease
ⓔ **F** Suggests primary biliary cirrhosis

30
- **A** F Defer biopsy if possible for 6 months
- **B** T Most ultimately develop cirrhosis
- **C** F About 10% of patients die within 5 years despite treatment
- **D** T Azathioprine also facilitates a reduction in corticosteroid therapy
- **E** F Also of limited value in chronic type B viral hepatitis

31
- **A** F Liver size reduces as disease progresses
- **B** F Mild splenomegaly due to portal hypertension
- **C** T Particularly in alcoholic liver disease
- **D** T Particularly in alcoholic cirrhosis
- **E** T Hepatopulmonary syndrome associated with pulmonary telangiectasia

32
- **A** F The majority of cases in the UK are alcohol related
- **B** T Or a later complication of chronic infection
- **C** F May cause acute massive hepatic necrosis
- **D** T More than 5–10 years of steady drinking
- **E** F Produces a fatty liver (macrovesicular steatosis)

33
- **A** F Refractory hypoxaemia due to intrapulmonary shunting
- **B** T As does falling serum albumin and rising prothrombin time
- **C** F Peripheral vasodilatation occurs
- **D** T Visceral blood flow is generally reduced
- **E** T As may splenomegaly and ascites

34
- **A** T
- **B** T
- **C** F Common and benign
- **D** F Only HBV, HCV, HDV infections
- **E** T

35
- **A** T And a flapping tremor
- **B** F Highly atypical—suggests other pathology
- **C** T Sometimes sleep reversal
- **D** F Transaminase level does not correlate with severity
- **E** T And other neuropsychiatric problems

36
- **A** T Spontaneous bacterial peritonitis should not be overlooked
- **B** T Often aggravated by diuretic use
- **C** T Or trauma
- **D** T Increased protein load in gut
- **E** F Reduces colonic ammonia absorption

37
- **A** F Restriction < 40 mmol/day is usually required
- **B** F A palliative, symptomatic measure with no prognostic value
- **C** F Calorie restriction is not required
- **D** F Weight loss > 1 kg/day may precipitate renal impairment and/or encephalopathy
- **E** T Restriction may be necessary to control encephalopathy

38
- **A** T Or reduced below 20 g/day
- **B** F May worsen or precipitate encephalopathy
- **C** T Avoid in uraemia
- **D** F May be required for coexistent ascites but may worsen encephalopathy
- **E** T Hypoglycaemia may coexist

39
- **A** F No intrinsic renal damage
- **B** F Suggests glomerular disease
- **C** T Normal renal response to secondary hyperaldosteronism
- **D** F Ratio > 1.5
- **E** F Hypovolaemia is more common

40
- **A** T Intrahepatic parenchymal
- **B** T Intrahepatic presinusoidal
- **C** T Intrahepatic presinusoidal; also sarcoidosis
- **D** T Extrahepatic presinusoidal (portal vein thrombosis)
- **E** T Extrahepatic postsinusoidal

41
- **A** T Oesophageal, gastric and rectal
- **B** T Associated with hypergastrinaemia
- **C** T Associated with reduced renal blood flow
- **D** T
- **E** T And hypersplenism

42
- **A** T May be higher in presence of encephalopathy and ascites
- **B** F Stop bleeding in 80% of cases
- **C** T Constrict splanchnic arterioles; give GTN to combat arterial vasoconstriction
- **D** T Unless exsanguinating, 20% are bleeding from non-variceal sources
- **E** F TIPSS has replaced emergency shunt surgery

43
- **A** F Somatostatin may be useful in acute bleeds
- **B** T Also used in acute bleeds
- **C** T β-blockers reduce portal pressure
- **D** T Better than sclerotherapy in the elective situation
- **E** T Easier than banding in the emergency situation

44
- **A** T Also constrictive pericarditis—transudate
- **B** T Also protein-losing enteropathy—transudate
- **C** T Also carcinomatosis—exudate
- **D** T Chylous effusion
- **E** T Transudate associated with hepatic vein occlusion

45
- **A** F Middle-aged females
- **B** F May precede jaundice by months or years
- **C** T Vitamin D malabsorption and hepatic osteodystrophy
- **D** F Suggests obstruction of large bile duct
- **E** F High titres of antimitochondrial antibody

46
- **A** T And on elbows, knees and buttocks
- **B** F Prognosis excellent in the absence of symptoms or signs
- **C** T Splenomegaly occurs as portal hypertension develops
- **D** F Suggests biliary obstruction
- **E** F None proven to be effective

47
- **A** T Inherited as an autosomal recessive
- **B** T Typically over 40 years of age
- **C** T 'Bronzed diabetes'
- **D** F May be a congestive cardiomyopathy
- **E** F Melanin not iron deposition

48
- **A** T Sometimes accompanying an acute hepatitis in children
- **B** T Or acute hepatic failure or cirrhosis
- **C** T A variety of extrapyramidal syndromes may be seen
- **D** F Serum copper falls, hepatic copper is increased
- **E** T Kayser–Fleischer rings are an important diagnostic clue

49
- **A** T Earliest stage with good prognosis
- **B** T 33% mortality if liver dysfunction is severe
- **C** T 50% 5-year survival after the initial presentation if abstinent
- **D** T Often associated with tender hepatomegaly and abdominal pain
- **E** T Usually associated with at least 50 g/day for at least 10 years

50
- **A** T Often associated with intractable pruritus
- **B** T Unless the patient has HIV infection
- **C** T Contraindicated if abstinence is impossible
- **D** T
- **E** T But contraindicated due to poor prognosis if the hepatoma is extensive

51
- **A** T Most commonly alcoholic cirrhosis
- **B** T A fungal poison
- **C** T Occurs in 30% of those with cirrhosis
- **D** F Associated with HBV, HCV, HDV chronic hepatitis
- **E** T And anabolic steroids

52
- **A** T Pain in a cirrhotic should be suggestive
- **B** T Tumours are vascular and spread locally
- **C** F May be a hepatic bruit
- **D** T Rises in 90% of cases
- **E** F 10% are suitable for surgery

53
- **A** T Secondary to biliary obstruction
- **B** T Secondary to portal pyaemia
- **C** T Acute pancreatitis
- **D** T Infection via hepatic artery
- **E** T Direct local spread

54
- **A** F Jaundice is usually mild and uncommonly obstructive
- **B** T Splenomegaly suggests coexistent pathology
- **C** T May be right shoulder tip pain
- **D** T Single lesions are more common in the right liver
- **E** T Multiple organisms in one-third of cases

55
- **A** F Common hepatic duct
- **B** F Normal common bile duct < 8 mm in diameter
- **C** F Distal common bile duct usually joins pancreatic duct
- **D** F Principally vagal tone controls the gallbladder muscle wall
- **E** T

56
- **A** F Commoner in North America, Europe and Australia
- **B** F 40% of patients > 60 years old
- **C** T But pigment stones are the more common in the developing countries
- **D** T Usually calcium bilirubinate
- **E** F Hepatic hypersecretion of cholesterol more important

57
- **A** T Increased hepatic cholesterol secretion
- **B** T Increased hepatic cholesterol secretion and impaired gallbladder motility
- **C** T Pigment stones
- **D** T Pigment stones
- **E** T Increased hepatic cholesterol secretion

58
- **A** F Cystic duct or gallbladder neck are obstructed in 90%
- **B** F 50% are infected
- **C** F May be acalculous
- **D** F Even though intrabiliary pressure may rise
- **E** F Most gallstones are radiolucent

59
- **A** F Jaundice occurs in less than 20% even in the absence of stones (Mirizzi's syndrome)
- **B** F Pain is typically continuous for up to 6 hours
- **C** T Murphy's sign
- **D** F May follow passage of a gallstone into intestine or biliary surgery
- **E** T May be absent in the elderly

60

Ⓐ T Less common in patients with previous typical biliary colic and gallstones

Ⓑ T Associated with the irritable bowel syndrome and functional dyspepsia

Ⓒ T Hence the need to investigate this possibility

Ⓓ F This abnormality may not be causal and may in fact result from cholecystectomy

Ⓔ T Suggests the possibility of a biliary stricture

61

Ⓐ F Associated with gallstones and ulcerative colitis

Ⓑ T Often with weight loss

Ⓒ F Suggests hepatocellular carcinoma

Ⓓ T But not a specific finding

Ⓔ F Commonest treatment is palliative stenting

62

Ⓐ F Female preponderance—most aged > 70 years

Ⓑ F Adenocarcinoma

Ⓒ T Can also be suspected by the findings on ultrasound scanning

Ⓓ T Usually diagnosed at routine cholecystectomy for gallstones

Ⓔ F Often advanced at diagnosis since presentation is usually late

11 DISEASES OF THE BLOOD

1

Ⓐ F Bone marrow is functional by 5 months in utero

Ⓑ T Some migrate to the thymus

Ⓒ T At birth most of the bone marrow is haemopoietically active

Ⓓ T Proerythroblast is earliest identifiable red cell precursor

Ⓔ F Produced by renal tubular cells

2

Ⓐ F Membrane antigens

Ⓑ F Reticulocytes stain in this way

Ⓒ T Required to maintain biconcave morphology

Ⓓ T Shorter (25–35 days) if measured by chromium labelling

Ⓔ T By conversion to carbonic acid which then dissociates

3

Ⓐ F Two alpha and two gamma chains

Ⓑ F Two alpha and two delta chains

Ⓒ T Methaemoglobin contains a ferric ion

Ⓓ T H^+ generated in dissociation buffered by deoxyhaemoglobin

Ⓔ F Decreased

4

Ⓐ T Ranges from 40% to 70%; under the age of 7 years, lymphocytes predominate

Ⓑ T Around 8 hours in the circulation

Ⓒ F Less nuclear segmentation—a shift to the left in the Arneth count

Ⓓ F Both derive from granulocyte-macrophage colony-forming cells

Ⓔ T Hence high serum vitamin B_{12} levels in chronic myeloid leukaemia

5

Ⓐ T Their granules contain peroxidase to generate reactive oxygen

Ⓑ T Resemble tissue mast cells

Ⓒ T Long-lived cells with major phagocytic functions

Ⓓ F T lymphocytes (80% of all lymphocytes) mediate cellular immunity

Ⓔ F T lymphocytes comprise CD4 positive helper cells and CD8 positive suppressor cells

6

Ⓐ T And in viral infections, salmonellosis, alcohol and adverse effect of many drugs

Ⓑ T An effect of excess corticosteroids and catecholamines

Ⓒ T

Ⓓ T And in lymphoma and systemic lupus erythematosus

Ⓔ T Also occurs in iron deficiency

7

Ⓐ T Often with neutropenia

Ⓑ F Polymorphonuclear leucocytosis

Ⓒ T Non-specific feature of many viral infections

Ⓓ F Non-Hodgkin's lymphoma

Ⓔ T Predominantly small lymphocytes

8

Ⓐ T Or may be neutropenia in systemic lupus erythematosus

Ⓑ T And lithium therapy

Ⓒ T Variable, increases at delivery

Ⓓ F Typically lymphocytosis

Ⓔ T And myocardial infarction

9
Ⓐ F 10-day lifespan
Ⓑ T By the megakaryocytes
Ⓒ F Found in red blood cells
Ⓓ F May increase
Ⓔ T Serotonin (delta granules) and vWF and fibrinogen (alpha granules)

10
Ⓐ F Seen in other disorders of haemoglobin synthesis (e.g. thalassaemia)
Ⓑ T Residual ribosomal material is stained faintly
Ⓒ T Sign of dyserythropoiesis
Ⓓ T And lead poisoning
Ⓔ T And haemoglobinopathies

11
Ⓐ T Average menstrual loss is 30 mg per month
Ⓑ F Males lose 1 mg per day, females lose 2 mg per day
Ⓒ T 60–70% resides in the haemoglobin molecule
Ⓓ F Stored as ferritin
Ⓔ T Normally about 15% of which is absorbed

12
Ⓐ T Microcytosis is the first sign
Ⓑ T Sometimes poikilocytosis
Ⓒ F Only in severe anaemia; hypochromia is due to microcytosis
Ⓓ F Suggests hyposplenism
Ⓔ T Thrombocytosis occurs even in the absence of bleeding

13
Ⓐ F Only if coexistent deficiency demonstrated
Ⓑ F Continue for 3 months to replenish stores
Ⓒ F 10 g/L 10 days unless malabsorption, bleeding or poor compliance
Ⓓ F Peak reticulocyte count at 7–10 days
Ⓔ F Oral iron is usually effective

14
Ⓐ F Macrocytic with polychromasia
Ⓑ T Typically a dimorphic red cell population
Ⓒ F Typically macrocytic
Ⓓ T And other thalassaemias
Ⓔ T Or a normochromic normocytic picture

15
Ⓐ F Typically macrocytic
Ⓑ T Erythropoietin deficiency
Ⓒ T Typically macrocytic
Ⓓ T Protein energy malnutrition
Ⓔ F Anaemia is rare in modest reductions of dietary vitamin B_{12} intake

16
Ⓐ T With megaloblastic marrow
Ⓑ T With polychromasia
Ⓒ T With or without cirrhosis
Ⓓ F Dimorphic, with microcytic population
Ⓔ T But variable red cell morphology

17
Ⓐ T Commonly due to vitamin B_{12} deficiency
Ⓑ T Shift to the right in the nuclear segmentation count (Arneth count)
Ⓒ T And red cell fragmentation
Ⓓ F Features of bleeding or haemolysis
Ⓔ F Bilirubinuria is not a feature of any anaemia

18
Ⓐ F Feature of vitamin B_{12} deficiency only
Ⓑ T Glossitis less common in folate deficiency
Ⓒ T Mild haemolysis
Ⓓ T
Ⓔ T Partially dependent on underlying cause

19
- **A** F Typically 45–65 years
- **B** T Found in 90% and < 50% respectively
- **C** T Mild haemolysis occurs
- **D** T Associated gastric atrophy
- **E** T Failure to correct suggests terminal ileal disease

20
- **A** F Caused by inadequate vegetable intake
- **B** T Characteristic finding
- **C** T Increased requirements
- **D** T Increased requirements
- **E** F Methotrexate and phenytoin may cause folate deficiency

21
- **A** F Typically elderly patients
- **B** T Usually with hypercellular dysplastic marrow
- **C** T Normoblasts with interrupted perinuclear iron ring
- **D** T Particularly of chromosomes 5 and 7
- **E** T Risk is dependent on the precise type of myelodysplastic syndrome

22
- **A** T Sometimes haemolytic anaemia alone
- **B** T Or penicillamine
- **C** T Rare but also associated with other viral hepatitides
- **D** T Occurs with both folate and vitamin B_{12} deficiency
- **E** T Sometimes with sideroblastic marrow change

23
- **A** F Peaks about 30 years of age
- **B** F Thrombocytopenia
- **C** T Diagnosis cannot be made on peripheral blood film alone
- **D** F Splenomegaly occurs in under 10% of cases
- **E** T Typical

24
- **A** F Bilirubin is unconjugated therefore not found in urine
- **B** T The latter always indicating intravascular haemolysis
- **C** F Decreased serum haptoglobin
- **D** T Most is bound to serum haptoglobin
- **E** T Often with reticulocytosis

25
- **A** T Red cells are rich in LDH
- **B** F Unconjugated hyperbilirubinaemia and excess urobilinogen in the urine
- **C** T Also red cell abnormalities (e.g. spherocytes)
- **D** T Reflects reticulocytosis
- **E** T With megaloblastic change if folate deficiency is also present

26
- **A** T Mechanical intravascular haemolysis
- **B** T Associated with cold agglutinins
- **C** T Low-grade haemolysis
- **D** T Severe in blackwater fever
- **E** F Occurs with dapsone and salazopyrine therapy in G6PD-deficient patients

27
- **A** T Also pigment gallstones
- **B** F Red blood cell destruction occurs in the spleen
- **C** F Osmotic fragility is increased
- **D** T Often in association with parvovirus infection
- **E** T Red blood cell membrane protein

28
- **A** T Often precipitated by viral infection
- **B** F Not until HbF levels fall after the age of 3 months
- **C** T Causing pleuritic pain and also renal infarcts
- **D** F Splenic atrophy and functional hyposplenism
- **E** T Painful bone infarcts

29
- **A** T Decreased PaO_2
- **B** T May present as pseudo-toxaemia syndrome
- **C** T Rehydration is an essential component of therapy
- **D** T Treat promptly to prevent sickle-cell crises
- **E** T

30
- **A** F Typically hypochromic microcytic anaemia
- **B** T In the 'major' (homozygous) form
- **C** T Pigment gallstones can be associated with chronic haemolysis
- **D** F Not until HbF synthesis declines
- **E** T particularly in the 'minor' (heterozygous) form

31
- **A** T Characteristic
- **B** T Suggesting intravascular haemolysis
- **C** F Decreased serum haptoglobin concentration
- **D** T Warm usually IgG, cold usually IgM
- **E** T Chronic lymphatic leukaemia, lymphoma and also systemic lupus erythematosus

32
- **A** F Males > 40 years
- **B** T And elevated red cell mass
- **C** T But may be asymptomatic
- **D** F A feature of chronic myeloid leukaemia
- **E** T E.g. increased risk of stroke

33
- **A** T Usually with demonstrable marrow infiltration
- **B** T An ominous finding
- **C** T And tear-drop poikilocytosis of the red blood cells
- **D** F Lymphocytosis
- **E** T Also rare after acute bleeding

34
- **A** T Fever even without underlying infection
- **B** T Infection and infiltration contribute
- **C** T Particularly purpura
- **D** F Normocytic or macrocytic anaemia, with primitive white cells
- **E** F Hypercellular with leukaemic blast cells

35
- **A** F Peaks in childhood
- **B** F Acute myeloblastic leukaemia (AML)
- **C** T AML has a 40% 5-year survival with chemotherapy
- **D** F AML is four times more common than ALL
- **E** F May complicate myelofibrosis

36
- **A** T Splenomegaly in 90% of cases
- **B** T Hyperuricaemia is often asymptomatic
- **C** F Atypical feature
- **D** T Variable platelet dysfunction
- **E** F Median survival 5 years

37
- **A** T Platelet count falls after blast transformation
- **B** T
- **C** T Philadelphia chromosome
- **D** F Usually decreased LAP score
- **E** T Transformation results to either ALL (30%) or acute myeloid leukaemia (AML) (70%)

38
- **A** F Peak age 65 years
- **B** T Typically warm antibody
- **C** F Mild organomegaly only
- **D** T Bacterial more than viral
- **E** F Overall median survival 6 years

39
Ⓐ F Mild thrombocytopenia with usually normal urate
Ⓑ T Associated with a paraproteinaemia in 5%
Ⓒ T Total WCC typically 50–200 × 10⁹/L
Ⓓ T May be associated with haemolysis
Ⓔ F Transformation is rare

40
Ⓐ F But useful in acute myelofibrosis
Ⓑ T
Ⓒ T All severe thalassaemias
Ⓓ T
Ⓔ F But useful in most other acute and chronic leukaemias

41
Ⓐ T Usually occurs 2–3 weeks after the graft and associated with infection
Ⓑ T A major problem, especially with viruses and atypical microorganisms
Ⓒ T Important given the age of many of the patients
Ⓓ T
Ⓔ T

42
Ⓐ F Neither is characteristic
Ⓑ T Mild splenomegaly, generalised lymphadenopathy
Ⓒ F Moderate to massive splenomegaly, no lymphadenopathy
Ⓓ T Usually both mild
Ⓔ F Splenomegaly without lymphadenopathy

43
Ⓐ F Massive splenomegaly can occur
Ⓑ T Characteristic finding
Ⓒ T In contrast to chronic myeloid leukaemia
Ⓓ T Increased cell turnover
Ⓔ F Excess of megakaryocytes

44
Ⓐ F Peak prevalence in males aged 60–70 years
Ⓑ T Amyloidosis occurs in 10% of cases
Ⓒ T Median survival of 40 months
Ⓓ T Reduction of normal plasma cells causes immunodeficiency
Ⓔ T All of which may be asymptomatic

45
Ⓐ F Myeloma produces suppression of the other serum immunoglobulins
Ⓑ T A diagnostic prerequisite
Ⓒ T Amyloidosis also causes a restrictive cardiomyopathy
Ⓓ T But the serum paraprotein may be undetectable
Ⓔ T Malignant infiltration typically associated with a normal isotope bone scan

46
Ⓐ T Advanced disease
Ⓑ F High serum beta₂-microglobulin concentration suggests poor prognosis
Ⓒ T Also severe hypoalbuminaemia
Ⓓ F No prognostic significance
Ⓔ T And plasma cell leukaemia

47
Ⓐ T A pathological hallmark
Ⓑ T Mixed cellularity type occurs especially in the elderly
Ⓒ T 70% of cases; especially common in the young and in females
Ⓓ F In contrast to non-Hodgkin's lymphoma
Ⓔ F Usually involved though without palpable splenomegaly

48
Ⓐ T Usually painless
Ⓑ F Unlike non-Hodgkin's lymphoma
Ⓒ T Lymphopenia suggests poor prognosis
Ⓓ T And fever
Ⓔ T Dependent on staging at presentation

49
- **A** F Indolent and often asymptomatic course with low cell proliferation rates
- **B** T Typically extra-nodal at diagnosis
- **C** T MALToma may be cured by *H. pylori* eradication
- **D** F 70% are B cell tumours
- **E** T Prognosis is also stage- and age-dependent

50
- **A** T Haemorrhagic tendency with nosebleeds and bruising
- **B** F IgM paraproteinaemia
- **C** T Cryoglobulinaemia occurs in 30% of patients
- **D** T Characteristic
- **E** T

51
- **A** T Associated with the hyperviscosity syndrome
- **B** T
- **C** T Vitamin C deficiency—scurvy
- **D** F
- **E** F Thrombotic thrombocytopenic purpura (DIC)

52
- **A** T Failure to synthesize von Willebrand Factor
- **B** T Impaired collagen synthesis impairs capillary support
- **C** T Endothelial damage
- **D** F Factor IX deficiency
- **E** T Platelet dysfunction may also occur in severe renal failure

53
- **A** T E.g. myelofibrosis
- **B** T Even in absence of blood loss
- **C** F Thrombocytopenia
- **D** T With marrow infiltration
- **E** T Non-specific inflammatory response

54
- **A** T Often with leucopenia
- **B** T Primary, or secondary to superimposed infections
- **C** T Increased peripheral consumption of platelets
- **D** F The platelet count is normal
- **E** T Also many commonly used drugs including heparin and beta-blockers

55
- **A** T Can therefore be transmitted transplacentally
- **B** F Usually the young and commoner in females
- **C** T Other clotting tests normal
- **D** F Suggests others causes of thrombocytopenia
- **E** T Particularly in children

56
- **A** F The extrinsic pathway
- **B** T The Stuart–Prower factor
- **C** T First factor in extrinsic pathway
- **D** T Also affects the activated partial thromboplastin time
- **E** F Disorder of the intrinsic pathway

57
- **A** F The intrinsic pathway
- **B** F Detected by prothrombin time
- **C** T Factor X also influences prothrombin time
- **D** F Specific assay to measure
- **E** T Initial factors in the intrinsic system

58
- **A** T Initiated by thromboplastin
- **B** T An unusual complication
- **C** T Endothelial injury
- **D** T Exogenous endotoxins
- **E** T Commonly bronchial carcinoma

59

Ⓐ T Microangiopathic platelet destruction

Ⓑ T These red cell fragments may be absent in mild cases

Ⓒ F Increased FDPs and increased levels of D-dimer

Ⓓ F Both are prolonged due to factor V and fibrinogen deficiency

Ⓔ T Due to factors V, VIII and fibrinogen deficiency

60

Ⓐ F Bleeding time is normal but petechial haemorrhages may occur

Ⓑ T Irrespective of its cause

Ⓒ F No vessel wall or platelet defect

Ⓓ F

Ⓔ T Secondary decrease in factor VIII level with a qualitative platelet defect

61

Ⓐ F A primary vascular defect

Ⓑ T Factor IX deficiency

Ⓒ F Reduced cutaneous capillary integrity

Ⓓ F Vasculitis without thrombocytopenia

Ⓔ T Factor VIII deficiency

62

Ⓐ T Prenatal diagnosis is possible

Ⓑ T Usually not apparent until the age of 6 months

Ⓒ F Only the activated partial thromboplastin time is prolonged

Ⓓ F Half-life is 12 hours

Ⓔ T Desmopressin (DDAVP) therapy is useful to limit exposure to blood products

63

Ⓐ F Autosomal dominant—gene locus on chromosome 12

Ⓑ T And secondary reduction in factor VIII levels

Ⓒ T

Ⓓ F Half-life is 12 hours

Ⓔ T Desmopressin (DDAVP) therapy increases vWF concentrations

64

Ⓐ F Also by the platelets and endothelial cells

Ⓑ T And secondary reduction in factor VIII levels

Ⓒ T Hence deficiency is often first suspected on finding resistance to heparin therapy

Ⓓ T Hence the effectiveness of low-dose heparin therapy

Ⓔ F Inhibits vitamin K epoxide reductase necessary to maintain vitamin K-dependent carboxylase activity

65

Ⓐ T May present with recurrent spontaneous abortion

Ⓑ T Decreased inactivation of factors IIa, VIIa, IXa, Xa, XIa, causing heparin resistance

Ⓒ T Prolonged factor V activation; factor II Leiden increases plasma prothrombin levels

Ⓓ T And chronic myeloid leukaemia—both are associated thrombocytosis

Ⓔ T And protein S deficiency—reduced inactivation of factors Va and VIIIa

66

Ⓐ T Interferes with the coagulation reactions that are enhanced by platelet membranes

Ⓑ F Both may occur and can affect every organ system

Ⓒ T Prolongs the APTT due to an in vitro interaction with phospholipids

Ⓓ F Characteristically one or both are positive

Ⓔ F Thrombocytopenia is typical; autoimmune haemolytic anaemia may also occur

67

Ⓐ T Maintain the prothrombin ratio in the range 2.0–4.0

Ⓑ T Less effective in non-embolic peripheral vascular disease

Ⓒ F Unless associated with mural thrombus

Ⓓ T Reduces the risk of arterial embolism

Ⓔ T Reduces the risk of embolic clots and possibly endocarditis

68

Ⓐ T High risk of DVT (deep venous thrombosis)

Ⓑ T High risk of DVT

Ⓒ T High risk of DVT

Ⓓ F Minimal risk of recurrent DVT if mobility is unimpaired

Ⓔ F Moderate risk—use compression stockings; the risk of intracerebral haemorrhage outweighs the benefits from low-dose heparin

69

Ⓐ T Allergic reaction

Ⓑ T Volume overload—in patients with previous CCF, give prophylactic diuretic therapy

Ⓒ T Particularly important in women of child-bearing age

Ⓓ T Allergic reaction to one or more of the constituents of the transfusion

Ⓔ T Major ABO incompatibility is the likeliest cause

70

Ⓐ T Delayed haemolytic transfusion reaction occurs 5–7 days after the transfusion

Ⓑ T Stop the transfusion immediately

Ⓒ T

Ⓓ F Unlikely in the absence of other premonitory changes

Ⓔ T May be problematic in anaesthetised patients

12 DISEASES OF THE CONNECTIVE TISSUES, JOINTS AND BONES

1
- **ⓐ T** Plus a collagen framework which entraps proteoglycans
- **ⓑ F** Avascular
- **ⓒ T** Key constituent comprising a protein core with keratin and chondroitin sidechains
- **ⓓ T**
- **ⓔ F** Aggrecan turnover rather than collagen turnover is rapid and critical to repair mechanisms

2
- **ⓐ T**
- **ⓑ F** Fluid is secreted by type B fibroblasts
- **ⓒ F** It provides the blood supply to the cartilage
- **ⓓ T**
- **ⓔ T** Together with type VI collagen

3
- **ⓐ T**
- **ⓑ F** Cortical bone predominates in the diaphyses, trabecular bone in the epiphyses
- **ⓒ T** Which, together with minerals, provides mechanical rigidity
- **ⓓ T** Organised as concentric lamellae of collagen
- **ⓔ T** In cortical bone, the lamellae are concentric

4
- **ⓐ T** Chronic infections (e.g. tuberculosis, leishmaniasis and schistosomiasis)
- **ⓑ T** Also found in myasthenia gravis
- **ⓒ T** And systemic lupus erythematosus, dermatomyositis and progressive systemic sclerosis
- **ⓓ T** And autoimmune hepatitis and sarcoidosis
- **ⓔ F** And, by definition, all the seronegative spondyloarthritides

5
- **ⓐ T** And systemic lupus erythematosus, progressive systemic sclerosis and autoimmune hepatitis
- **ⓑ T**
- **ⓒ T** Also associated with anti-SSB (anti-La)
- **ⓓ F** Associated with CREST syndrome
- **ⓔ F** Associated with Wegener's granulomatosis and systemic vasculitides

6
- **ⓐ T** Positive ANA is, however, found in many other conditions
- **ⓑ T** High anti-ds-DNA titre is highly suggestive of SLE
- **ⓒ T** Rising titre may precede clinical deterioration
- **ⓓ F** Low titres are commonly found, particularly in the elderly
- **ⓔ F** There are no auto-antibodies of diagnostic value in polyarteritis nodosa

7

Ⓐ F All three are normal in osteoporosis

Ⓑ T Occasionally the serum calcium may be elevated if immobilisation is prolonged

Ⓒ F All three may be normal (see **Ⓔ**)

Ⓓ F Increased calcium, normal or low phosphate and high serum alkaline phosphatase

Ⓔ T But all three may be normal

8

Ⓐ F At least 30% of bone mineral needs to have been lost from the skeleton

Ⓑ T Effective dose equivalent is about 20 microsieverts

Ⓒ T

Ⓓ T Osteoporotic patients typically have a low T-score and low Z-score

Ⓔ T Osteopenia T-score values between −1 and −2.5; osteoporosis T-score values below −2.5

9

Ⓐ T Gout and pseudogout

Ⓑ T Trauma usually obvious

Ⓒ T

Ⓓ F Usually polyarticular in onset

Ⓔ T Reactive arthritis following enterically or sexually acquired infection

10

Ⓐ F Onset usually acute, but less so in the elderly or the immunocompromised

Ⓑ T Also occurs after trauma or surgery

Ⓒ F Large joints are most frequently affected

Ⓓ F *H. influenzae* is the main cause in children, streptococci and staphylococci in adults

Ⓔ F Early joint aspiration is vital if the diagnosis is not to be delayed

11

Ⓐ F More common in females

Ⓑ T A macular rash may also be seen

Ⓒ T Joint involvement is additive rather than flitting

Ⓓ F Positive in only 20% of cases; always check blood and genital tract cultures

Ⓔ F Unusual

12

Ⓐ F A rare complication

Ⓑ F X-ray change may be minimal in early infection

Ⓒ T Typically ensues 3–5 years post primary tuberculosis

Ⓓ F Synovial biopsy adds to diagnostic yield

Ⓔ F Systemic antituberculous therapy must be given

13

Ⓐ T Especially in rubella in adults

Ⓑ T Somatic presentations are common

Ⓒ T Can cause muscle aches and pains

Ⓓ T Aches and pains are prominent in osteomalacia

Ⓔ F

14

Ⓐ T Relapsing pauciarticular large joint involvement

Ⓑ T Small and large joint involvement with hypertrophic spondylosis

Ⓒ T Pseudogout

Ⓓ T Small joint involvement

Ⓔ T Small joint involvement like rheumatoid arthritis

15

Ⓐ T

Ⓑ T

Ⓒ T And Reiter's disease

Ⓓ T Also photosensitive skin rashes

Ⓔ F

16
- **A** T Suggests lumbar nerve root compression
- **B** F Suggests an active inflammatory pathology
- **C** T Suggests lumbar nerve root compression
- **D** F Suggests significant pathology even if there are no physical signs
- **E** F Suggests inflammatory disease

17
- **A** F Typically asymptomatic
- **B** F A non-specific finding in back pain of many causes
- **C** F Exercise typically ameliorates pain in sacroiliitis
- **D** T Especially oil-based contrast media
- **E** T Only about 3% of cases persist for more than 3 months

18
- **A** F A high ESR suggests another diagnosis
- **B** T Typical of most psychosomatic disorders
- **C** T
- **D** F Often very chronic
- **E** F Multiple tender points are characteristic

19
- **A** F Often better during activity
- **B** F Continuous but aggravated by movement
- **C** F Loss of normal function may be the only feature
- **D** F
- **E** F Typically relieved by rest

20
- **A** T Disc prolapse may also produce upper or lower limb neurological signs
- **B** T Common in tension headache
- **C** F Suggest cervical radiculopathy
- **D** F Rheumatoid arthritis typically involves atlantoaxial articulations
- **E** T

21
- **A** T Either alone or associated with central chest pain
- **B** T With characteristic painful arc on shoulder abduction
- **C** T Suggests extra-pleural spread or bony metastases
- **D** T Classically due to diaphragmatic irritation secondary to pleurisy
- **E** T Due to cervical nerve root compression

22
- **A** T As for infraspinatus tendinitis
- **B** F The bicipital groove may be tender
- **C** F Suggests acromioclavicular joint disease
- **D** T 'frozen shoulder'
- **E** F Pain worsens on resisted internal rotation

23
- **A** T Definitive radiological criteria
- **B** F In the elderly; Scheuermann's osteochondritis is typically seen in the adolescent spine
- **C** F Caused by excessive proteoglycan synthesis at entheses
- **D** T And with gout, obesity and hypertension
- **E** F Typically absent, though heel pain and hypertrophic hip osteoarthrosis may occur

24
- **A** T Often symptomatic
- **B** F Females are more severely affected
- **C** F Synovial inflammation is mild; proliferation of new bone and cartilage is typical
- **D** T Collagen turnover is increased as total collagen declines
- **E** F Simple analgesics are equally effective and have fewer adverse effects than NSAIDs

25

A F More suggestive of an inflammatory arthritis such as rheumatoid arthritis

B F Typically distal interphalangeal joint involvement

C T

D T

E T

26

A T

B T And any joint previously traumatised

C T Also chondrocalcinosis and Wilson's disease

D T And most hip dysplasias

E T Also other causes of hypermobility

27

A T Diminished renal excretion of uric acid

B T Increased purine turnover

C T Diminished renal excretion of uric acid

D T Increased purine turnover

E T Diminished renal excretion of uric acid

28

A T Enzyme induction induces an acute attack

B T Non-articular signs may predominate

C T Onset may be explosively sudden

D F Serum urate is usually elevated but may be normal

E T Urate urolithiasis

29

A F Uricosuric drugs include probenecid, sulphinpyrazone and the NSAID azapropazone

B F Aspirin may worsen an acute attack by reducing renal urate excretion

C T

D T

E F Delay hypouricaemic therapy unless concomitant colchicine therapy is given

30

A F Crystals are deposited in articular cartilage then shed into the joint space

B T

C T Hence 'pseudogout'

D F Characteristic appearances of calcium pyrophosphate dihydrate (CPPD) crystals under polarising light microscopy

E F Such injections are often highly effective

31

A T

B T May cause severe calcific periarthritis

C T Also occurs in Paget's disease

D T

E T Apatite-associated destructive arthropathy seen in elderly women

32

A F Age of onset follows a normal distribution (no age group is exempt)

B T After the age of 55, affects 5% of women and 2% of men

C T In 50–75% of affected Caucasians

D T

E F Large and small joints can be affected

33

A T One of the American Rheumatism Association criteria (1988)

B F Arthritis affecting both hands and/or 3 or more joints

C T Pathognomonic

D T

E T In significant titres

34

A T Especially in patients with nodules and positive rheumatoid factor

B F CH50, C3 and C4 levels are low (activation of the classical pathway)

C F Characteristic feature is central fibrinoid necrosis

D T Nodes are typically non-tender

E T Reflects chronic immune stimulation

35

Ⓐ T These also occur with minimal joint symptoms, making diagnosis difficult

Ⓑ F Anaemia is classically normochromic and normocytic

Ⓒ F Anterior uveitis is specifically associated with the seronegative spondyloarthritides

Ⓓ F Modest elevation in platelet count is common

Ⓔ T Most obvious in nodes draining actively inflamed joints

36

Ⓐ F More suggestive of a seronegative spondyloarthritis such as ankylosing spondylitis

Ⓑ T Characteristic pattern of onset

Ⓒ T Involvement of the proximal interphalangeal and metatarsophalangeal respectively

Ⓓ F More suggestive of osteoarthrosis or psoriatic arthritis

Ⓔ T Often not obvious clinically but can produce cord compression

37

Ⓐ T Due to vasculitis or ulceration of nodules

Ⓑ T The fluid is an exudate not a transudate

Ⓒ T Commonly becomes apparent as unexplained proteinuria

Ⓓ T Due to arteritis of the vasa nervorum, and can be sensory, motor or mixed

Ⓔ T Relatively rare (Felty's syndrome)

38

Ⓐ T Early morning stiffness is a characteristic feature of all inflammatory arthritides

Ⓑ T May be absent at disease onset and is not specific to rheumatoid arthritis

Ⓒ T The usual pattern; in palindromic arthritis flitting episodes are typical

Ⓓ F Scleromalacia is a painless wasting of the sclera unlike the rarer scleritis

Ⓔ F Both features can occur in rheumatoid arthritis

39

Ⓐ F Peak prevalence in the age group 50–70 years

Ⓑ T

Ⓒ F Positive rheumatoid factor test

Ⓓ T Characteristic

Ⓔ T Characteristic

40

Ⓐ F Bed rest is of great value and without risk of bony ankylosis

Ⓑ T Reduces joint pain and may reduce contractures

Ⓒ F Not usually iron-deficient and reflects disease activity

Ⓓ F Low dose steroids may lessen disease progression with only a small risk of side-effects

Ⓔ F Not disease-modifying drugs, unlike gold, penicillamine and immunosuppressants

41

Ⓐ T 50% of patients respond in 3–6 months

Ⓑ F None of the NSAIDs are DMARDs

Ⓒ T Benefit may not be apparent for 3 months

Ⓓ T Adverse effects are common (e.g. proteinuria and marrow suppression)

Ⓔ T Reserved for life-threatening or unresponsive disease

42

Ⓐ T An explosive onset confers a relatively better prognosis

Ⓑ T Especially within 12 months of onset

Ⓒ T Indicates seropositive disease

Ⓓ T

Ⓔ F The presence of periods of remission is a favourable sign

43

Ⓐ T

Ⓑ T

Ⓒ T Demonstrable with the Shirmer's test

Ⓓ F More females than males

Ⓔ T Not diagnostic of primary Sjögren's (sicca) syndrome

44

Ⓐ T Axial joints are involved initially, only 10% of cases present with a peripheral arthritis

Ⓑ T E.g. the sacroiliac joints, involvement is rare in seropositive arthritides

Ⓒ T Achilles tendonitis

Ⓓ F Typical ocular problem is acute anterior uveitis

Ⓔ F An aortitis usually causing aortic regurgitation

45

Ⓐ T

Ⓑ F Nodules suggest seropositive arthritis, especially rheumatoid arthritis

Ⓒ T Identical twins homozygous for HLA-B27 may, however, be discordant for the disease

Ⓓ T *Klebsiella* carry an antigen similar to HLA-B27, suggesting a possible aetiology

Ⓔ T Familial aggregation of overlapping seronegative spondyloarthritides

46

Ⓐ T Due to sacroiliitis and sometimes mistaken for lumbar disc disease

Ⓑ T Lumbar lordosis may be lost in advanced disease

Ⓒ T Due to involvement of the costovertebral joints

Ⓓ T Leading to the 'bamboo' spine appearance

Ⓔ T Involvement of cartilaginous joints is a hallmark of the disease

47

Ⓐ F Can be invaluable in acute iritis

Ⓑ F In contrast to rheumatoid arthritis, the patient with ankylosing spondylitis stiffens with bed rest

Ⓒ F Only to improve symptoms

Ⓓ T Education regarding appropriate back exercises is vital

Ⓔ T As does extra-articular disease

48

Ⓐ F Conjunctivitis is the classical ocular manifestation

Ⓑ T Causes dysuria, frequency and suprapubic discomfort

Ⓒ F Arthritis is asymmetrical, involving large or small joints

Ⓓ T Similar delay following sexually acquired infections

Ⓔ T Similar to psoriatic skin and nail disease

49

Ⓐ F Polymorphonuclear leucocytosis is typical in the acute phase

Ⓑ F Occur in only 15% of patients

Ⓒ F Organisms cause the preceding dysenteric illness

Ⓓ F Appear on X-ray as a periostitis

Ⓔ F 10% of patients have chronic active arthritis 20 years after onset

50

Ⓐ T Occasionally there is no evidence of skin disease at onset

Ⓑ F Occurs in around 7% of patients

Ⓒ T Such as pitting and onycholysis

Ⓓ F Except for patients with arthritis mutilans

Ⓔ F Should be avoided due to precipitation of an exfoliative dermatitis

51

Ⓐ T Occurs in 70% of patients

Ⓑ T Occurs in 15% of patients

Ⓒ T Develops in 40% of patients—may be indistinguishable from ankylosing spondylitis

Ⓓ T Occurs in 15% of patients

Ⓔ T Occurs in 5% of patients

52

Ⓐ F Either as a primary disorder or in association with some connective tissue diseases

Ⓑ T Rare condition

Ⓒ F An association between coeliac disease and HLA-B8, DR17 and OQ2 but not HLA-B27

Ⓓ T Arthritis may precede evidence of ulcerative colitis or Crohn's disease

Ⓔ T Suggested by orogenital ulceration and iritis (more common in Japan)

53

Ⓐ T Associated with bone infarcts

Ⓑ T Reactive arthritis

Ⓒ T

Ⓓ T Purpura, abdominal pain and arthritis suggest Henoch–Schönlein vasculitis

Ⓔ T Either a purulent monoarthritis or transient polyarthritis may occur

54

Ⓐ F Systemic features predominate

Ⓑ T 10% of all juvenile polyarthritis; usually present over the age of 8

Ⓒ T Especially if ANA test is positive; chronic iritis is HLA-DR5 associated

Ⓓ T Enthesitis-related arthritis; 75% are HLA-B27 positive

Ⓔ F Oligoarticular disease (four or fewer joints affected) predominates

55

Ⓐ F Afro-Caribbean females are particularly susceptible

Ⓑ F Most commonly in the 2nd and 3rd decades

Ⓒ T Associated with polyclonal B lymphocyte activation

Ⓓ T Genetic factors appear to be of importance in aetiology

Ⓔ T Oestrogens appear to be important in disease expression

56

Ⓐ T Not, however, specific to SLE

Ⓑ T Occurs in at least 50% of patients

Ⓒ T Characteristic

Ⓓ F Renal involvement is not infrequent and heralds a poor prognosis

Ⓔ T Especially depression and organic psychosis

57

Ⓐ F Leucopenia and thrombocytopenia are typical

Ⓑ T Associated with an anticardiolipin antibody (antiphospholipid syndrome)

Ⓒ T Positive tests in low titre are however common and diagnostically unhelpful

Ⓓ F Depressed, suggesting activation of the classical complement pathway

Ⓔ F Rarely elevated unless coincidental infection is present

58

Ⓐ F

Ⓑ T Associated with slow acetylator status and HLA-DR4

Ⓒ T Cerebral and renal manifestations are typically absent

Ⓓ T

Ⓔ T And procainamide therapy

59

Ⓐ F NSAIDs may worsen renal function

Ⓑ T High doses are often used initially, then reduced to as low a dose as possible on remission of disease

Ⓒ T Especially when combined with immunosuppressant drugs

Ⓓ T Beware retinal complications

Ⓔ F Little evidence to suggest that this improves the long-term prognosis

60

Ⓐ T Associated with polymyositis

Ⓑ T

Ⓒ T Anti-ENA are usually present in high titres

Ⓓ F Rare

Ⓔ F Muscle enzymes may be elevated

61

A T Raynaud's may precede other features by years

B T Gastrointestinal tract is involved in most patients

C T Occurs in the majority of cases

D T 'Sausaging' of the fingers and sclerodactyly are also seen

E F ANA only in 50%; anti-DNA antibodies are not seen and complement is normal

62

A T

B F ANA and rheumatoid factor are often positive

C T

D F Weight loss may occur in the absence of malignancy

E T Cutaneous features suggest dermatomyositis

63

A T

B T Due to claudication of the masseters

C F Histological involvement is characteristically patchy

D T Due to proximal myopathy

E T

64

A F This finding would suggest an alternative diagnosis

B F Biopsy is positive in < 40% of patients

C T No such response should prompt a review of the diagnosis

D F Most patients require steroids for a minimum of 2 years

E F Suggests acute ischaemic optic neuritis due to vasculitis and is a medical emergency

65

A T Male to female ratio is 2:1

B T HBV markers may only become apparent on follow-up

C F Systemic vasculitis affecting medium sized arteries

D T Due to arteritis of the vasa nervorum

E T Especially in association with renal involvement

66

A F PMN leucocytosis is typical, eosinophilia suggests Churg-Strauss vasculitis

B F Raises the suspicion of a connective tissue disorder

C T P-ANCA; C-ANCA suggests Wegener's granulomatosis

D F Typically normochromic and normocytic

E T Renal involvement is common

67

A T Also produces vestibular damage

B T And keratitis and uveitis

C T Usually presents with pain and swelling of the pinna of the ear or nose

D T Renal biopsy may show proliferative glomerulonephritis

E T Also A-V conduction defects due to small vessel vasculitis

68

A T

B T More often transient coronary artery dilatation

C T

D T Followed by desquamation

E T

69

Ⓐ T Serum alkaline phosphatase may rise if fractures occur

Ⓑ T Accelerated bone loss occurs with oestrogen withdrawal

Ⓒ T Pain only occurs after fracture

Ⓓ F Occurs in states of corticosteroid excess

Ⓔ T Also associated with cigarette smoking

70

Ⓐ T All causes of malabsorption including liver disease

Ⓑ T And ankylosing spondylitis

Ⓒ T Multifactorial

Ⓓ T Multifactorial

Ⓔ T Improved by androgen replacement therapy

71

Ⓐ T Excessive exercise may be associated with low body weight and osteoporosis

Ⓑ F Unless the patient is hypophosphataemic from severe malnutrition

Ⓒ T Bisphosphonate therapy is the most effective and best evaluated

Ⓓ T But this is less effective than bisphosphonate therapy

Ⓔ F Causes osteoporosis; androgen or oestrogen therapy are both effective

72

Ⓐ F Characteristic; patients may have difficulty in standing up or in climbing stairs

Ⓑ F Pain may be generalised and severe

Ⓒ F Hypocalcaemia increases neuromuscular excitability (latent tetany)

Ⓓ F Give 1-α-hydroxycholecalciferol; renal 1-α-hydroxylation is impaired

Ⓔ T Looser's zones are translucent bands seen on X-ray

73

Ⓐ F Onset usually over the age of 60 years

Ⓑ T Increased bone turnover and osteoblast activity

Ⓒ F Insidious asymptomatic progression; with nerve root and spinal cord compression

Ⓓ F Fractures occur more commonly but usually heal normally

Ⓔ T Rare complication suggested by bony expansion and localised pain

74

Ⓐ F Prostatic secondaries are typically osteosclerotic

Ⓑ F Serum calcium is usually normal

Ⓒ F Asymptomatic disease may be detected coincidentally on X-ray

Ⓓ F Serum alkaline phosphatase is frequently elevated due to osteoblast activation

Ⓔ T Androgen deprivation therapy is of proven value in prostatic cancer

DISEASES OF THE SKIN

13

1
Ⓐ T
Ⓑ T
Ⓒ F   They comprise 90% of epidermal cells
Ⓓ F   These are modified macrophages; keratinocytes synthesise vitamin D
Ⓔ F   Sweat is also produced by apocrine sweat glands

2
Ⓐ F   Papules < 5 mm in diameter
Ⓑ T   Larger than papules
Ⓒ F   Vesicles < 5 mm in diameter
Ⓓ T   They are not palpable
Ⓔ F   Macules are flat, with altered skin colour or texture

3
Ⓐ T
Ⓑ T   Important in the differential diagnosis
Ⓒ T
Ⓓ T   Typically on the extremities of young adults
Ⓔ T   Usually facial in site

4
Ⓐ T   There may also be purpura
Ⓑ T   The skin is thin and fragile
Ⓒ F   Systemic absorption can occur
Ⓓ F   Hirsutism may rarely occur
Ⓔ T   Local and systemic immune function may be compromised

5
Ⓐ T   Epidermal oedema (spongiosis) and epidermal thickening (acanthosis)
Ⓑ F   This is a feature of allergic contact eczema
Ⓒ F   Serum IgE concentrations are elevated
Ⓓ T   The initial eruption occurs at the contact site
Ⓔ F   Occurs only in about one-third of subjects

6
Ⓐ F   Nickel may cause problems
Ⓑ T   In sticking plasters
Ⓒ T   Due to wool alcohols
Ⓓ T   In clothing or shoes
Ⓔ F

7
Ⓐ T   Often starts in first 2 years of life
Ⓑ T   But may occur anywhere
Ⓒ F   Pityriasis rosea
Ⓓ T   In contrast to eczema
Ⓔ F   Intensely itchy

8
Ⓐ T
Ⓑ T
Ⓒ T
Ⓓ T
Ⓔ T

9
Ⓐ F
Ⓑ F
Ⓒ T
Ⓓ T
Ⓔ F

10
Ⓐ F
Ⓑ F Coeliac disease
Ⓒ T And on the limbs
Ⓓ T
Ⓔ F Dermatitis herpetiformis

11
Ⓐ T Typically painless
Ⓑ T And also cryoglobulinaemia
Ⓒ T Arterial and neuropathic aetiology
Ⓓ T Associated with inflammatory bowel disease
Ⓔ T

12
Ⓐ F
Ⓑ F
Ⓒ T Typically patchy
Ⓓ F
Ⓔ F Male-pattern baldness

13
Ⓐ F 15% if there is one affected parent
Ⓑ T Of helper type in the dermis
Ⓒ T Typically throat infection
Ⓓ T And onycholysis
Ⓔ T

14
Ⓐ T Typically on the elbows, knees and lower back
Ⓑ T Also a dermal T lymphocyte infiltrate
Ⓒ T Including surgical wounds (Köbner phenomenon)
Ⓓ T Inheritance is probably polygenic
Ⓔ T Also antimalarial drugs

15
Ⓐ F The scalp is frequently involved
Ⓑ F Usually seen in children
Ⓒ T Also subungual hyperkeratosis
Ⓓ T Perhaps mimicking rheumatoid arthritis
Ⓔ T Axillary folds may be similarly affected

16
Ⓐ F This irritates and therefore is best avoided on these skin areas
Ⓑ T
Ⓒ T Reduce the risk of rapid relapse
Ⓓ F UVA are long waves
Ⓔ T Or PUVA and methotrexate

17
Ⓐ T Ducts may be obstructed
Ⓑ T Lesions elsewhere suggest an alternative diagnosis
Ⓒ T Antibiotics are helpful
Ⓓ T Largely hormonally mediated
Ⓔ T Seborrhoea (greasy skin) is often present also

18
Ⓐ T And tar, oils and oily cosmetics
Ⓑ T Also associated with late-onset 21-hydroxylase deficiency
Ⓒ T Also associated with androgen-secreting tumours
Ⓓ T
Ⓔ T

19
Ⓐ T For a minimum of 3 months
Ⓑ T Antibacterials such as chlorhexidine may also help
Ⓒ F Unless given with cyproterone acetate
Ⓓ T Anti-androgen therapy often in combination with an oestrogen
Ⓔ T Reduces sebum secretion; highly teratogenic

20
Ⓐ T Slate grey in exposed areas
Ⓑ T
Ⓒ F
Ⓓ T Yellow pigmentation
Ⓔ F

21
Ⓐ F Commonest in middle age
Ⓑ F Sebum secretion is normal
Ⓒ T
Ⓓ T
Ⓔ F Repeated courses may be necessary

22
- **A** T But the nails are usually normal
- **B** T With hyperkeratosis and basal cell degeneration
- **C** T Perhaps with Wickham's striae
- **D** F Post-inflammatory pigmentation occurs
- **E** F But topical steroids may aid symptoms

23
- **A** T
- **B** T Also caused by biliary obstruction
- **C** T
- **D** T Also caused by chronic renal failure
- **E** T

24
- **A** F The rash is non-pruritic
- **B** T Usually intensely itchy
- **C** T Classically pruritic
- **D** F Non-pruritic
- **E** T Associated with coeliac disease

25
- **A** T Perhaps with target lesions
- **B** T Typically on extensor surfaces
- **C** T Tense blood-filled lesions
- **D** T Superficial flaccid lesions
- **E** F Small scaly raised lesions

26
- **A** T Disordered haem metabolism
- **B** T Perhaps progressing to chronic actinic dermatitis
- **C** T And also to amiodarone and sulphonamides
- **D** F Associated with inflammatory bowel disease
- **E** F Unaffected by sunlight

27
- **A** T 'Bull's eye' lesions
- **B** F The eruption rapidly resolves
- **C** F Classical features of the condition
- **D** T May be severe systemic upset
- **E** T Radiotherapy may precipitate such lesions

28
- **A** T Also orf and other viruses
- **B** T Classical
- **C** T Also penicillins and barbiturates
- **D** T And other connective tissue disorders
- **E** T And oral contraceptives

29
- **A** T Lesions are painful
- **B** F Resolve over several weeks leaving bruises
- **C** T Mild systemic upset is typical
- **D** F Suggests an alternative diagnosis
- **E** F More common in younger individuals

30
- **A** T Also brucellosis
- **B** T Also mycoplasmal and chlamydial infections
- **C** T Also leukaemias and Hodgkin's disease
- **D** T Also leprosy
- **E** T Erythema nodosum can also be caused by some drugs e.g. iodides and sulphonamides

31
- **A** T Typically Hodgkin's disease or other lymphoma
- **B** T Especially intra-abdominal carcinomas
- **C** T Ovarian, gastric and nasopharyngeal carcinoma
- **D** T Also caused by some chemotherapy
- **E** F Especially common in HIV infection

32
- **A** F Most appear in early childhood
- **B** F Should raise suspicion of malignancy
- **C** F Not hairy and are macular
- **D** F They are nodular
- **E** F 6% in congenital melanocytic naevi

33
- **A** T 30–50% develop in this way
- **B** T But smaller lesions may be malignant
- **C** T Typically asymmetrical
- **D** T Risk is also increased with fair skin and blonde hair
- **E** T Characteristically painless

34

Ⓐ T **A**symmetry
Ⓑ T **B**order
Ⓒ T **C**olour
Ⓓ T **D**iameter
Ⓔ T **E**levation (viz. the **ABCDE** rule)

35

Ⓐ T Doubled in the past 10 years
Ⓑ F Rare before puberty
Ⓒ F Female to male ratio is 2:1
Ⓓ F Truly amelanotic lesions are rare
Ⓔ F < 10% survive in stage III

36

Ⓐ F Tend to occur in later life
Ⓑ F Light exposure is not a factor
Ⓒ T Pedunculated or sessile
Ⓓ T With variable pigmentation
Ⓔ F Not pre-malignant

37

Ⓐ T Rare in young adults
Ⓑ F Spread by local invasion
Ⓒ T Typically on the face or head
Ⓓ T With a rolled, pearly edge
Ⓔ F Radiosensitive but surgery is preferred

38

Ⓐ T Typically in Caucasians living in equatorial regions
Ⓑ F Tumour comprises differentiated suprabasal cells
Ⓒ T Or actinic keratosis on the skin
Ⓓ F Haematogenous dissemination is rare
Ⓔ F Radiosensitive, but surgery is preferred

39

Ⓐ F A feature of iron deficiency
Ⓑ T Also nail pitting and subungual hyperkeratosis
Ⓒ T A non-specific sign of hypoalbuminaemia
Ⓓ F May be associated with trauma
Ⓔ T Fingernails grow faster than toenails

DISEASES OF THE NERVOUS SYSTEM

14

1
- **Ⓐ T** Lower frequencies predominate during sleep
- **Ⓑ F** It disappears
- **Ⓒ F** Normal in 50%
- **Ⓓ F** 50–60 m/s
- **Ⓔ T** There is no change in muscle fibre structure

2
- **Ⓐ T** And temporal lobe
- **Ⓑ F** Better for both
- **Ⓒ F** MRI provides more detail
- **Ⓓ T** In contrast to CT
- **Ⓔ F** Highly operator dependent

3
- **Ⓐ T** Increased in subarachnoid haemorrhage
- **Ⓑ F** > 60% of blood level
- **Ⓒ T**
- **Ⓓ T**
- **Ⓔ T** When present, oligo IgG bands suggest multiple sclerosis

4
- **Ⓐ T** Typically intermittent
- **Ⓑ T** With dysarthria and dysphagia
- **Ⓒ T** Soft rapid indistinct speech
- **Ⓓ F** Scanning dysarthria
- **Ⓔ F** Expressive dysphasia

5
- **Ⓐ F** Dysphonia
- **Ⓑ T** Often due to cerebrovascular disease
- **Ⓒ T** 'Scanning' dysarthria
- **Ⓓ T** In addition to dysphonia
- **Ⓔ F** Receptive dysphasia

6
- **Ⓐ T** Flexor or absent in lower motor neuron lesion
- **Ⓑ T** Segmental level T8–T12
- **Ⓒ F** Lower motor neuron sign
- **Ⓓ T** 'Clasp-knife' rigidity is typical
- **Ⓔ T** Rossolimo's sign

7
- **Ⓐ T** Increased in upper motor neuron lesions
- **Ⓑ T** Disuse atrophy may follow prolonged paralysis from any cause
- **Ⓒ T** With flexor or absent plantar response
- **Ⓓ F** Upper motor neuron sign
- **Ⓔ F** Pattern entirely dependent on site of lesion(s)

8
- **Ⓐ F** Resting tremor
- **Ⓑ F** 'Lead pipe' or 'cog-wheel' rigidity
- **Ⓒ T** Also other involuntary movements
- **Ⓓ F** Hypothyroidism
- **Ⓔ T** Hypokinesis

9
- **Ⓐ F** Opposite side
- **Ⓑ F** Decussate below this level
- **Ⓒ T** And temperature sensation
- **Ⓓ F** Lowest segments outermost
- **Ⓔ F** No decussation at this level

10
- **Ⓐ F** Reflexes preserved
- **Ⓑ T** Sensory or motor
- **Ⓒ T** In upper limbs
- **Ⓓ F** Reflexes preserved
- **Ⓔ T** With sensory ataxia

11

Ⓐ T

Ⓑ T Finger flexion jerk—C8–T1

Ⓒ T Same as the biceps jerk

Ⓓ T

Ⓔ T

12

Ⓐ T Parasympathetic innervation impaired

Ⓑ T And incomplete bladder emptying

Ⓒ T Internal sphincter relaxation and detrusor contraction

Ⓓ F Feature of spinal cord lesions

Ⓔ T And internal sphincter contraction

13

Ⓐ T 'Past pointing'

Ⓑ T With loss of normal rhythm

Ⓒ T Absent at rest

Ⓓ F Hypotonia

Ⓔ F Jerking nystagmus

14

Ⓐ T The optic tract runs between optic chiasma and lateral geniculate body

Ⓑ T Upper fibre damage causes lower field defect

Ⓒ F Midline lesions cause bitemporal hemianopia

Ⓓ F Left lateral geniculate body

Ⓔ F Left monocular visual loss

15

Ⓐ F Suggests sixth cranial nerve palsy

Ⓑ F Occurs in Horner's syndrome

Ⓒ T Paralysis of levator palpebrae superioris

Ⓓ T Impaired parasympathetic flow

Ⓔ T And direct light response impaired

16

Ⓐ F Superior oblique

Ⓑ F No pupillary change

Ⓒ T May be difficult to detect clinically

Ⓓ T Head may tilt towards normal side

Ⓔ F Suggests internuclear ophthalmoplegia

17

Ⓐ F Impaired abduction

Ⓑ F May be a feature of Horner's syndrome

Ⓒ T Usually bilateral, perhaps other ocular nerves also involved

Ⓓ T Infarction, haemorrhage or demyelination typically

Ⓔ T May be 'false localising sign' in raised intracranial pressure

18

Ⓐ T Partial or complete ptosis

Ⓑ T With pupillary dilatation

Ⓒ T With pupillary constriction

Ⓓ F Orbicularis oculi may be affected

Ⓔ F No ptosis occurs

19

Ⓐ T Accommodation preserved

Ⓑ T Defect is probably in the ciliary ganglia

Ⓒ T An afferent defect

Ⓓ F Reaction in right eye may be impaired

Ⓔ T Both pupils may be small but response preserved

20

Ⓐ T Ophthalmic and maxillary divisions of fifth nerve

Ⓑ F Facial pain

Ⓒ T In cerebellopontine angle

Ⓓ T Contralateral to site of loss

Ⓔ T Unilateral or bilateral

21

Ⓐ T Frontalis weakness

Ⓑ F Decreased due to involvement of nervus intermedius

Ⓒ T Bell's sign

Ⓓ F Produces hyperacusis

Ⓔ T Involvement of the chorda tympani

22
- Ⓐ T   With dysphonia
- Ⓑ T   Often with aspiration
- Ⓒ T   Particularly in cerebrovascular disease
- Ⓓ F   Suggest lower motor neuron lesion twelfth nerve
- Ⓔ F   Jaw jerk is typically brisk

23
- Ⓐ T   Test at least twice
- Ⓑ T   No response to pain = 1
- Ⓒ T   No eye opening = 1
- Ⓓ T   No speech = 1
- Ⓔ T   Maximum score = 15

24
- Ⓐ F   Dilated and unreactive to light
- Ⓑ T   A brain stem reflex
- Ⓒ T   20 ml ice cold water into each ear in turn
- Ⓓ T   With $PaCO_2 > 6.7$ kPa
- Ⓔ F   All brain stem reflexes absent

25
- Ⓐ T   And other 'primitive' reflexes
- Ⓑ F   Suggests a parietal lobe lesion
- Ⓒ F   Posterior temporoparietal lesion (Wernicke's area)
- Ⓓ F   Temporal lobe sign
- Ⓔ T   Perhaps with antisocial behaviour

26
- Ⓐ T   Contralateral to lesion
- Ⓑ T   Non-dominant hemisphere
- Ⓒ T   Perhaps with sensory neglect
- Ⓓ F   Broca's area in the inferior frontal lobe
- Ⓔ T   Gerstmann's syndrome of the dominant angular gyral region

27
- Ⓐ F   Suggests more sinister cause for headache
- Ⓑ T   Perhaps in polycythaemia rubra vera
- Ⓒ T   Central retinal artery occlusion
- Ⓓ T   With hypercapnia
- Ⓔ F   May cause optic atrophy

28
- Ⓐ F   Only associated with 1 in 8 patients
- Ⓑ F   Meningism less common than in bacterial infection
- Ⓒ F   Migrainous hemiparesis is well recognised
- Ⓓ F   Tension headaches are typically poorly responsive
- Ⓔ T   As does morning vomiting

29
- Ⓐ F   Male to female ratio is 5:1
- Ⓑ F   10–50 times less common
- Ⓒ T   And unilateral lacrimation
- Ⓓ F   Prophylaxis may not be helpful
- Ⓔ T

30
- Ⓐ T   Persistent vertigo is more often central
- Ⓑ F   Often present although transient
- Ⓒ T   Exclude acoustic neuroma
- Ⓓ F   Tends to persist
- Ⓔ T   But a rare cause

31
- Ⓐ F   But many patients are aware that something is about to happen
- Ⓑ F
- Ⓒ F   Also absence of injury or tongue-biting
- Ⓓ F
- Ⓔ F   Also pallor rather than central cyanosis suggests fainting

32
- Ⓐ T   Often with dragging of the affected foot
- Ⓑ T   Perhaps with slapping steps
- Ⓒ T   Classically of the vermis
- Ⓓ T   Associated with festination
- Ⓔ T   Usually myopathic in nature

33
- **A T** Maximal on gaze towards lesion if cerebellar disease is unilateral
- **B T** May be more marked in the abducting eye with disruption of the MLB
- **C F** Typically present only when looking away from side of lesion
- **D F** Suggests vestibulocochlear disease
- **E T** Demonstrable using electronystagmography

34
- **A F** Lancinating paroxysms lasting a few seconds
- **B T** 'Trigger areas' may exist
- **C F** No abnormal signs
- **D F** Occurs in elderly subjects
- **E T** E.g. carbamazepine

35
- **A T** May be disabling
- **B T** Usually unilateral
- **C T** Typically during attacks
- **D F** Suggests benign positional vertigo
- **E F** May delay progression but cannot restore auditory loss

36
- **A F** Postural instability and syncopal symptoms
- **B T** Or other pathology of the eighth nerve
- **C T** Usually associated with vertebral artery ischaemia
- **D T** And other ototoxic drugs
- **E T** With secondary labyrinthine inflammation

37
- **A F** Bilateral supranuclear lesions cause a spastic tongue
- **B F** But can cause dysarthria, dysphonia and dysphagia
- **C T** Without any sensory involvement from bulbar palsy
- **D T** Invasion of the base of the skull
- **E T** Causes stenosis of hypoglossal canal

38
- **A T** May follow focal EEG abnormality and symptoms—partial seizures
- **B F** Often absent
- **C F** Usually no obvious abnormality
- **D T** TV or computer games may induce fits
- **E T** Often used during the recording of an EEG

39
- **A T** With vague irritability or lethargy
- **B F** Audible cry may occur at the onset of the tonic phase
- **C T** Tonic phase
- **D T** Clonic phase
- **E T** Variable duration

40
- **A T** Sometimes with loss of posture
- **B F** Typically in childhood
- **C T** May be detected inter-ictally
- **D T** May not occur until adulthood
- **E F** Rapid recovery although may occur very frequently

41
- **A T** With automatic movements (e.g. lip-smacking)
- **B T** May be detailed with graphic descriptions
- **C T** Or *jamais vu* (unreality)
- **D T** In the minority
- **E F** Todd's paresis suggests focal motor seizures

42
- **A F** Await evidence of recurrent seizures
- **B F** 70%, mostly in first 2 months
- **C T** Also febrile illnesses and metabolic disturbances
- **D F** 2%
- **E T** Only one in 1000 are false positives

43
- **Ⓐ T**
- **Ⓑ T** Providing no potentially epileptogenic brain lesion identified
- **Ⓒ F** Should stop driving for 6 months after their withdrawal
- **Ⓓ F** 10 years
- **Ⓔ T**

44
- **Ⓐ F** Phenytoin and carbamazepine
- **Ⓑ F** Megaloblastic anaemia
- **Ⓒ F** Ethosuximide
- **Ⓓ T**
- **Ⓔ T** Particularly in older patients

45
- **Ⓐ F** Indicated if rapid recurrence
- **Ⓑ T** Or 3 years of nocturnal seizures only
- **Ⓒ T** Unless no seizures since the age of five
- **Ⓓ F** Primidone is metabolised to phenobarbitone
- **Ⓔ T** Monotherapy is preferable

46
- **Ⓐ F** Suggests syncope
- **Ⓑ T** Not specific, especially in the elderly
- **Ⓒ T** An eye-witness is vital but jerking movements are common in simple faints
- **Ⓓ F** Suggests vasovagal syncope
- **Ⓔ T** Can also feature in blackouts due to bradycardias

47
- **Ⓐ F** Bradycardia and hypertension
- **Ⓑ T** And vomiting
- **Ⓒ T** And coughing
- **Ⓓ T** And impairment of conscious level
- **Ⓔ T** 'False localising signs'

48
- **Ⓐ T** 10% of all cerebral tumours
- **Ⓑ F** 40% of all cerebral tumours
- **Ⓒ T** They are usually cerebellar tumours
- **Ⓓ T** Indication for CT scanning
- **Ⓔ F** 4th and 5th decade

49
- **Ⓐ F** Suggests an optic neuritis
- **Ⓑ F** Suggests chronic glaucoma
- **Ⓒ F** Suggests optic neuritis
- **Ⓓ T** Causes visual impairment
- **Ⓔ T** Foster Kennedy syndrome

50
- **Ⓐ T** In 50% of sufferers
- **Ⓑ F** Typically post-pubertal
- **Ⓒ F** May become generalised
- **Ⓓ T** Visual scintillations and also fortification spectra and scotomas
- **Ⓔ T** Focal deficits may persist > 24 hours

51
- **Ⓐ F** Rare paradoxical embolism occurs if there is a right to left cardiac shunt
- **Ⓑ T** Risk dependent on other cardiac factors
- **Ⓒ T** With left atrial myxoma
- **Ⓓ T** And cerebral abscess
- **Ⓔ F** Occasionally if there is atrial fibrillation

52
- **Ⓐ T** Usually contralateral motor, sensory, speech disturbance
- **Ⓑ T** Bilateral events may occur
- **Ⓒ T** Associated with standing
- **Ⓓ F** Fixed deficit stroke
- **Ⓔ F** Slowly progressive typically

53
- **Ⓐ F** The optic pathway is only affected by larger lesions
- **Ⓑ F** Suggests cortical damage
- **Ⓒ T** Internal capsule lacuna
- **Ⓓ T** Internal capsule lacuna
- **Ⓔ T** Account for > 80% of lacunar strokes

54
- **Ⓐ T** Headache is not specific to haemorrhage
- **Ⓑ T** In midbrain haemorrhage
- **Ⓒ T** With subhyaloid retinal haemorrhage
- **Ⓓ F** More suggestive of infarction
- **Ⓔ F** Suggest peripheral eighth nerve lesion

55
- **Ⓐ F** 85%
- **Ⓑ T** Minority 'stutter' over a longer period
- **Ⓒ T** Another 20% are lacunar infarcts
- **Ⓓ T** 75–150 mg daily
- **Ⓔ T** Carotid endarterectomy may then be beneficial

56
- **Ⓐ T** Especially pontine lesions
- **Ⓑ T** With demonstrable third, fourth or sixth nerve lesions
- **Ⓒ F** A cortical sign
- **Ⓓ T** Often with vomiting
- **Ⓔ T** Central type of jerking nystagmus

57
- **Ⓐ T** Worse if the coma is prolonged for more than 24 hours
- **Ⓑ T** Early mortality is higher
- **Ⓒ T** Suggests raised intracranial pressure or brain stem involvement
- **Ⓓ T** Especially if sustained
- **Ⓔ T** Functional outcome is worse with strokes of the non-dominant hemisphere

58
- **Ⓐ F** Most have no history of trauma
- **Ⓑ T** Slowly progressive
- **Ⓒ F** Late-onset epilepsy suggests intracerebral disease
- **Ⓓ F** Suggests cerebral infarction or haemorrhage
- **Ⓔ T** And impairment of consciousness

59
- **Ⓐ T** Often streptococcal in origin
- **Ⓑ T** Usually staphylococcal in origin
- **Ⓒ T** Typically affects the frontal lobe
- **Ⓓ T** Cerebellar or temporal
- **Ⓔ T** Typically staphylococcal in origin

60
- **Ⓐ F** Usually there is no suggestion of infection
- **Ⓑ T** Prophylactic anticonvulsants should be considered
- **Ⓒ T** Raised intracranial pressure
- **Ⓓ T** With focal hemispheric signs
- **Ⓔ F** Lumbar puncture may be hazardous

61
- **Ⓐ T** And general malaise
- **Ⓑ T** Fever often low-grade
- **Ⓒ T** Cranial nerve lesions in 25% of cases
- **Ⓓ T** Usual source of infection
- **Ⓔ F** Lymphocytic meningitis

62
- **Ⓐ F** Intrathecal penicillin is both unnecessary and dangerous
- **Ⓑ T** Covers meningococci, pneumococci and haemophilus
- **Ⓒ F** Start therapy if the diagnosis is likely given the mortality and morbidity
- **Ⓓ T** Septicaemic shock often complicates the disease
- **Ⓔ F** Suggests meningococcaemia

63
- **Ⓐ T** Sometimes with encephalitis
- **Ⓑ T** With subsequent anterior horn cell infection
- **Ⓒ T** Lymphocytic choriomeningitis
- **Ⓓ T** Common cause in UK
- **Ⓔ T** Usually self-limiting

64
- **Ⓐ T** Usually no prodrome
- **Ⓑ T** Occasionally a mild impairment of consciousness
- **Ⓒ F** Suggests pyogenic infection
- **Ⓓ F** Other viruses may cause this
- **Ⓔ T** In 75% of patients

65

Ⓐ F Marked post inflammatory depigmentation may occur

Ⓑ T Sometimes with dysaesthesia

Ⓒ F Rarely anterior (motor) ganglia involved

Ⓓ T Rash follows in 3–4 days; initial diagnosis may be difficult

Ⓔ F May limit severity and duration of initial illness

66

Ⓐ T Neurosyphilis can mimic many conditions

Ⓑ T Remember HIV infection

Ⓒ T Secondary syphilis

Ⓓ T Tabes dorsalis

Ⓔ T Secondary syphilis

67

Ⓐ T 'Lightning pains'

Ⓑ T With trophic ulceration and Charcot joints

Ⓒ T And optic atrophy

Ⓓ T Plantar responses may be extensor with taboparesis

Ⓔ T Sensory ataxia

68

Ⓐ F More women than men are affected

Ⓑ T Different haplotypes in countries outside UK

Ⓒ T Highest prevalence in the UK is in north-east Scotland and Shetland

Ⓓ F The converse applies

Ⓔ F Central white matter

69

Ⓐ F Only 25% of cases have a chronically progressive course

Ⓑ F Rare in childhood

Ⓒ F No extrapyramidal features

Ⓓ T In spinal involvement

Ⓔ F Epilepsy and hemiplegia are unusual

70

Ⓐ T Can detect clinically silent lesions in 75% of patients

Ⓑ T MRI more sensitive than CT scanning

Ⓒ T Occurs in 70–90% of patients between attacks

Ⓓ F Non-specific abnormalities

Ⓔ F Test of lower motor neuronal disease

71

Ⓐ T Impaired fine finger movements

Ⓑ F May coexist in the elderly

Ⓒ F Resting tremor

Ⓓ T Also 'cogwheel' rigidity if a tremor is prominent

Ⓔ T And convergence

72

Ⓐ F Typically arm tremor

Ⓑ T Suggests underlying cerebrovascular disease

Ⓒ T Suggests drug-induced extrapyramidal disease

Ⓓ T Suggests possible multisystem atrophy

Ⓔ F Impairment of upgaze is also common

73

Ⓐ T Initial illness frequently unrecognised

Ⓑ T Other involuntary movement disorders

Ⓒ T And dementia

Ⓓ T 'Punch drunk' syndrome

Ⓔ T Used in some herbicides

74

Ⓐ F Principally useful for tremor

Ⓑ F Early introduction means earlier waning of effect

Ⓒ F May be a sign of undertreatment also

Ⓓ F Neuropsychiatric problems occur with both types of therapy

Ⓔ T Sustained-release preparations sometimes help

75
Ⓐ F Autosomal dominant transmission
Ⓑ F Onset in middle-aged subjects
Ⓒ F May help chorea
Ⓓ T But becomes generalised
Ⓔ F Suggests Friedreich's ataxia

76
Ⓐ T Prevalence of 4 per 100 000
Ⓑ T Typically with absent reflexes
Ⓒ T Particularly tongue fasciculation
Ⓓ T Or in the upper limbs
Ⓔ T Or in the lower limbs

77
Ⓐ T But no sensory signs in MND
Ⓑ T Look for evidence of diabetes mellitus
Ⓒ T Treatment may limit progression
Ⓓ T Protean manifestations of a number of tumours
Ⓔ T Check syphilis serology

78
Ⓐ F Changes are usually degenerative and non-specific
Ⓑ T Follows the distribution of nerve root(s)
Ⓒ T Only if due to disc prolapse or destructive pathology
Ⓓ T Or C5–C7 involvement with appropriate reflex loss
Ⓔ F Conservative management is usually adequate

79
Ⓐ T Usually extradural deposits
Ⓑ F Typically elevated with xanthochromia (Froin's syndrome)
Ⓒ T Pain may follow nerve root distribution
Ⓓ F A late feature
Ⓔ T MRI now invaluable

80
Ⓐ T Important to remember if spinal investigations are normal
Ⓑ T Rare in UK in this severity
Ⓒ T Associated with vertebral collapse (Pott's disease)
Ⓓ T Sudden onset typically
Ⓔ T Intradural pathology accounts for 20% cases of cord compression

81
Ⓐ T Spinothalamic tracts decussate after entering the spinal cord
Ⓑ T Dorsal column involvement
Ⓒ T Pyramidal tract involvement
Ⓓ F No contralateral pyramidal signs
Ⓔ F Ipsilateral dermatomal sensory changes

82
Ⓐ T Guided by sensitivities of colonising organisms
Ⓑ F Immobility in itself predisposes to sore formation
Ⓒ F Intermittent catheterisation is usually preferrable
Ⓓ F Good posturing and passive movement can minimise risk
Ⓔ T Manual evacuation may be necessary

83
Ⓐ T Onset in 3rd or 4th decade
Ⓑ T Leading to trophic ulceration
Ⓒ T Damage to anterior horn cells
Ⓓ T A common early feature
Ⓔ T Pyramidal tract damage

84
Ⓐ T Central and peripheral forms occur
Ⓑ T And axillary skin freckling
Ⓒ T E.g. phaeochromocytoma
Ⓓ T At almost any site
Ⓔ T Acoustic neuroma

85
- **A** T Most commonly Alzheimer's disease
- **B** F Risk of Alzheimer's increased four-fold
- **C** T Particularly in Alzheimer's
- **D** T And amyloid rich plaques
- **E** T Patients often made worse by L-dopa therapy

86
- **A** F Causes peripheral neuropathy
- **B** T Typically bilateral and associated with abnormal cyanide metabolism
- **C** T Often reversible
- **D** T Pyramidal tract degeneration
- **E** T Proprioceptive loss due to dorsal column disease (SACD)

87
- **A** F Often develops or worsens with pregnancy
- **B** F Supplied by the ulnar nerve
- **C** T Radiates up the arm even to the shoulder
- **D** T Compression of the tunnel
- **E** T And previous wrist fracture

88
- **A** T Usually arthropathy apparent
- **B** T Check chest X-ray and tuberculin test
- **C** T Occurs in 40–50%
- **D** T Check glucose tolerance test (GTT)
- **E** T Vasculitis of the vasa nervora

89
- **A** F Median nerve
- **B** F Ulnar nerve
- **C** T Often with weakness of wrist extension
- **D** T Often with foot drop
- **E** F Lateral cutaneous nerve of thigh

90
- **A** T Typically sensory
- **B** T And systemic lupus erythematosus; also cause mononeuritis multiplex
- **C** T Also vitamin B_1, B_2, B_6, A and E deficiency
- **D** T And numerous drugs
- **E** T And myxoedema

91
- **A** T Look for haematological clues
- **B** F Motor weakness predominates
- **C** T Also autonomic neuropathy with local sympathetic neural dysfunction
- **D** F The seventh nerve especially is commonly involved in neurosarcoid
- **E** T Suggests autonomic involvement

92
- **A** T Suggests lead poisoning
- **B** T Suggests B_{12} or folate deficiency
- **C** T Inappropriate production of antidiuretic hormone (SIADH) bronchial carcinoma
- **D** F Wilson's disease does not cause a peripheral neuropathy
- **E** F Not associated with a peripheral neuropathy

93
- **A** T 1–4 weeks, usually after viral infection
- **B** T Paraesthesiae spread proximally
- **C** T Muscle wasting is usually absent
- **D** F Cranial nerves involved in 30–40%
- **E** F CSF protein is elevated, cell count is normal

94
- **A** F Compression of the lateral cutaneous nerve of thigh
- **B** F Look for an endocrine abnormality
- **C** T A common non-metastatic syndrome
- **D** T May be rapid in onset
- **E** T Lambert–Eaton syndrome

95

Ⓐ F Dysphonia, dysarthria and dysphagia
Ⓑ T 80% have ACh receptor antibodies
Ⓒ T Especially occurs in females more than males
Ⓓ F Only in chronic severe cases
Ⓔ T Often more marked in the evenings or following exercise

96

Ⓐ T 'Cholinergic crisis'
Ⓑ F Best given every 3–6 hours
Ⓒ T Unless disease established for more than 7 years
Ⓓ T Initiation of therapy is best undertaken in hospital
Ⓔ T Even after the thymoma is removed

97

Ⓐ T As late as 10 years of age
Ⓑ T With preserved tendon reflexes
Ⓒ T Characteristic finding—Gowers' sign
Ⓓ F Serum CK is raised from birth
Ⓔ T Often before the age of 20 years

98

Ⓐ T And also hyperthyroidism; both resolve with treatment
Ⓑ F Causes a variety of different peripheral nerve disorders
Ⓒ T And also acromegaly
Ⓓ F Causes a peripheral neuropathy and spinal cord degeneration
Ⓔ T Often with a peripheral neuropathy

PRINCIPLES OF CRITICAL CARE MEDICINE

1
- **A** T Inspired oxygen content
- **B** F 5 L/min
- **C** T Arterial oxygen saturation
- **D** T Alveolar oxygen saturation is less than that of air (21 kPa)
- **E** T Q_t $(CaO_2 - CvO_2)$

2
- **A** F Hb carriage accounts for the majority
- **B** T Bohr effect— facilitates unloading of O_2 to tissues
- **C** F 10–11 g/dl to minimise hyperviscosity problems
- **D** F Around 50%
- **E** T Hb concentration and saturation are major determinants of O_2 content

3
- **A** F Calculated from inspiratory/expiratory gas analysis
- **B** T Equates to DO_2 (oxygen delivery) $-VO_2$ (global oxygen consumption)
- **C** T
- **D** F Varies depending on metabolic rate
- **E** T Sepsis and trauma also increase VO_2

4
- **A** T
- **B** F High, contributing to metabolic acidosis
- **C** F The reverse occurs—myocardial failure
- **D** T
- **E** F Consumption rises even at very high levels

5
- **A** F Bleeding may be internal
- **B** F Peripheral cyanosis is characteristic
- **C** T Due to central vessel obstruction
- **D** F Vasodilatation occurs
- **E** T Capillary damage and vasodilatation also occur

6
- **A** F Suggests cardiogenic shock
- **B** F Suggests septic shock
- **C** T
- **D** T Due to cerebral hypoperfusion
- **E** F Causes oliguria

7
- **A** F Hypovolaemic shock occurs
- **B** T Acute right ventricular failure
- **C** F
- **D** T
- **E** T

8
- **A** F Useful if CVP < 1 cm and hypovolaemia is suspected
- **B** F Suggests shock secondary to fluid loss
- **C** F A pulmonary artery catheter is needed to judge left heart pressures
- **D** F May be necessary in metabolic acidosis
- **E** F Frequently negative

9
- **A** T Sepsis may cause hypothermia as well as fever
- **B** F > 20/min
- **C** T
- **D** T
- **E** T

10

Ⓐ F Relatively uncommon but check urine culture

Ⓑ F Transoesophageal echo is more sensitive

Ⓒ F Change if in situ for more than 4 days

Ⓓ T

Ⓔ T

11

Ⓐ F Hypoxaemia is a cardinal feature

Ⓑ F Compliance decreases

Ⓒ F Diffuse infiltrates are typical

Ⓓ F Typically normal or slightly elevated

Ⓔ T Pulmonary hypertension is common

12

Ⓐ F There is a protein-rich pulmonary exudate

Ⓑ T A systemic upset and multiorgan failure

Ⓒ F Crepitations are typical

Ⓓ T 'Ground glass' appearance on chest X-ray due to alveolar oedema

Ⓔ T But not in all cases

13

Ⓐ T May improve gas exchange

Ⓑ F

Ⓒ F

Ⓓ F Avoid $FiO_2 > 0.8$

Ⓔ T

14

Ⓐ T

Ⓑ F 6–12 mmHg

Ⓒ F Increased, often > 35 mmHg

Ⓓ T Also pneumothorax, air embolism, sepsis and arrhythmias

Ⓔ T

15

Ⓐ F Maintain above > 90%

Ⓑ T As is alveolar arterial oxygen gradient

Ⓒ T As is $PaCO_2$

Ⓓ F Finger or earlobe spectrophotometry are satisfactory in most instances

Ⓔ T

16

Ⓐ T Q_t is determined by the preload, afterload, heart rate and myocardial contractility

Ⓑ F Venous return determines the preload

Ⓒ F SVR = 1440 dyn sec cm^{-5} , PVR = 80 dyn.sec.cm^{-5}

Ⓓ T

Ⓔ T Assumes flow to be linear and non-pulsatile

17

Ⓐ T Blood pressure typically falls

Ⓑ F Reduces PVR

Ⓒ T And moderate increase in myocardial contractility

Ⓓ F Usually tachycardia

Ⓔ F Typically declines

18

Ⓐ T

Ⓑ T

Ⓒ F Decreases pulmonary compliance

Ⓓ T As in ARDS

Ⓔ T Dependent on the reversibility of airways obstruction

19

Ⓐ F

Ⓑ F May be volume controlled

Ⓒ T Recruits areas of atelectatic lung

Ⓓ T With PEEP of 5–10 cmH$_2$O

Ⓔ F Risk of aspiration is increased

20

Ⓐ T A sustained pressure > 30 mmHg suggests a poor prognosis

Ⓑ T Should be > 65 mmHg

Ⓒ F Glycaemic control should be strict

Ⓓ T Target $PaCO_2$ of 4 kPa for 24 hours

Ⓔ T And avoid excessive neck flexion

21

A **F** Cardiac output often falls

B **T** Improves oxygenation in atelectatic areas

C **F** A tightly-fitting face or nasal mask can be used

D **F** Can occur with all forms of mechanical ventilation

E **T**

16 PRINCIPLES OF ONCOLOGICAL AND PALLIATIVE CARE

1
- **A** T
- **B** T
- **C** T Increases with cell proliferation rate
- **D** T Evidence of metastatic spread
- **E** F

2
- **A** F Useful in testicular germ cell tumours
- **B** T And testicular germ cell tumours
- **C** F Metastatic colorectal carcinoma
- **D** F There are no useful serum markers for cervical carcinoma
- **E** F Useful in ovarian carcinoma

3
- **A** T Expresses the value of a positive test (i.e. the sensitivity)
- **B** T Expresses the value of a negative test (i.e. the specificity)
- **C** T A limitation in all screening
- **D** F Sensitivity
- **E** F Specificity

4
- **A** F Small cell carcinoma
- **B** T And renal and ovarian carcinoma
- **C** T And ovarian and nasopharyngeal carcinoma
- **D** T Lambert–Eaton syndrome
- **E** T And other gastrointestinal malignancy

5
- **A** F Also records the presence or absence of lymph node involvement
- **B** F T0 = excised tumour
- **C** T And permits assessment of treatment
- **D** T Without new lesions appearing
- **E** F No response to therapy = < 25% reduction in tumour size

6
- **A** T And stage IIIE if there was also extra-lymphatic involvement
- **B** F Disease would be classified as stage IIE
- **C** T Or other diffuse extra-lymphatic involvement
- **D** F Classified as stage IISE
- **E** T A = asymptomatic

7
- **A** T TX, N0, M0 = occult carcinoma
- **B** T Or extension to visceral pleura/partial attelectasis
- **C** T Or spread to heart, great vessels, mediastinum
- **D** F Peribronchial or ipsilateral hilar
- **E** T M1 = metastases present

8
- **A** T Impairing cell reproduction
- **B** F 1 joule per kilogram
- **C** F That is teletherapy; brachytherapy is the use of sealed sources implanted internally
- **D** F Low energy radiation (50–100 kVp)
- **E** F Hypoxia renders tissue less sensitive to irradiation

9
- **A** T An antimetabolite
- **B** F A plant alkaloid
- **C** F An antibiotic anticancer drug which causes breaks in DNA strands
- **D** F Naturally-derived agents which stabilise mitotic spindles
- **E** T And also blocks DNA transcription

10
- **A** F As different as possible
- **B** F Differing modes of action
- **C** T Against the treated tumour type
- **D** T Or toxicity may limit benefit
- **E** F Some reduction from optimal dose may be necessary

11
- **A** F Refractory to chemotherapy
- **B** F Refractory to chemotherapy
- **C** T Also testicular teratoma
- **D** F Resistant
- **E** F Resistant

12
- **A** F Chemotherapy can be curative
- **B** F Chemotherapy can be curative
- **C** F Chemotherapy can be curative
- **D** F Chemotherapy can be curative
- **E** F Chemotherapy can be curative

13
- **A** T Usually reversible
- **B** F Usually alkylating agents
- **C** T Usually dilated (congestive)
- **D** F Bleomycin and busulphan
- **E** T Peripheral sensorimotor

14
- **A** T Testosterone suppression
- **B** T Suppresses TSH
- **C** T Particularly the well-differentiated tumours
- **D** F Used in breast carcinoma
- **E** T Blocks oestrogen binding

15
- **A** F Should be given regularly
- **B** T Affects prostaglandin metabolism
- **C** F Diamorphine can also be given in smaller volumes
- **D** F Dihydrocodeine is more potent
- **E** F Occasionally valuable pre-terminally

16
- **A** T A benzodiazepine
- **B** T Blocks dopaminergic receptors
- **C** T $5HT_3$ receptor antagonist
- **D** T Given parenterally with chemotherapy
- **E** F Chemotherapeutic agent which causes nausea and vomiting

17 PRINCIPLES OF GERIATRIC MEDICINE

1

Ⓐ F Bone mass declines (osteoporosis) but mineralisation is normal

Ⓑ F Reduced insulin sensitivity and glucose tolerance declines

Ⓒ T Limits ability to mount a tachycardia

Ⓓ F Decreased number of nephrons, GFR and medullary function

Ⓔ T May contribute to increase in autoimmune disease

2

Ⓐ T But not to the extent of producing dementia of clinical significance

Ⓑ T High tone hearing loss and presbyacusis

Ⓒ T Promotes muscle wasting and weakness

Ⓓ T One of many reasons for increased risk of falls

Ⓔ T Contributing to impaired balance, especially if also visually impaired

3

Ⓐ T Unable to reach the toilet in time

Ⓑ T Urge incontinence—short-acting diuretics may help avoid nocturnal incontinence

Ⓒ T Faecal impaction inhibits bladder motility and produces overflow incontinence

Ⓓ F Typically frontal lobe disease impairs the mechanisms initiating micturition

Ⓔ T Causes urge incontinence

4

Ⓐ F This problem is typical of urge incontinence

Ⓑ F More helpful in managing urge incontinence

Ⓒ F This problem is typical of stress incontinence

Ⓓ F This finding suggests denervation of the bladder or outflow obstruction

Ⓔ F Typical symptoms of prostatism

5

Ⓐ F Opiates can induce urinary retention directly and via constipating effect

Ⓑ T Blocks muscarinic cholinergic receptors and reduces detrusor instability

Ⓒ T Faecal impaction may cause overflow urinary incontinence

Ⓓ T Used topically to ameliorate atrophic vaginitis and reduce stress incontinence

Ⓔ T Selective α_1-adrenoreceptor blocker useful in benign prostatic hypertrophy

6

Ⓐ T Exacerbated by poor mobility

Ⓑ T Often drug induced

Ⓒ F More common in the young

Ⓓ T Multiple factors involved

Ⓔ T Absence of loss of consciousness and difficulty in regaining the upright position

7

Ⓐ F Decreased below normal (normal value 4°C)

Ⓑ T The elderly can only detect changes > 2°C (compare detection of 1°C change in younger people)

Ⓒ T Metabolic heat production is 50% < than younger people

Ⓓ F Thyroid function is normal

Ⓔ T The elderly are less able to maintain a constant core temperature

8

Ⓐ F Increased step length variability

Ⓑ T A slower gait

Ⓒ T A broader-based gait

Ⓓ F Shorter steps

Ⓔ T Sway exhibits gender differences at all ages

9

Ⓐ T May be fluctuant

Ⓑ T May find simple mental arithmetic taxing

Ⓒ T Usually with disorientation in time and place

Ⓓ T Perceptual disturbances

Ⓔ T Apathy in some cases

10

Ⓐ T E.g. opiates, L-dopa

Ⓑ T Check core temperature with a low-reading thermometer

Ⓒ T Consider the possibility of meningitis

Ⓓ T More often asymptomatic in the elderly

Ⓔ T CT scan to exclude subdural haematoma or tumour

11

Ⓐ T Impaired consciousness suggests delirium

Ⓑ T Logical reasoning is impaired

Ⓒ F The converse occurs

Ⓓ T Volition and interest decline

Ⓔ T Mimicks depressive illness

12

Ⓐ T Especially if associated with postural hypotension

Ⓑ T Absence of attacks when lying in bed is suggestive

Ⓒ T Rare in the absence of hearing loss

Ⓓ T Common and may be reproduced by head movements

Ⓔ T Dizziness is more likely to occur with bradycardias than tachycardias

18 PRINCIPLES OF MEDICAL PSYCHIATRY

1
- **Ⓐ F** 15–20%
- **Ⓑ F** 30%
- **Ⓒ T** Range 20–30%
- **Ⓓ T** Range 25–40%
- **Ⓔ F** Schizophrenia occurs in 1%

2
- **Ⓐ T** Rarely, single gene disorder identified
- **Ⓑ T** Especially physical or sexual abuse
- **Ⓒ T** E.g. bereavement, redundancy, retirement
- **Ⓓ T** Also acute severe physical illness
- **Ⓔ T** Particularly lack of a close relationship

3
- **Ⓐ T** Including motor retardation
- **Ⓑ T** E.g. suicidal ideation
- **Ⓒ T** Paranoid, grandiose or depressive
- **Ⓓ T** Depersonalisation, illusions and hallucinations
- **Ⓔ T** Concentration, memory and orientation

4
- **Ⓐ F**
- **Ⓑ F**
- **Ⓒ F** Suggests affective disorder
- **Ⓓ T** Often with short-term memory loss
- **Ⓔ T** Impaired concentration

5
- **Ⓐ T** Suggestive of psychosis
- **Ⓑ T** Compare hallucinations
- **Ⓒ T** Suggests psychosis
- **Ⓓ T** Often with derealisation
- **Ⓔ T** Typical pattern in neurosis

6
- **Ⓐ T** Useful in the treatment of phobias
- **Ⓑ T** Exposure of the patient to maximal stress
- **Ⓒ T** With positive and negative reinforcement
- **Ⓓ F** Undertaken in interpretative psychotherapy
- **Ⓔ F** Feature of cognitive therapy

7
- **Ⓐ F** Undertaken in psychotherapy
- **Ⓑ T** E.g. in depression
- **Ⓒ T** Altering thoughts may alter behaviour
- **Ⓓ T** And development of positive views
- **Ⓔ F** Features of psychotherapy

8
- **Ⓐ F** Blocks 5 HT_2 receptors more than D_2 receptors (hence fewer parkinsonian features)
- **Ⓑ T** SSRIs such as fluoxetine have fewer adverse effects but are more expensive
- **Ⓒ T** Dry mouth, constipation, tachycardia etc.
- **Ⓓ F** Less potent and with potentially more serious drug interactions
- **Ⓔ F** Inhibitor of neurotransmitter-induced phosphoinositide hydrolysis

9

A T Hence the extra-pyramidal features of parkinsonism

B F These side-effects are due to dopamine receptor blockade

C T Thioridazine may produce a retinitis pigmentosa-like syndome

D F Like gynaecomastia, a typical side-effect of dopamine receptor blockade

E T Neutropenia occurs in 3% and requires careful monitoring

10

A T But diurnal variation may occur

B T Or early morning wakening

C T 'anhedonism'—loss of sense of enjoyment

D T Perhaps with other somatic symptoms

E T With delusions of worthlessness

11

A F Suggest depression

B T May be seen in affective disorders

C T With irritability

D T Typical somatic symptoms

E F Features of phobic anxiety states

12

A T Delirium may also occur

B T Exclude biochemically

C T Measure blood glucose

D T EEG may be necessary

E T Rare—measure urinary catecholamines

13

A T Occasionally with malabsorption

B T Heart failure may occur

C T Or asymptomatic hyperuricaemia

D T Or cerebellar degeneration

E T Or amenorrhoea

14

A F Narrowing of choices of alcoholic beverages

B F Decreasing tolerance

C T

D T Classical

E T

15

A T Provoking early morning drinking

B T Typically persecutory if auditory

C T With acute confusion

D F Suggest alcohol dependence

E F Suggest Wernicke's encephalopathy

16

A T Perhaps with depersonalisation

B T And other perceptual disorders

C T Particularly in acute withdrawal

D F Affect not typically disturbed

E F Agitation rather than retardation

17

A F No conscious motivation in hysteria

B T E.g. chest pain, altered bowel habit

C T May be present in up to 50% of cases

D T With relatively few or no physical signs

E T Pseudo-seizures are commonest in epileptic patients

18

A T Psychological explanations are often firmly rejected

B T May become delusional (e.g. delusional parasitosis)

C T Also hyperventilation, palpitation and functional chest pain

D T Often pain is an isolated symptom

E T

19

A F Either sex, rarely non-adolescent

B T With avoidance of high calorie foods

C T In contrast to bulimia nervosa

D F Emaciation is unrecognised by the patient

E F And psychosexual retardation

20

A F Typically post-pubertal

B F Body weight maintained

C T With recurrent bouts of binging

D T Or dieting after binges

E F Rarely necessary

21
- **Ⓐ T** Most often young females
- **Ⓑ T** More common in socioeconomic groups 3–5
- **Ⓒ T** Associated with poverty and overcrowding
- **Ⓓ T** Either from death or from separation
- **Ⓔ T** Especially common in deliberate self-harm

22
- **Ⓐ F** Older males
- **Ⓑ F** Self-poisoning is frequently parasuicidal
- **Ⓒ F** Suicide note often left and usually a history of previous attempts
- **Ⓓ T** And drug or alcohol abuse
- **Ⓔ T** Or bereavement

23
- **Ⓐ F** Suggests organic brain disease
- **Ⓑ T** Especially depressive illnesses
- **Ⓒ F** Favours organic brain disorder
- **Ⓓ T** Common precipitants of psychiatric illness
- **Ⓔ F** Strongly suggest organic brain syndrome

24
- **Ⓐ T** Patient has no right of appeal
- **Ⓑ T** Patient can appeal to the Tribunal within 14 days
- **Ⓒ T** Patient has no right of appeal
- **Ⓓ T** Patient has no right of appeal
- **Ⓔ T** Patient has no right of appeal

25
- **Ⓐ T** Also permits an emergency admission to hospital under section 24
- **Ⓑ T** For the purpose of assessment and treatment; patient can appeal within 14 days
- **Ⓒ T** Patient can appeal to the Mental Welfare Commission or the Sheriff
- **Ⓓ T** Patient can appeal to the Mental Welfare Commission or the Sheriff
- **Ⓔ T** Patient has no right of appeal

PRINCIPLES OF DRUG THERAPY AND MANAGEMENT OF POISONING

19

1

Ⓐ F Volume varies with extent of tissue distribution

Ⓑ T

Ⓒ F Volume of distribution cleared of drug per unit time

Ⓓ T Drug clearance during the first passage through the liver

Ⓔ F Amount of drug reaching the circulation when given by any route other than i.v.

2

Ⓐ T Definition of drug half life

Ⓑ T

Ⓒ T

Ⓓ T Drugs in an ionised state are not reabsorbed

Ⓔ T Bioavailability is measured as ratio of plasma drug concentrations after oral/i.v. administration

3

Ⓐ T Both sensations delay gastric emptying and hence the rate of drug absorption

Ⓑ T But can be increased to 30% using a spacer device

Ⓒ T Hence value in administration of nitrates in angina

Ⓓ F Passes through the liver and lungs before entering systemic circulation

Ⓔ F No significant quantity of any drug is absorbed through the gastric mucosa

4

Ⓐ T Drugs like propranolol also reach the plasma in chylomicrons via the thoracic duct

Ⓑ F Increases bioavailability due to impaired first-pass hepatic metabolism

Ⓒ F Lower plasma protein concentrations means less binding and greater clearance rates

Ⓓ T 'Grey baby' syndrome in neonates

Ⓔ F Reduces gut flora and enterohepatic recirculation of the drug lowering drug concentrations

5

Ⓐ T And 6-mercaptopurine; both are metabolised by xanthine oxidase

Ⓑ T Anticholinergic effect

Ⓒ T Similarly, quinidine and amiodarone compete with digoxin for renal excretion

Ⓓ F Increased effect due to inhibition of renal tubular secretion of methotrexate

Ⓔ T Recommend a barrier method as well for patients on the contraceptive pill and taking antibiotics

6

Ⓐ F Causes hepatic enzyme induction

Ⓑ T Also true for norfloxacin and erythromycin

Ⓒ T Also true for fluconazole

Ⓓ T Also true for isoniazid, 6-mercatopurine and azathioprine

Ⓔ T Also true for rifampicin and clarithromycin

7
- **Ⓐ F** Reduce dose frequency and measure plasma concentrations daily
- **Ⓑ T** Induces protein catabolism and rapidly increasing uraemia
- **Ⓒ F** Reduce both dose and dose frequency
- **Ⓓ T** Like all NSAIDs, reduces renal blood flow by prostaglandin inhibition
- **Ⓔ T** Causes lactic acidosis

8
- **Ⓐ F** Similar to paracetamol in this respect
- **Ⓑ F** Low rates of clearance during its first passage through the liver
- **Ⓒ T** Lignocaine is also rapidly cleared during its first passage through the liver ('first-pass' effect)
- **Ⓓ T**
- **Ⓔ F**

9
- **Ⓐ T** Reduces the synthesis of clotting factors
- **Ⓑ T** Produces lactic acidosis
- **Ⓒ T** Induces bone marrow suppression
- **Ⓓ T** Increases the risk of hypoglycaemia
- **Ⓔ T** Like other NSAIDs, increases the risk of gastrointestinal bleeding

10
- **Ⓐ F** Error rates of up to 60% can be found in patients over the age of 60 years
- **Ⓑ T** Adverse drug reactions are 2–3 times more common
- **Ⓒ T** Propranolol accumulation is also increased by reduced drug metabolism
- **Ⓓ F** Impaired renal clearance associated with reduced GFR is common
- **Ⓔ T** As with other drugs (e.g. theophylline and sedative drugs) doses should be reduced

11
- **Ⓐ F** Prescriptions must be written entirely in the prescriber's own handwriting, in ink
- **Ⓑ T**
- **Ⓒ T**
- **Ⓓ T** Including the total quantity, number of doses, form and strength of the drug
- **Ⓔ T**

12
- **Ⓐ T**
- **Ⓑ T** 60% of males, 40% of females
- **Ⓒ F** Most are parasuicidal and are best considered as a cry for help
- **Ⓓ F** Most patients are aged 12–35 years
- **Ⓔ F** 20% repeat within 1 year (50% of patients have a previous history of self-poisoning)

13
- **Ⓐ T** Commonest cause of unconsciousness in this age group
- **Ⓑ T** E.g. tricyclics, carbamazepine or phenytoin
- **Ⓒ T** A feature of a behavioural disorder often associated with abuse in childhood
- **Ⓓ T** Suggesting drug abuse, typically opiate abuse
- **Ⓔ T** Suggesting solvent abuse, often with a characteristic odour

14
- **Ⓐ F** Assess need for supportive treatment first
- **Ⓑ T** Patients may require intubation and ventilation
- **Ⓒ T** Look for hypovolaemia, arrhythmias and acid-base disturbances
- **Ⓓ F** May result in aspiration and even induce hypernatraemia
- **Ⓔ T** Naloxone ± flumazenil if opioids and/or benzodiazepines are suspected

15

Ⓐ F Only considered if a potentially toxic dose has been consumed within the previous 2 hours

Ⓑ F Check by aspiration or insufflation and auscultation

Ⓒ T Protect the airway at all times

Ⓓ F No significant role in the management of poisoning

Ⓔ T Reduces further drug absorption, especially if given within 2 hours of self-poisoning

16

Ⓐ T More effective if given early

Ⓑ T More effective if given early and repeated 4-hourly ('gut dialysis')

Ⓒ F Not absorbed by activated charcoal

Ⓓ F Not absorbed by activated charcoal

Ⓔ F Not absorbed by activated charcoal

17

Ⓐ F Value is outweighed by the risks

Ⓑ T Useful in arsenic, gold and mercury poisoning

Ⓒ F Used in benzodiazepine overdose

Ⓓ T As indicated by plasma paracetamol concentrations post-ingestion

Ⓔ T

18

Ⓐ T Abdominal pain may develop

Ⓑ F Late features suggesting hepatic encephalopathy (after 3–5 days)

Ⓒ F Rare before 24 hours

Ⓓ F Consequence of hepatic necrosis (after 36 hours)

Ⓔ T But not useful beyond 15 hours

19

Ⓐ F Coma is more common in children

Ⓑ T Common features

Ⓒ T Metabolic acidosis is particularly common in children

Ⓓ T

Ⓔ F Gastric emptying is delayed

20

Ⓐ T

Ⓑ F Severe cardiorespiratory depression is rare

Ⓒ F Suspect mixed overdose

Ⓓ F Suspect alternative or mixed overdose

Ⓔ F Drowsiness is often prolonged

21

Ⓐ T Ectasy is also an amphetamine derivative

Ⓑ F Tachycardia and hypertension; hypotension can occur but is rare

Ⓒ F Bullous lesions develop in 6% of patients poisoned with barbiturates

Ⓓ T Also occur following withdrawal from chronic barbiturate usage

Ⓔ F Characteristic of severe opioid toxicity

22

Ⓐ T Deep coma is unusual

Ⓑ T Anticholinergic features

Ⓒ F Dilated pupils from the anticholinergic effects

Ⓓ T Stimulatory CNS effects may precede depressant effects

Ⓔ T Particularly ventricular tachycardia

23

Ⓐ F Hypoventilation and sedation

Ⓑ T Convulsions in children

Ⓒ T May be early and marked

Ⓓ T Typically drug is combined with paracetamol (e.g. co-proxamol)

Ⓔ F Rapid but short acting opioid antagonist

24

Ⓐ T

Ⓑ F Pin-point pupils

Ⓒ T

Ⓓ T Use naloxone

Ⓔ T Characteristic and the commonest mode of death

25
Ⓐ T Early features
Ⓑ T Resolve many hours after ingestion
Ⓒ T An early feature
Ⓓ T Usually after 3–4 days
Ⓔ T Pyloric and small bowel strictures occur particularly in children

26
Ⓐ T Common early features
Ⓑ T Develop later due to neurological toxicity
Ⓒ F Of no value; haemodialysis may be required for patients with neurological features
Ⓓ T Associated with nephrogenic diabetes insipidus
Ⓔ T And ST segment and T wave changes

27
Ⓐ F Common features include agitation, headache and confusion
Ⓑ F Usually skin pallor; patients may appear 'pink' due to carboxyhaemoglobin
Ⓒ T Especially in patients whose coma is prolonged
Ⓓ T Due to the effects of cerebral oedema and cerebral anoxia
Ⓔ T Neuropsychiatric sequelae occur in 10% 2–4 weeks following recovery

28
Ⓐ T
Ⓑ T Ethanol inhibits gluconeogenesis; hepatic glycogen is also often depleted
Ⓒ T Hypothermia can be profound
Ⓓ T Even in moderate poisoning
Ⓔ T Depressed gag reflex

29
Ⓐ F Much more toxic than ethanol
Ⓑ T Often develop 8 hours or more after ingestion
Ⓒ T With progressive visual loss
Ⓓ T And marked overproduction of formic acid
Ⓔ F With as little as 10 ml

30
Ⓐ F Metabolised to aldehydes and glycolates
Ⓑ T And subsequent optic atrophy
Ⓒ T Renal failure 24 hours post-ingestion
Ⓓ F Hyperkalaemia and hypocalcaemia
Ⓔ T Inhibits the metabolism of ethylene glycol